MW01128367

The Principles and Practice
of Narrative Medicine

The Principles and Practice of Narrative Medicine

RITA CHARON

SAYANTANI DASGUPTA

NELLIE HERMANN

CRAIG IRVINE

ERIC R. MARCUS

EDGAR RIVERA COLÓN

DANIELLE SPENCER

MAURA SPIEGEL

OXFORD
UNIVERSITY PRESS

OXFORD
UNIVERSITY PRESS

Oxford University Press is a department of the University of Oxford. It furthers
the University's objective of excellence in research, scholarship, and education
by publishing worldwide. Oxford is a registered trade mark of Oxford University
Press in the UK and certain other countries.

Published in the United States of America by Oxford University Press
198 Madison Avenue, New York, NY 10016, United States of America.

Library of Congress Cataloging-in-Publication Data
Names: Charon, Rita, author.
Title: The principles and practice of narrative medicine / Rita Charon [and seven others].
Description: New York, NY : Oxford University Press, [2017] |
Includes bibliographical references and index.
Identifiers: LCCN 2016013641 | ISBN 9780199360192 (hardcover : alk. paper)
Subjects: | MESH: Narration | Clinical Medicine—methods | Professional-Patient Relations
Classification: LCC RC65 | NLM WB 102 | DDC 616—dc23 LC record available
at http://lccn.loc.gov/2016013641

9

Printed by Sheridan Books, Inc., United States of America

TABLE OF CONTENTS

PART VI ▪ **QUALITATIVE WAYS OF KNOWING**

PART VII ▪ **CLINICAL PRACTICE**

ACKNOWLEDGMENTS

This book reflects the work of many persons over many years. Our ideas about narrative medicine have grown from our engagement with colleagues and students in literary and narrative studies, philosophy, and healthcare practice—at Columbia, in individual friendships, and in our wide circles of professional societies. We offer our deep gratitude to all the workshop participants, students, colleagues, and national and international partners who have been our fellow learners through the years.

We thank the students and faculty of the Columbia University Medical Center for their willingness to work with us through our years of developing these principles and practices. We especially are indebted to the "K07" group of Foundations of Clinical Medicine preceptors at College of Physicians and Surgeons of Columbia and to the students and faculty who joined us in the Columbia/Macy Interprofessional Education project. We acknowledge the Columbia University Center for Psychoanalytic Training and Research, the Center for Family Medicine and the Department of Medicine at the Columbia University Medical Center, and the Columbia University School of Professional Studies. We thank the National Endowment for the Humanities, the National Institutes of Health, and Dr. George Thibault and the Josiah Macy, Jr. Foundation for their generous support of our research through these years.

Many ongoing projects have nourished our work through the years, including the Editorial Board of *Literature and Medicine,* the International Society for the Study of Narrative, the American Society for Bioethics and Humanities, and the Health Humanities organizations in the United States and abroad.

Thanks to the many colleagues and friends who have contributed to the development of this work. To name just a few: Marsha Hurst, Paul Browde, Murray Nossel, Ephraim Rubenstein, Ann Burack-Weiss, Michael Davidovits, and Paul McNeil, in the growth of the Master of Science in Narrative Medicine program; Deepthiman Gowda, Chris Adrian, Craig Blinderman, Michael Devlin, Delphine Taylor, Hetty Cunningham, Mindy Fullilove, Ronald Drusin, Jonathan Amiel, Boyd Richards, and Dorene Balmer at the medical school; Helena Hansen, Jack Saul, Rachel Adams, Mary Marshall Clark, Bradley Lewis, Rebecca Garden, Brian Hurwitz, Ann Jurecic, Catherine Belling, John Launer, Arthur Frank, David Morris, Priscilla Wald, Jens Brockmeier, and Jim Phelan for inspiration and partnership. Without Elliot Mishler and Steven Marcus at the very beginnings, this work would not have been possible.

We are indebted to Anna Fenton-Hathaway for her expert editorial assistance. Thanks to our chapter readers for their invaluable reflections: Kris Slesar, Lynne Sharon Schwartz, Shannon Wooden, and Gayatri Devi.

Thanks to the Program in Narrative Medicine administration in years past and present: Gillian Graham, Tressie LaFay, Scott Alderman, Rachel Rampil, Cindy Smalletz, Wanda O'Connell, and Donna Bulseco.

Thanks to all those who granted permission for their writing to be excerpted in this book. Specific passages are not credited by name, but all such inclusion has been specifically approved by the authors: Stephanie Adler Yuan, Aubrie Ann-Jones, James Belarde, Katelyn Connor, Anne Cunney, Adam De Fazio, Cameron Donald, Denzil Douglas, Lauren Edwards, Chelsea Garnett, Barbara Hirsch, Sarah Keesecker, Eleanor Kim, Angela Lloyd, Lauren Mautner, Catherine Rogers, Rebekah Ruppe, Bridget Sheehy, Anoushka Sinha, Cindy Smalletz, Leyla Vural, Nikhil Suneel Wadhwani, Patrick Walsh, James Wendt, Abigail Ford Winkel, Erica Zorn Wrightson, and Jane Zhao.

* * *

Lucille Clifton, "the death of fred clifton" from *Collected Poems of Lucille Clifton*. Copyright ©1987 by Lucille Clifton. Reprinted with the permission of The Permissions Company, Inc., on behalf of BOA Editions, Ltd., www.boaeditions.org.

David Ferry, "Soul" from *Bewilderment: New Poems and Translations*. Copyright ©2012 by David Ferry. Reprinted with the permission of University of Chicago Press.

"Wait" from *MORTAL ACTS MORTAL WORDS* by Galway Kinnell. Copyright ©1980, renewed 2008 by Galway Kinnell. Reprinted by permission of Houghton Mifflin Harcourt Publishing Company. All rights reserved.

Tsevat, R. K., Sinha, A. A., Gutierrez, K. J., & DasGupta, S. Bringing Home the Health Humanities: Narrative Humility, Structural Competency, and Engaged Pedagogy. *Academic Medicine* 90(11) (2015): 1462–1465. Permission to reprint portions of this essay in Chapter 6, "The Politics of the Pedagogy: Cripping, Queering and Un-homing Health Humanities" is granted by Walters Kluwer Health, Inc., of Lippincott Williams & Wilkins for *Academic Medicine*.

Introduction

Narrative medicine began as a rigorous intellectual and clinical discipline to fortify healthcare with the capacity to skillfully receive the accounts persons give of themselves—to recognize, absorb, interpret, and be moved to action by the stories of others. It emerged to challenge a reductionist, fragmented medicine that holds little regard for the singular aspects of a patient's life and to protest the social injustice of a global healthcare system that countenances tremendous health disparities and discriminatory policies and practices. We clinicians, scholars, and creative writers who began this work together were convinced that narrative knowledge and skills have the power to improve healthcare by increasing the accuracy and scope of clinicians' knowledge of their patients and deepening the therapeutic partnerships they are able to form. A healthcare that recognizes and affiliates with patients, that exists to serve and not to profit, will assure justice while it promotes health for all.

From a confluence of narrative studies and clinical practices, we have developed an increasingly nuanced view of the workings of the narrative, relational, and reflexive processes of healthcare. Literary theory, narratology, continental philosophies, aesthetic theory, and cultural studies provide the intellectual foundations of narrative medicine. Informing our work are the 1980s' revolutionary upheavals in linguistic, narrative, and postmodern theory that led to profound questioning of certainty and a realization of language's ever-shifting representations of reality.[1] Reading became recognized as an ethical act joining reader and writer in transformative engagement, leading to singular consequences for each reader instead of an orderly plotting toward an inevitable and shared conclusion.[2] Primary care medicine, collaborative team-based healthcare, narrative ethics, the qualitative social science studies of healthcare, and psychoanalysis supply the clinical foundations of our work.[3] From these sources come our commitments to relationships in patient-centered care and our conviction that narrative competence can widen the clinical gaze to include personal and social elements of patients' lives vital to the tasks of healing.

The goal of narrative medicine from its start has been to improve health-care. This accounts for the title we have chosen for our book, *The Principles and Practice of Narrative Medicine*. Echoing William Osler's 1892 *The Principles and Practice of Medicine* that set the standards for the practice of internal medicine, we believe the work that has emerged in narrative medicine has the potential to help move an impersonal and increasingly revenue-hungry healthcare toward a care that recognizes, that attunes to the singular, and that flows from the interior resources of the participants in encounters of care. We want to bring to clinical practice much that has been learned or hypothesized about the relationships between narrativity and identity, about the co-construction that takes place in any serious narrative telling, and about the discovery potential of creative acts. We want clinicians to come to appreciate the importance of the emotion and intersubjective relation borne of the telling and listening that occur in any clinical encounter. And we hope for patients that our work might open up healthcare to more trust, more accurate knowledge about one another, and more justice.

The History of Narrative Medicine

A group of scholars and clinicians teaching and practicing at Columbia University in New York gathered at the millennium to take up questions that had engaged each of us in our work. By 2000, there were already decades of discovery in fields in which many of the founding participants of narrative medicine were active—including literature and medicine, narrative ethics, medical humanities, healthcare communication, and primary care medicine. With funding from the National Endowment for the Humanities, we established an intensive collaborative learning seminar at Columbia. For over two years, we gathered to pose and grapple with foundational questions about the consequences of bringing literary and creative practices into the realms of healthcare.[4]

The authors of this book include those founding faculty members—Sayantani DasGupta of pediatrics and activism, Craig Irvine of philosophy and family medicine, Eric R. Marcus of the psychoanalytic institute, Maura Spiegel of English and cinema studies, and Rita Charon of medicine and English. One founding member, novelist David Plante, moved some years later to London, and we invited fiction writer Nellie Hermann to join us in his stead. Our group included then-graduate-students Rebecca Garden and Tara McGann and student-intern Patricia Stanley. The seventh and eighth coauthors of this book—Edgar Rivera-Colón of anthropology and Danielle Spencer of literary studies—are newer members of our group who bring critical elements to the book.

Our inaugural efforts in narrative medicine began with questions of narrativity in the clinic: why was it helpful for clinicians and trainees in healthcare to read and write? We had already been inviting health professions students, clinicians of many disciplines, patients, and family caregivers to read and write with us in various literature and medicine classes and medical humanities settings, but we wanted to think through the mechanisms and intermediates by which such narrative work might be helpful. The nature of the clinical work itself would be transformed if narrative skills and methods could become part of the fabric of clinical thought and care. And so our goal was to find ways to directly, irreversibly alter the ways that persons seeking healthcare were received.

What crystallized was a dynamic and questing set of findings and concerns about the discovery nature of writing, the relational substrate of reading, the affective processes of narrating, the ethical complexities of the accounts of self, and how they all influence the wide, wide ground of health. We early recognized *attention, representation,* and *affiliation* as the three movements of narrative medicine that emerged from our commitment to skilled listening, the power of representation to perceive the other, and the value of the partnerships that result from narrative contact. By *attention* we mean the state of heightened focus and commitment that a listener can donate to a teller—a patient, a student, a colleague, a friend. Rare, demanding, and rewarding, attention uses the listening self as a vessel to capture and reveal that which a teller has to tell. *Representation,* usually in writing but also in visual media, confers form on what is heard or perceived, thereby making it newly visible to both the listener and the teller. And *affiliation,* which results from deep attentive listening and the knowledge achieved through representation, binds patients and clinicians, students and teachers, self and other into relationships that support recognition and action as one stays the course with the other through whatever is to be faced.

Many of those who are today active in narrative medicine joined us for ensuing Narrative Medicine workshops, whose design arose from our initial NEH project. With the contributions of persons who attended these workshops— since 2006 we have hosted almost 40 NM workshops engaging some 2,000 participants—the practices that we describe in this volume emerged. Many others studied with us in the required narrative medicine curriculum at the College of Physicians and Surgeons of Columbia University or in wide-ranging work internationally; all of these partners also have contributed to the current shape of narrative medicine.

In 2009 we inaugurated the Master of Science in Narrative Medicine at Columbia University, a program that equips graduate students with foundational literary, philosophical, and cultural theories in the context of complex relational and emotional processes of teaching and learning. We admit a small number of students each year into the graduate program, including recent college graduates on their way to health professions schools, mid-career clinicians committed to strengthening their practice with narrative skills, and writers and artists who want to share with patients and clinicians these new ways of healing. Teaching and learning with our graduate students have revealed fresh dimensions of narrative medicine to us, things we could not have seen on our own. Some graduates from our Master's program are now directing projects in narrative medicine themselves and have been appointed to faculties of colleges and professional schools. Many are enrolled in health professions schools or are attending graduate school in the humanities. Our graduates join us in teaching and spreading narrative medicine and in studying the outcomes of our work.

The teaching methods of narrative medicine range widely, as you will see in the many pedagogic demonstrations offered in this volume. Wherever and with whomever the teaching occurs, it is marked by attention to the principles we present in this volume—intersubjectivity, relationality, personhood and embodiment, action toward justice, close reading (or slow looking), and creativity. Over the years of our work, we have taught narrative medicine to patients in oncology, in trauma care, in physical therapy, in long-term care facilities, and in day programs for persons with dementia and mental illness. Our work has spread to VA hospitals and clinics as means to help address the traumas suffered by military personnel. We and our trainees have brought narrative medicine seminars to children and adults at Gilda's Club, a support site for persons who live with cancer, and to high school students envisioning health professions for themselves. Professional narrative medicine training occurs in scores of hospitals and health systems, often with interprofessional groups of learners, in settings of geriatrics, obstetrics and gynecology, family medicine, pediatrics, internal medicine, dentistry, surgery, and hospice care.

In all these places we engage learners in telling and listening to stories, reading and talking about literary and visual texts, doing creative writing together, and sharing with one another what they have written.

Beyond healthcare settings, our work has spread to law schools, grammar schools, and corporate headquarters. Whether in an ongoing seminar or a single session on a special visit, participants open up aspects of themselves for view—so many who think they cannot write learn that they can, so many who have worked together for years discover new dimensions of one another. All who engage in this work discover things about themselves.

Narrative medicine work has also developed internationally; we and our trainees have developed scholarly and teaching practices widely in the Americas, Western and Eastern Europe, the United Kingdom, Asia, and Africa. For example, an Italian collaborative with a nationwide reach gathers teachers in health professions schools, clinicians caring for chronically ill children, and scholars in university settings for ongoing consultation and joint projects. With Open Society collaboration and funding, narrative medicine methods provided an intensive training for clinicians and activists committed to improving healthcare for the Roma population in Eastern Europe. A children's hospital in Buenos Aires is benefitting from rigorous narrative medicine consultation to enrich pediatric care with methods of visual and textual arts teaching and practice for patients and clinicians. Ongoing intensive narrative medicine workshops are being offered in Tokyo and Kyoto for clinicians in social work, medicine, nursing, and psychotherapy.

The field of narrative medicine is now embarked on an international effort to research the outcomes of the work we do. We and others have surveyed students who had been exposed to narrative medicine curricula to gather their evaluations of the courses' teaching and salience to their studies.[5] We are learning more and more about the long-term implications of developing narrative competence in healthcare. Such outcomes as recognition of emotion, perceptual sharpness, tolerating uncertainty, decreasing burnout, improving healthcare team function, and deepening individual clinicians' knowledge of individual patients' situations are all being demonstrated as consequences of narrative training.[6]

One thing we have all consistently learned over the years is that clearings open up wherever we bring the methods of narrative medicine for teaching and learning. Not unlike the open spaces in a forest, these clearings function as sites of protection and safety, welcoming persons to join and work together without the encumbrance of hierarchy or status differentials. An egality that emits from storytelling itself levels even hard-bitten power asymmetries, so that members of interprofessional healthcare teams or groups of teachers and students or clinicians and patients can meet one another as equals, bent on reflexively giving and receiving, teaching and learning. Overtones, or harmonics, of care and unity are achievable in a healthcare that becomes a service at the command of patients rather than a professional monopoly that serves the interests of the institutions who deliver it. All who seek care and all who seek to give care can unite in a clearing of safety, of purpose, of vision, and unconditional commitment to the interests of patients. This is the vision of narrative medicine.

The Shape of the Book

In the Preface to *The Ambassadors*, Henry James distinguishes between the two "stories" of his novel: "There is the story of one's hero and then, thanks to the intimate connexion of things, the story of one's story itself."[7] The hero or heroine of this volume is the set of ideas and practices that has emerged from the development of narrative medicine. The story of the book is how these ideas and practices guided the architecture of this volume, saying beyond its content what we hope to convey by virtue of having written it.

We organically discovered a shape for this book through the writing of it. The principles, we learned, can be best articulated in concert with a detailed description of how they are actually practiced. Accordingly, most of the parts of this book pair a theoretical chapter or chapters with a detailed description of how these principles are practiced in teaching or clinical work. Faithful to our commitment to participatory learning and to the particularity of narrative itself, we provide singular scenes of learning throughout the volume. You will read particular texts that are being taught in particular settings. You will read the creative writing produced by some of our learners, all of whom gave us enthusiastic permission to publish their writing. Finally, you will hear our pedagogic rationale for the shape of the learning experience. In the clinical sections, you will accompany us as we care for particular patients with narrative methods of care. We find the reflexive resonance between principles and practice results in both directions of influence—the principles inform the practice while the ongoing practice feeds back to clarify or amend or sometimes challenge the principles on which they are based. As befits a new field of inquiry and practice, this reflexivity assures that teachers and learners mutually co-instruct, that clinicians and patients share insight and power, and that the ideas and the real, together, design the work.

We begin our study with two persons—a teller and a listener—as the germ of the care of the sick. This dyad demonstrates the human capacity for the radical humility to recognize and hail and value the other, while reciprocally being recognized and hailed and valued. In "Part I: Intersubjectivity," Maura Spiegel and Danielle Spencer describe the literary and critical bases of relationality through the study of literature. In Chapter 1, "Accounts of Self: Exploring Relationality through Literature," they present a selected number of first-person accounts in works of fiction with which to model and probe the processes of self-revelation in words. A very close examination of their chosen works exposes the characters' and narrators' voices and the relationships formed among them and the readers. Their teaching "thickens the story" for the students, showing how the worlds of these texts are co-constructed by those within and outside of the spaces of the story. Accounting for the self becomes not an autonomous act but a relational one, accomplished through experiential and creative contact with the stories of others.

In Chapter 2, "This Is What We Do and These Things Happen: Experience, Emotion, and Relationality in the Classroom," Maura and Danielle proceed to show *how* these concepts may be actualized in a narrative medicine classroom.

Using the teaching of Alice Munro's short story "Floating Bridge" as an instance, they dramatize the process of the narrative medicine classroom, complete with writing by the students that emerged in the study of this short story. Paying exquisite attention to the responses of the student-readers of these texts enables Maura and Danielle to reveal the role of personal awareness in one's capacity to receive the account of self of another. Concepts from sources as varied as John Dewey's *Art as Experience*, Derald Wing Sue's writing on race talk, and Stephen Mitchell's relational theories of attachment inform their interpretation of the classroom experiences that incarnate or embody the principles articulated in Chapter 1.

We look next at some of the powerful impediments to intersubjective relation in healthcare. Paramount among these is the concept of mind–body dualism. For over 2000 years, Western philosophy has asserted complex negations of the unity of the individual subject, subjecting him or her to fragmentation into mind and body or body and soul. Part II, "Dualism, Personhood, and Embodiment" provides three chapters delineating the divisions of dualism and the reversal of dualism through phenomenological attention to the body/self continuum. In Chapter 3, "Dualism and Its Discontents I: Philosophy, Literature, and Medicine," Craig Irvine and Danielle Spencer provide a robust history and critique of mind–body dualism. They perform close readings of the seminal texts of Plato and Descartes, among others, that established dualism as, for centuries, the primary means of conceptualizing the human subject. In Chapter 4, "Dualism and Its Discontents II: Philosophical Tinctures," Craig and Danielle assert that the theories of the phenomenology of the body, stretching from Merleau-Ponty to such contemporary philosophers as Richard Zaner and Havi Carel, offer an alternative conceptual approach to the situation of embodiment. Through these chapters runs a sustained and generous effort to provide readers with frameworks of mind/body/soul unity as powerful as those that produced dualism.

Following these two chapters on dualism and its challenges is a chapter that treats the concepts of the phenomenology of embodiment in contemporary clinical practice. In narrative ethics, clinicians and consultants put into practice an awareness of the unities of narrative and identity in which body and self—of both patient and clinician—are one. In Chapter 5, "Deliver Us from Certainty: Training for Narrative Ethics," Craig Irvine and Rita Charon describe the rise of narrative ethics from within literary studies and simultaneously from within clinical ethics, where it functioned as one of several challenges to principlism, the dominant rule-based approach to ethical conflicts in healthcare. Craig and Rita's study of narrative ethics reveals the commonalities between the ethics of reading and the ethics of clinical practice and the fruitfulness of putting them side by side. Finally, they suggest that close reading of literature may be the optimal training for those who would practice narrative ethics in clinical settings, for the major tools of the narrative ethicist are those fortified by serious literary work: use of the imagination, radical humility, and the capacity to represent situations so as to fully perceive them.

Part III, "Identities in Pedagogy," takes up urgent questions about individual identities within settings of teaching and learning. Having rehearsed the narrative foundations of intersubjectivity and relation in Part I and having reviewed the philosophical currents of dualism in the face of embodiment in Part II, we take up the particulars of the situated subject in teaching and learning. How do narrativity and identity inflect the classroom space? How can teachers and learners keep space open and safe in which all persons have a voice? These questions are considered by Sayantani DasGupta in Chapter 6, "The Politics of Pedagogy: Cripping, Queering and Un-Homing Health Humanities." These pedagogical questions frame the teaching enterprise itself—no learning will take place in a classroom in which some participants are made less welcome than others. Texts must be introduced into that space that represent marginalized or silenced voices, while assumptions and perspectives of all in the learning experience are submitted to self-critique. To uphold narrative medicine's commitment to social justice in healthcare, its teaching has to guarantee inclusivity of those who do and those who do not feel "at home" within healthcare, within the academy, and within the clearing we are trying to open in this field.

Once we have considered the rules of engagement for serious narrative work in the classroom or workshop, we turn in Part IV to consider the nature of close reading. In Chapter 7, "Close Reading: The Signature Method of Narrative Medicine," Rita Charon traces the origins and conceptual foundations of what came in the 1920s to be called *close reading*, that form of reading in which every word counts, in which no textual feature is squandered for its contribution to the meaning of the words. As our signature method, close reading reflects and articulates the foundational principles of narrative medicine: (1) action toward social justice, (2) disciplinary rigor, (3) inclusivity, (4) tolerance of ambiguity, (5) participatory and nonhierarchical methods, and (6) relational and intersubjective processes. Reflexive, the relation between these foundational principles and the nature and process of close reading continues to reveal to us the deep elements of this work on which we have embarked. We hope readers will join us in recognizing close reading's exquisitely attentive reading practice to be the laboratory for the exquisitely attentive listening practice that is our goal in clinical work.

Chapter 8, "A Framework for Teaching Close Reading," provides practical guidance in how one might go about teaching the skills and methods of close reading. Rita offers a conceptual map for the elements of narrative or poetic texts that repay attention in the classroom. Her choice to concentrate on time, space, voice, and metaphor in this chapter does not rule out attention to other textual features, of course. Some of the texts discussed, reprinted in the chapter, have been used in classrooms and hospital seminars that support close examinations of one or another of these narrative features—among them Lucille Clifton's poem "the death of fred clifton" in teaching about time, and a paragraph from James' *Portrait of a Lady* in teaching about space in narrative texts. The texts produced by students in various settings reveal the potentials of this kind of teaching and, ultimately, the gifts of this kind of reading.

Part V, "Creativity," takes up both theoretical aspects of creativity and the pedagogical means to encourage persons in clinical settings to release their own creative spark. Fiction writer Nellie Hermann has inspired our growing realization that creativity is at the center of the work of narrative medicine. From her own experience in writing her first novel *The Cure for Grief*, which represented in fiction her own lived losses, she has committed herself to developing a conceptual understanding of the consequences of creative writing in the individual writer's life.[8] In Chapter 9, "Creativity: What, Why, and Where?," she describes creativity as an openness to uncertainty and doubt, an expansion of the mind, a welcoming of the unexpected. It is a way of being in the world that quickens the spirit. With the help of a variety of texts written by narrative medicine students and by noted creative writers and scholars, Nellie explains the interior processes of writing about one's own life and the consequences in the subsequent life of having written. Without distinguishing between "great writers" and the rest of us, she expresses plainly and deeply the human necessity for bringing forth from within the self the unsaid experiences of life.

Chapter 10, "Can Creativity Be Taught?" is a practical manual for teaching writing in unusual places. Relying on her experiences teaching writing at Columbia University's health sciences campus and arts & sciences campus, Nellie shows how to encourage writing and how to respond to the writing that results. The "Reading Guide" included in the chapter gives guidance to those new to the task of reading and commenting on students' creative writing. The chapter also provides practical guidelines for structuring writing seminars, choosing texts to study, and crafting the writing prompt that invites participants to write. Through extensive quotation and close reading of students' writing, Nellie leads readers toward a creative insight into the creativity of others.

Part VI takes up the questions of assessing the consequences of this work. How do we know that our work in narrative medicine is useful? What happens as an outcome of teaching writing to hospital staff members or of writing about one's patients in forms different from the hospital chart? We have asked medical anthropologist Edgar Rivera Colón to help us answer these questions.

Having taught the Qualitative Research Methods course in the Master of Science in Narrative Medicine graduate program for years, he is in the ideal position to consider the means of learning from social activity as an ethnographer and participant/observer. Rather than soliciting a research manual, we invited Edgar to meditate on the ways of the ethnographer. Chapter 11, "From Fire Escapes to Qualitative Data: Pedagogical Urging, Embodied Research, and Narrative Medicine's Ear of the Heart," demystifies qualitative research, encouraging readers to recognize their own experiences in attentively hearing and watching and trying to make sense of the activities that surround them. Edgar describes the necessity for the researcher to identify his or her position—race, class, gender, ideological beliefs—to achieve a reflexive practice of ethnographic enquiry. Providing a stark critique of the US healthcare system's corporatization and its focus on increasing productivity in a context of alarming wealth and health disparities, he suggests that narrative medicine's commitment to "slow down" is a powerful and corrective response to the healthcare-industrial complex that threatens to diminish the good that healthcare can do.

Part VII turns to clinical practice. Throughout our work, the premium has been on means by which narrative medicine can improve routine healthcare, aligning clinician and patient in a stronger affiliation and providing fresh means by which they can come to recognize one another's concerns. Eric R. Marcus and Rita Charon join in writing Chapter 12, "A Narrative Transformation of Health and Healthcare." As Director of Columbia University's Center for Psychoanalytic Training and Research and member of narrative medicine's founding faculty, Eric has contributed deeply to the development of our conceptual understanding of the healing relationship. His work as a psychoanalyst and scholar of psychoanalytic methods has enabled narrative medicine to recognize the interior processes of intersubjectivity in the care of the sick. Eric and Rita focus on one clinical case in this chapter, of a patient from Rita's internal medicine practice whose care included extensive narrative work. Both patient and doctor wrote about the events of care, read one another's writing, and thereby achieved a complex and helpful insight into the patient's situation. The patient graciously and enthusiastically gave permission to publish the considerations that arose from her care. Through a detailed examination of the events of a few months of care, Eric and Rita each discuss cardinal elements in the clinical relationships with medically ill patients, from the psychoanalytic literature and the narrative literature. Eric focuses on the unusual form of transference found in the care of the medically ill and the opening up of a transitional space in the long process of their care. Rita examines three concepts—creativity, reflexivity, and reciprocity—that illuminate the events that befall patients and their caregivers.

In Chapter 13, "Clinical Contributions of Narrative Medicine," Rita summarizes clinical methods or practices that have been developed by those trained in narrative medicine. She reviews several categories of clinical inventions with examples of work spanning continents. Starting with innovations in individual interviewing techniques toward developing narratively fortified clinical relationships, she moves to narrative means of improving the effectiveness of the healthcare team and then to such novel practices in clinical narrative medicine as transforming the ways in which clinicians write in clinical charts, including electronic health records, and means of bearing witness in busy clinic schedules. This chapter is conceived as the opening of a conversation that, we hope, will continue forward as our work grows.

As we wrote singly or in pairs, together reading and commenting on each developing chapter, we appreciated the emerging patterns in our work. Individual topics intersected with others in ways we had not yet perceived, offering fresh means of deepening the work and suggesting new answers to puzzling questions. We are more convinced than ever that there is a future for a narrative vision of healthcare, that the care of the sick can proceed on the grounds of dignity and recognition, and that those who commit their lives to healthcare can be nourished personally in return. To this vision, we commit our work.

Rita Charon, on behalf of this book's co-authors

Notes

1. For some of the canonical contributions to this revolutionary theory, see Derrida, *Of Grammatology*; Barthes, *Rustle of Language*; Lacan, *Écrits*; Lyotard, *Postmodern Condition*; Foucault, *Order of Things*; Cixous, "Laugh of the Medusa." See also Krieswirth, "Trusting the Tale," on the turn toward narrative studies in many disciplines; and Hayden White, *Metahistory*, questioning the capacity of historical writing to display "objective" historical facts.
2. See J. Hillis Miller, *Ethics of Reading*; Culler, *On Deconstruction*; Iser, *Act of Reading*; W.J.T. Mitchell, *On Narrative*; Peter Brooks, *Reading for the Plot*; and Tompkins, *Reader-Response*, for a few examples of the extensive body of scholarship on the nature of reading that emerged during the rise of theory.
3. See Engel, "Need for a New Medical Model"; Kleinman, *Illness Narratives*; Cassell, "Nature of Suffering"; and Schafer, *Retelling a Life*, for some of the landmarks of the clinical turn toward the patient.
4. The National Endowment for the Humanities (NEH) celebrated its 50th Anniversary in 2015. To commemorate, the NEH chose the 50 grants they have given that best exemplify the missions of the NEH, grants that have "changed the landscape of the humanities." The grant they awarded to us to start narrative medicine is one of the 50 out of 63,000 grants awarded over 50 years to receive this distinction.
5. See, for example, Miller et al., "Sounding Narrative Medicine"; Arntfield et al., "Narrative Medicine"; Winkel et al., "No Time to Think"; Hellerstein, "City of the Hospital"; Pearson,

McTige, and Tarpley, "Narrative Medicine in Surgical Education"; Garrison et al., "Qualitative Analysis."
6. For a sample of studies in clinical settings of methods of narrative medicine, see Olson, "Narrative Medicine: Recovery"; Nowaczyk, "Narrative Medicine in Clinical Genetics"; Sarah Chambers and Glickstein, "Making a Case"; Lövtrup, "Here Is the Patient"; and Sands, Stanley, and Charon, "Narrative Pediatric Oncology."
7. James, Preface to the *Ambassadors*, x.
8. Hermann, *Cure for Grief.*

INTERSUBJECTIVITY

CHAPTER 1

Accounts of Self: Exploring Relationality Through Literature

Maura Spiegel and Danielle Spencer

Introduction

> We are so much embedded in our relations with others that those very relations are
> difficult to discern clearly. We are so in the thick of relationality that it is almost im-
> possible to fully appreciate its contours and inner workings, a little like the eye trying
> to see itself.
>
> —Stephen A. Mitchell[1]

We turn our attention to what literature has to teach us about relationality, about the ordinary yet surprisingly complex occurrence of human interaction. It has been through working with literary texts—alongside literary, philosophical, and psychoanalytic theories—that we have developed many of our principles and some of our practices. In these pages we explore the theme of relationality in a few works on the syllabus of the Giving and Receiving Accounts of Self course in our Master's degree program. Investigating literature, film, and critical texts, the course in some ways resembles a traditional academic approach, except that narrative medicine teaches the skills of close and attentive reading in order to better understand narrative competence and relationality and to explore their implications for healthcare.

Literature opens a bottomless resource for observing, thinking, and talking together about human interactions at a level of depth and complexity that other worthy approaches (such as "professionalism" or communication skills training) cannot match. Instead of instructing clinicians and caregivers with a list of correct attitudes and affects, we explore the clinical applications of literary knowledge. A recent study published in *Science* found that subjects performed better on tests measuring theory of mind, social perception, and emotional intelligence after reading literary fiction.[2] Notably, those who read nonfiction or popular fiction did not perform as well. To explain these findings, the researchers, citing philosopher and literary critic Roland Barthes, pointed to the fact that literary fiction engages readers in a creative experience, positioning us to fill in gaps, draw inferences about characters, and become sensitive to nuance and complexity. In this kind of reading we "must draw on more flexible interpretive resources to infer the feelings and thoughts of characters."[3]

The creative texts under discussion here are all first-person accounts, both fiction and nonfiction. In our approach we look closely at literary texts instead of medical notes or transcripts. Such clinical materials offer crucial information, and a glimpse or trace of an experience, to be sure. A literary text, however, takes as its subject the nuances and intricacies of character, context, and circumstance. It draws the reader into a complex relation, inscribing her into its world in a way that a transcript does not. Furthermore, the texts we choose are not primarily about medical experiences. We read stories that address themes of loss, memory, identity, and the construction of personal history, studying the operations of narrative. With an eye to different forms of relationality, we—as readers and as listeners—take in the relationships between characters, between narrator and character, narrator and reader, and between an individual and society. By reading works that are not explicitly *about* healthcare, the connections *with* health, illness, care, and mortality must be made—and in this way yet one more relation takes form.

In order to explore different perspectives on narrative and relationality, we assign works of literary theory and criticism, psychoanalysis, philosophy, memory and trauma studies, including Mikhail Bakhtin's study of dialogism, Rita Felski's work on the reader's experiences of "recognition" and "enchantment," Judith Butler's excavations into our ethical relation to the Other, Stephen A. Mitchell's building blocks in relational psychoanalysis, Michael White's breakthroughs in Narrative Therapy, and many others. Our scope of practice here is to open a discussion of selected texts, exploring the ways that literary narrative and concepts from these different analytical disciplines deepen our understanding of relationality. These are not prescriptive interpretations but examples of how such a discussion might begin—and, of course, the form and content depend on the pedagogical context. This chapter examines how literary texts can offer access to and strategies for exploring the many facets of relationality, with particular relevance to the clinical encounter.

Self-Telling: Colm Tóibín and the *Need* to Tell

> If I called, I could go over everything that happened six years ago. Because that is what is on my mind tonight, as though no time had elapsed, as though the strength of the moonlight had by some fierce magic chosen tonight to carry me back to the last real thing that happened to me. On the phone to you across the Atlantic, I could go over the days surrounding my mother's funeral. I could go over all the details, as though I were in danger of forgetting them.
>
> —"One Minus One" by Colm Tóibín[4]

On the sixth anniversary of his mother's death, the narrator of Colm Tóibín's short story, "One Minus One," finds himself recounting the details of her dying. Walking alone on a moonlit Texas night, he is carried back to the past as if "by some fierce magic," and he grapples with the urge to call a past lover, one who always demanded honesty from him, "the only person who shakes his head in exasperation when I insist on making jokes and small talk, when I refuse to be direct."[5] But he does not phone him, and instead the story unfolds as a hypothetical telephone call to this former intimate ("If I called . . .") in which he gives voice to long-ago experiences that are perhaps registering with him for the first time, or landing at a new depth. As memories unfold, he observes the half-known connections between his mother's aloofness, his regrets about not trying harder with her, and his own solitary peripatetic existence.

All stories can be said to exist in a hypothetical space, but in this one the "as if" is given a *relational* emphasis. It is in an imagined conversation with a particular person that the narrator finds the register in which to speak, to become intelligible to himself; this unfolding of memory is shaped by the person to whom it is addressed, despite his physical absence. What appears to be a kind of monologue is in fact a dialogue with a silent addressee or interlocutor. The reader can feel the presence and particularity of "the listener" in the intimate and confiding nature of the narration, and through the many comments directly addressed to "you" by the narrator ("I could remind you . . . that you wore a white shirt at the funeral . . . I could see you when I spoke about her from the altar"—". . . you are alone in wanting me always to say something that is true"[6]—"I wish that I had not called you all those other times when I did not need to as much as I do now."[7]) The story's quiet urgency builds on the onrush of delayed feeling and the narrator's *need* to tell and to be heard, even if the listener is merely imagined. Indeed, the presence of the absent listener, so far from the speaker in place and time, becomes palpably real to the reader over the course of the story.

"One Minus One" urges the reader to consider, among many things, the space a listener creates or fails to create, and how relationships from our past feature in our daily interactions, even those which appear singular. Moreover, this fine-grained work of literary fiction establishes a relationship with the reader who is positioned to "overhear" the tale and is also in some sense addressed by it. Of course different readers respond in quite different ways, and this variety enriches a group's discussion of the story. When asked to select a moment or passage that resonates particularly for them, readers discover in their choice a fresh locus of meaning. One reader might respond to the moment at the airport when the narrator recognizes the characteristic "tentative stance" of an Irish couple, finding comfort and familiarity in his compatriots, while another finds the story's deepest sadness in the narrator's night flight home when he begins to weep: "I was back then in the simple world . . . a world in which someone whose heartbeat had once been mine, and whose blood became my blood, and inside whose body I once lay curled, herself lay stricken in a hospital bed."[8] In every response the story locates the reader in a shaped world where we can feel the cumulative weight of things left unsaid, and it rouses us to give language to our experience of and reflections on the story—to linger in the intersubjective space created by the narrator's voice. It draws us into questions of connection and rupture, and of giving and receiving an account of self as a co-construction—ideas that might not be grasped in the abstract, might not be *felt* without the context of the story.

Within the clinical encounter, the therapeutic value for the patient of being listened to is widely recognized. Less considered is the co-constructed nature of the exchange, how the listener or clinician—as well as the context in which they confer—contributes to and even shapes what the teller is able to formulate or express.[9] Much of healthcare happens in interpersonal moments, and narrative medicine is attentive to the relational dynamics at work in every human encounter. In the medical context—and in any context—there is no such thing as a neutral human presence. As important as it is for clinicians to strive to present a benign, nonjudgmental composure and concern, an individual care provider carries a host of meanings to the patients she serves. These meanings are mutable, social, personal, and interpersonal. In all of their rich particularity, the clinician and patient are responding in complex ways to one another. In the examination room, as in any room, an atmosphere is created between two people.

Colm Tóibín's luminous and bittersweet "One Minus One" emphasizes loss and missed connections, yet the surprise of the story is that we gain a fresh, affirming appreciation for the complexities of human dynamics. Bringing the reader to a felt engagement with missed connections can help develop a new awareness of listening skills, but it can also remind us of the beauty of human encounters, a place where mysteries abound. Our experience in narrative medicine classrooms and clinic-based workshops teaches us that close reading can

bring readers to a fresh curiosity about and aliveness to what occurs in interactions between flesh and blood characters, between patient and healthcare
provider, family members, caregivers, between and among colleagues—all the
stakeholders in a given clinical situation. An alertness to what the psychoanalyst Stephen Mitchell calls the "relational space," we contend, is a crucial component of the delivery of effective care.

Monologue and Dialogue: Dostoevsky and Bakhtin

> I am a sick man. . . . I am a spiteful man. I am a most unpleasant man. I think my liver
> is diseased. Then again, I don't know a thing about my illness; I'm not even sure what
> hurts. I'm not being treated and never have been, though I respect both medicine
> and doctors. Besides, I'm extremely superstitious—well at least enough to respect
> medicine. (I'm sufficiently educated not to be superstitious; but I am, anyway.) No,
> gentlemen, it's out of spite that I don't wish to be treated. Now then, that's something
> you probably won't understand. Well, I do. Of course, I won't really be able to explain
> to you precisely who will be hurt by my spite in this case: I know perfectly well that
> I can't possibly "get even" with doctors by refusing their treatment; I know better than
> anyone that all this is going to hurt me alone, and no one else. Even so, if I refuse to be
> treated, it's out of spite. My liver hurts? Good, let it hurt, let it hurt even more![10]

The opening passage of the narrator's account—"I am a sick man . . ."—is rife
with paradox and contradiction, assertions which are belied and questioned.
Belief, knowledge, ignorance, superstition, respect, education, spite, lack of
understanding, understanding, incapacity, awareness—all are juxtaposed in a
manner that seems, oddly enough, both jarring and insouciant. The narrator's
relation to his listener/reader could hardly be more fraught. He acknowledges
the reader first through an accusation of misconstrual—". . . that's something
you probably won't understand"—while asserting his own understanding,
which we are, of course, then given to doubt. The Underground Man is our
paradigmatic "unreliable narrator," one who willfully lies and baits and spins
circles around us. In section I, he describes himself as spiteful and then explains: "I was lying about myself just now when I said that I was a nasty official.
I lied out of spite."[11] Here, lied to out of spite about being spiteful, we are caught
in a Liar's Paradox—but why?

One of the great works of nineteenth-century literature, *Notes from
Underground* has been analyzed from many perspectives. In a narrative medi
cine class we might first draw attention towards our own responses faced with
this ornery narrator—our irritation and resistance to his provocations. It is
natural to bracket the Underground Man as a ranting solipsist and to read

Notes as an extended monologue characterized by isolation, bitterness, and despair. Yet in this context we seize upon such strong readerly responses and hold them up to our scrutiny: how do the opening passages elicit such strong feelings; how are we invited into the text and inscribed within it, perhaps unwittingly?

As we become aware of our own complex relationship with the text, we think, too, about frustration—about annoyance and resistance—as readers and as listeners in different settings. Clinicians and medical educators struggle with "the difficult patient," the uncoöperative voice that embroils, that resists, that contradicts. A voice that does not hew easily to the rubric of a standard medical interview, that is "non-compliant" or "non-adherent," or one that simply refuses to speak. Refusal of treatment creates a tremendous practical and ethical challenge, as in the case of Mary C. Northern, an elderly woman in Tennessee who declined treatment for gangrene in her feet; the case went to trial in 1978 and has become a canonical case in bioethics. We are tempted to explain such cases by ascribing refusal to a lack of capacity, and that determination remains one of the most challenging areas of medical ethics. Yet how might we learn from our study of Dostoevsky— how might we "read" clinical encounters with more nuance, and explore the ways in which these stories are in dialogue with *us*?[12] Similarly, how might we understand the ways in which "resistant" patients are in fact in dialogue—how they have a need to tell, just like the narrator in Tóibín's story, and how their telling takes many different forms? How might we observe the ways in which speech is a kind of behavior, and behavior a kind of speech? And how can we remain attuned to all the myriad forms communication can take?

One of Dostoevsky's greatest literary critics, Mikhail Bakhtin, demonstrates that the Underground Man's monologue is a tortuously wrought interplay between isolation and relationality. As Bakhtin shows, the Underground Man can in fact only define himself *in opposition to* another, whether the other is (at any given moment) explicit, tacit, imputed, anticipated, ignored, or rejected. The Underground Man addresses his phantom audience:

> You probably think, gentlemen, that I want to amuse you. You're wrong about that, too. I'm not at all the cheerful fellow I seem to be, or that I may seem to be; however, if you're irritated by all this talk (and I can already sense that you are irritated), and if you decide to ask me just who I really am . . .[13]

As Bakhtin describes: "The hero's attitude toward himself is inseparably bound up with his attitude toward another, and with the attitude of another toward him. His consciousness of self is constantly perceived against the background of the other's consciousness of him . . ."[14] Bakhtin demonstrates that every phrase in the Underground Man's monologue is in fact relational, even the more abstract philosophical portions. As he explains, "Discourse about the world, just like discourse about oneself, is profoundly dialogic: the hero casts an energetic reproach at the world order, even at the mechanical necessity of nature, as if he were talking not about the world but with the world."[15] Thus at every level of the text "there is not a single monologic word."[16]

Philosopher Alisdair MacIntyre offers an example of this dynamic: ". . . what I feel is in large part a response to what I take others to feel or not feel. You are resentful of my lack of gratitude at your generosity in the face of my anger at your lack of sympathy for my depression over your sentimentality." Literary texts can *show* us this reciprocity with particular clarity, in contrast to the way we often experience the knotty character of interpersonal dynamics and every-day encounters. "Such chains of emotion are characteristic of the emotional life," explains MacIntyre, and "the plot of a novel often traces such a chain."[17]

How does understanding and awareness of relationality play out in the clin-ical encounter? Not long ago, a successful mid-career clinician was participat-ing in a narrative medicine class discussion which provoked an unexpected epiphany about a "difficult" patient. As he explained: "I've had this patient for 14 years, and for 14 years I've dreaded going into that room with him. I *just now realized* that if *I* behave differently towards *him*, he will behave dif-ferently towards me." His insight was into his own participation in a mutually frustrating dynamic, and his resolve was not merely to be nicer or more com-passionate, but—having identified his implication—to search for new ways to connect with his patient. Such realizations are distinguished from approaches which can be taught didactically, including "listening skills" and techniques of medical professionalism (though such efforts in healthcare education can indeed be beneficial). With a literary text, the connections drawn by the reader are *experiential* and are particular to her own history, associations, and cir-cumstances. Like the reader of Dostoevsky's *Notes*, the clinician or caregiver cannot disentangle her own responses from what occurs in the reading or in the listening. Our efforts to distance ourselves and to become neutral observ-ers are continually thwarted, are made *part of* the literary experience, and it is this realization which dawns in a new way in the practice of close reading.

Recognition in Bechdel's *Fun Home*: Thickening the Story

If with Dostoevsky we explore the dialogic nature of literature and become conscious of our own responses to the text, Alison Bechdel helps us take up a complementary set of relational issues, including the role of readerly recognition and different ways that a teller can "thicken" the story. Unlike Dostoevsky's tale, which specifies that it is fiction in the Author's Note (and complicates the statement by asserting that it reflects the reality of society), *Fun Home* is a memoir, enacting a narrative engagement with the often painful events of the author's own life. How do we experience the story differently with the knowledge that it is autobiographical—in what sense does its "contract" with the reader vary? How does this type of narrative encounter serve our understanding of relationality in other contexts, such as clinical encounters?

Unlike Dostoevsky's Undergound Man, a character who appears as eager to repel us as to hold us in his grip, Alison Bechdel invites her reader into this multifaceted, multilayered graphic memoir through many doors. On the front of the hardcover first edition of *Fun Home*, under the dust jacket, is a line drawing of Bechdel's childhood home with stark circular portals drawn into the house, each highlighting an isolated member of the family engaged in a different activity: father examining picture frames in the basement, mother playing the grand piano in the parlor, a young Alison drawing with a quill pen, and siblings playing the guitar and building model airplanes. What will we find as we enter the house? What draws these characters together, and what draws us into the tale? Turning to the flyleaf, we see a delicately painted pattern of wallpaper, and on the title page, 𝕱𝖚𝖓 𝕳𝖔𝖒𝖊, in Gothic script, is framed by a drawing of the eaves of the house doubling as photo corners.[18] The chapter title pages, too, feature line drawings of family snapshots placed as in a photo album. And so we find ourselves entering the physical space of the family manse as well as the album, and we will soon inhabit the leaves of diaries and novels and letters, exquisitely rendered on the page. As this opening suggests, *Fun Home* unfolds a many-layered and self-consciously "thickened" story. It is at once the story of a father's complex legacy, a coming-out story, and a *kunstlerroman*. At its center is the unsolved death of Alison's father—by suicide or accident—and the revelations that surround it, as well as this daughter's efforts to understand their shared history.

What does it mean, "to thicken a story?" And why is it pertinent to Alison Bechdel or to relationships within the medical context? The psychologist Michael White has proposed that many of the stories we live with about ourselves are *thin*, reductive descriptions of our own or others' identities. As he sees it, a thin story is often negatively charged, frequently characterized by "conclusions that one is 'hopeless', 'a failure', 'incompetent', 'unworthy', 'hateful', 'inadequate', and so on."[19] The "thin" version of Alison Bechdel's story could be that her father Bruce left her a legacy of his shame—his hidden sexual orientation and affairs and his probable suicide. To narrativize and thicken a story is to tell it in a new way to a responsive listener; not to change the events of the story but to discover novel significance in them so that the "thin" conclusion no longer appears fixed and essentialized. Indeed, *Fun Home* offers multiple perspectives and means of understanding, and it resists a neat resolution to the enigmas it explores.

Michael White draws upon the work of anthropologist Clifford Geertz, who proposes that thick description also has the power "to bring us in touch with the lives of strangers."[20] Geertz highlights the importance of enigmatic gestures such as facial expressions and argues that in order to provide an authentic analysis, the ethnographer must grasp, reflect upon, and represent nuance and context. For example: How does one distinguish between a wink and a twitch of the eye, the same physical act with two very different meanings? For Geertz, a thick description includes distinctions among "twitches, winks, fake-winks, parodies, rehearsals of parodies" so as to understand how they "are produced, perceived, and interpreted, and without which they would not in fact exist, no matter what anyone did or didn't do with his eyelids."[21] In other words, a gesture only exists within multiple relationships—to a particular moment, a particular person, and to other means of expression—and thick description begins to unpack such narrative elements. In this sense good literature *is* thick description.

In the clinical encounter such attentiveness is critical, as gestures, facial expressions, and body language can signal in such significant ways; patients will remember, for example, the exact posture of a clinician who sat and listened to them for the first time and can describe the scene in vivid detail, while a doctor, too, may seek to interpret a patient's facial expressions and posture in an effort to establish a rapport and to better understand the patient's story. Writer Anatole Broyard describes his own interpretation of the appearance and behavior of his doctors, bringing his critical literary sensibility to bear upon his experience as a patient. In describing a urologist's inelegant bearing in his surgical cap, Broyard writes: "He wore it like an American in France who affects a beret without understanding how to shape or cock it. To my eyes this doctor simply didn't have the charisma to overcome or assimilate those caps, and this completed my disaffection."[22] Acknowledging his own prejudices, Broyard enacts and reveals the critical importance of words and gestures in the context of a particular relationship, describing them in their rich singularity.

In Bechdel's *Fun Home* every scene contains a "thick" opulence of description and of different ways of depicting and understanding her family's experience. We are brought into such intimate knowledge of the characters that we come to understand the significance of their "twitches, winks, fake-winks, parodies, rehearsals of parodies". This is, after all, the essence of family life, in which no gesture is "thin" or neutral. To pick just one example, toward the end of the text is a scene of Alison and her father during her college years, when she has recently come out as lesbian to her parents. They are driving to the movies, and, in the dark, sitting side-by-side in the front seat of the car, they have an unprecedented exchange: "I wonder if you knew what you were doing when you gave me that Collette book," Alison says to her father—a way of indirectly asking him if he was aware that she was gay. "What?"—he says in the next panel—and then "Oh"—and then "I didn't, really"—followed by a panel where they stare ahead in silence. Alison's retrospective commentary appears in the next frame: "I kept still, like he was a splendid deer I didn't want to startle." Finally her father responds: "I guess there was some kind of . . . identification."[23] The cinematic repetition of frames, from the same angle—the only double-page spread in the book where the panels are all the same size—slows time, gives us the experience of the gaps and silences in this formative exchange. The alternation between dialogue and narration brings together the present-time of the image with the adult Alison's memory and perspective. As both Alison and her father are drawn in profile, watching the road ahead, they become two figures with certain parallels in their stories, heading into the darkness and an uncertain future. The knowledge Bechdel offers us—that this is one of the last conversations she will share with her father—endows it with a keen poignancy. With its rich, multilayered, "thickened" telling, the story becomes a type of homage, just as the book itself is an act of love.

RECOGNITION: THE READER IN THE TEXT

Many readers feel in this portrait of tentative yet significant father–daughter communication a deeply familiar experience of recognition. We read books and watch films in part to discover ourselves, to measure our own experience against fiction, to consider our lives from new and different perspectives—to thicken our own stories.

Readerly recognition plays a critical role within *Fun Home* as well. Alison sees herself in the Colette novel, recognizing her own sexual orientation in the text. Her father's comment, "I guess there was some kind of . . . identification" speaks to *their* shared identification as homosexuals through the fictional text. In a similar gesture, following the scene in the car, Alison invokes the encounter at the end of *Ulysses* when Stephen Dedalus and Leopold Bloom share cocoa, and this culminating "father–son" moment in Joyce's magisterial work leads Alison to ask which of them—she or Bruce—is the father/parent. As she explains, "I had felt distinctly parental listening to his shamefaced recitation."[24] Here Joyce provides her with a template for thinking through parent–child relations. Yet Alison also draws our attention to the differences, the ruptures between these influential texts and her experience, as well as the potential perils of readerly identification. For example, Bruce recognizes himself in fiction, particularly in a romanticized view of authors such as Fitzgerald and Camus—yet one might argue that such recognition allows him to preserve a false, alienated self, one which pulls him out of the reality of his life and family.

Indeed, the identificatory relationships we form with narratives are not always nourishing; they have their perils. Health humanities has long noted the negative impact of the narrative of "The Heroic Doctor," a staple of medical and popular culture. Ian Williams' moving graphic novel, *The Bad Doctor*, explores the negative self-assessments its protagonist undergoes on a daily basis, feeling that his service to his patients is inadequate, meager, fundamentally lacking. Perhaps this doctor's negative feelings can be in part attributed to the idealized image of the doctor and his or her retinue of grateful and admiring patients, against which he measures himself. As we are all well aware, narratives are not a good unto themselves—and even good ones can evoke unlooked-for responses. Finding and maintaining a functional critical stance is a crucial part of the work of narrative medicine.

What can we learn from this experience of readerly recognition in *Fun Home* and elsewhere? Literary theorist Rita Felski begins her *Uses of Literature* with the question: "What does it mean to recognize oneself in a book?"[25] Recognition in this sense includes the possibility for reflection upon one's circumstances or predicament, the conditions of one's life, and prevailing social forces. However, recognition—a form of relationality—opens longstanding debates about the status of the Subject, about our capacity for self-knowledge. Tracing the development of a "hermeneutics of suspicion" through 20th-century thinkers such as Derrida, Lacan, Althusser, and Foucault, Felski reviews the ways in which critics have derided the experience of self-recognition as illusory—as in the case of Lacan's mirror stage—or as a tool of suppression, as in the case of Althusser's subject who is thereby interpellated into the structure of social control. The "snare of a fictional subjectivity"—such as a character in a novel or film whom we encounter as reader or spectator—becomes a means of subjugation, and fiction itself perpetuates such misapprehension.[26] As Felski characterizes this critical wariness: ". . . identifying with characters is a key mechanism through which we are drawn into believing in the essential reality of persons. The role of criticism is to interrogate such fictions of selfhood . . ."[27]

Rather than wallow in what she sees as an epistemic quagmire, Felski suggests that we make a place for imperfect self-knowledge and also points toward a constructive role for recognition—specifically as a form of *acknowledgement*. As Felski argues, the desire for both knowledge and acknowledgement is ineluctably human, and reading is a dynamic lens through which this interplay of intersubjectivity can be brought in and out of focus. She argues for a nuanced understanding of the many multifaceted forms recognition can take, encompassing sameness and difference, the familiar and the strange—even including a modern reader's recognition of *failures* of recognition in literary texts. As she explains, "Recognition is about knowing, but also about the limits of knowing and knowability, and about how self-perception is mediated by the other, and the perception of otherness by the self."[28]

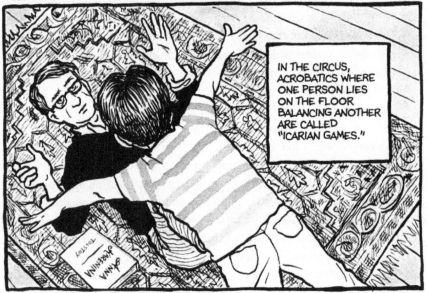

Source: Bechdel, *Fun Home,* 3.

Returning to *Fun Home*, we experience many different forms of recognition and misrecognition, from the particular to the broadly political, and from the events of the story to the very means of its telling. In the opening pages, Alison, as the adult narrator, describes her identification with Icarus; balancing on her father's upturned feet, "flying" on the metaphoric airplane of her father's making, it was "certainly worth the moment of perfect balance when I soared above him."[29] Yet she is aware that this is an experience both of recognition and *mis*recognition, and she explores the rupture between the myth and her experience. As she explains, "In our particular reënactment of this mythic relationship, it was not me but my father who was to plummet from the sky."[30] Moreover, she is not his son, though we perhaps do not realize that in these first few frames depicting the Icarus/Daedalus moment, as she has a haircut and clothing with male associations; such ambiguity introduces the vital issue of gender roles and social construction which both characters struggle to navigate throughout *Fun Home*. And, yet another rupture: when the young Alison seeks to repeat this moment of "perfect balance," her father is distracted by the dirty rug, which introduces the theme of his endless preoccupation with cleaning and renovating the family home. Following Felski, all such attempts and imperfections and *failures* of recognition here are integral to its operation, and Bechdel is busily unpacking its mechanics in her staging of the story.

Characters read and engage with a broad range of texts in *Fun Home*, from A. A. Milne to Proust, from Fitzgerald to the dictionary. The mutual recognition and lack of recognition between Alison and her father—knowledge and ignorance of themselves and one another, of themselves as constituted or misunderstood by one another—is also woven into their desire for broader social acknowledgment of their shared homosexuality, and this search is often conducted through reading. As a child the narrator sees her hometown parallel the map in *The Wind in the Willows*, and as a young woman she searches for acknowledgement of her lesbian identity in her avid consumption of what she terms the "Contemporary and Historical Perspectives on Homosexuality" genre. When she takes her school-teacher father's English class in high school, they experience a "novel" intimacy over their shared interest in the books he assigns, and when she leaves for college their exchange of authors such as Collette and Millett becomes part of "an ethical and political claim for acknowledgment," as Felski describes—a claim for a viable place and voice within society.[31] Felski discusses the vital role of such texts for groups that have been silenced and disenfranchised:

> We all seek in various ways to have our particularity recognized, to find echoes of our-selves in the world around us. The patent asymmetry and unevenness of structures of recognition ensure that books will often function as lifelines for those deprived of other forms of public acknowledgment. Until very recently, for example, such deprivation stamped the lives of women who desired other women; a yearning etched into the body and psyche functioned only as an absence, unmentionable at home or work, whited out in the media, invisible in public life, acknowledged only in the occasional furtive whisper or dirty joke.[32]

These texts shared and discussed between Alison and her father are also a shared mirror of sorts, an indirect means for them to acknowledge one another. Yet it is also a funhouse mirror that Bechdel uses to refract and explore their mutual recognition and misrecognition, bumping into false selves just as the "mirrors, distracting bronzes [and] multiple doorways" in the family home cause visitors to lose their way and walk into walls.[33] Never is there perfect transparency, neither between Alison and her father nor within their respective selves.[34] Yet the exchange of books and letters about books and about oneself-as-recognized-in-books speaks to an ongoing desire for both knowledge and acknowledgement.

Such varied examples of recognition and misrecognition permeate *Fun Home* as well as our lived experience, and they play a critical role in health-care. Anatole Broyard, describing his discontent with his urologist, writes, "I thought, I can't die with this man. He wouldn't understand what I was saying. I'm going to say something brilliant when I die."[35] In the clinical encounter, as in many relationships, we crave an experience of what Felski terms *acknowledgment*—to see and be seen in our own unique particularity.

RECOGNITION: RESISTING CLOSURE

At the end of *Fun Home*, Bechdel returns to the Dedalus/Icarus myth. "What if Icarus hadn't hurtled into the sea?" she asks. Having taken us through a story that calls attention to its own fissures, its own unconfirmed hypotheses, we are left in a hypothetical, up in the air. In the final frame of the book she is leaping from a diving board, her father waiting to catch her in the pool: "But in the tricky reverse narration that impels our entwined stories, he was there to catch me when I lept."[36] Relationships are thick stories, and thick stories are relationships—they are stories whose threads connect to so many other stories, and are not owned by any one of us. The "reverse narration" can mean so many things: that memory stretches into the past, while narrative reaches into the future; that we, as characters in one another's lives, and writers and readers, are forming one another's stories; that there are as many versions of stories as there are moments of reflection.

This gesture at the end of the memoir refuses a singular, univocal truth of Alison's family's experience, and the reader must allow for meanings to continue to emerge. There is a strong temptation to judge, to foreclose meaning, as a reader and as a listener. We want to solve riddles, to answer questions, to reach conclusions. We don't wish to wander endlessly in the labyrinth. And certainly answers and diagnoses are vitally important. But for Bechdel, and for the reader, there is a resonant truth to this ending in mid-air.

Identification and Refusal in Kazuo Ishiguro's *Never Let Me Go*

This chapter takes its title from Judith Butler's 2003 *Giving an Account of Oneself*, in which she makes a critical foray into moral philosophy. She poses the fundamental question: Who is this "I" who speaks, and what degree of self-knowledge can I possess? How is it possible to give an account of self that initiates and structures an *ethical* relation? Kazuo Ishiguro's 2005 novel *Never Let Me Go* offers an account of self that probes precisely these questions of self-knowledge, relationality, and ethical action, through the voice of its narrator Kathy H.

For Butler, and for many other contemporary theorists, there is no such thing as a purely autonomous self. Such a proposal might come as an affront to many, including those trained in clinical medicine and principlist bioethics who are taught that respect for "autonomy" is sacrosanct.[37] (See Chapter 5, Deliver us from Certainty: Training for Narrative Ethics.) Such "autonomy" presupposes a degree of self-knowledge and independence from others; yet, as Butler asks, how can we ever presume to completely know ourselves—our wishes and desires? Her enquiry draws upon broad-ranging contemporary critiques of "the Subject"—the human self. Theorists such as Michel Foucault, Jacques Lacan, Jacques Derrida, Julia Kristeva, and many others roundly interrogated the model of the Enlightenment subject, the rational, objective, self-determining individual who surveys the world from a distance. Such a critique leaves us—speaking quite broadly here—with a self who is inescapably formed *in relation* to others and formed *by* language and social structures.

With such a conception of the self, where do we locate the ground of moral responsibility? As Butler frames the question: How can I account for myself ethically—or at all? Can I offer an adequate narrative of myself if I am in some sense formed by my social being, the context and the conditions of my existence, or by the received language with which I construct my narrative? The ancient injunction to "Know thyself" is overthrown, and in its place Butler—drawing particularly on the work of philosophers Emmanuel Levinas and Adriana Cavarero—offers an ethics predicated on recognition of our own opacity to ourselves and the fundamental alterity between self and other. It is on this basis, one of humility and vulnerability, that a fragile ethic is urged.

In our work in narrative medicine we share Butler's conviction of the provisionality, relationality, co-constructedness of the "speaking I," and we see value in bringing these tumultuous vicissitudes into view. For where more than in the medical context, so rife with power inequities and rigid hierarchies, does one need to call out our social embeddedness and contingent identities; and where more than in the patient's unasked questions, unspoken anxieties, and unanswered phone calls does one recognize the fragility of communication in the medical encounter? Where more than in our technocentric era does one need to explore the limits of rationality and positivism? And, lastly, for the clinician or clinician-in-training, so loath to speak in the subjective voice, the question, "Who is this 'I' who speaks?" is an urgent one. And so we turn to philosophy as well as psychology and literary texts where these questions are so often given vibrant form, offering readers a fresh way to think about who we are and the relationships and contingencies we inhabit.

In this particular literary text—Ishiguro's *Never Let Me Go*—we find (spoiler alert) a gripping dystopic tale of clones living in an alternative post-Thatcher England, having been created solely for the purpose of donating their organs and forfeiting their lives to non-cloned humans. The novel is often read in bioethics courses, where it offers grist for discussion of public policy concerning such issues as organ transplantation, cloning, genetic engineering, healthcare inequities, and social justice. Readers often marvel at how fiction can mirror our predicament with uncanny precision, offering allegorical narratives, alternative presents, and possible futures, challenging us to examine the ways in which our world is not as dissimilar from such dystopian visions as we might like to believe. Likewise concerned with these urgent questions, our attention, in the context of narrative medicine, is also directed toward the relation between narrative decisions and ethical decisions: Where does the story begin? Who tells it, and to whom, and for what reasons? What is included in and excluded from "the story," and what do we learn from the means of its telling?

SCENE OF ADDRESS

Ishiguro's novel begins with an ordinariness that leaps out at the reader: "My name is Kathy H." Unaware, of course, of who is speaking or what world we are entering, we wonder what this stunningly bland opening portends. As we proceed, we realize that this formulation contains far more than the information of what the narrator is called. Where narrators often provide some personal background, something to orient us in relation to them, Kathy (we will later discover) has no familial history or identity—nothing except her name and the "school," Hailsham, and her memories of her peers and "guardians" to ground her story. On first reading we wonder, what does the H. signify? Is it the first letter of her last name, used by her to distinguish herself from other Kathys? Later, once we realize that she has no "family name," we will wonder whether the H. functions as a number might, such as *Kathy, model #8.*

Kathy's introduction takes us by surprise in its immediacy, and yet, pausing over this very first sentence of the novel, we find ourselves estranged by this most familiar of gestures, someone telling us her name. And here in the opening sentence our relationship with the narrative begins to take shape. We ponder whether Kathy H. is introducing herself to us, her "flesh-and-blood readers," or if we are to imagine a fictional receiver of her story—a narratee? Sure enough, we soon learn that Kathy H. is addressing herself to her fellow clones, those who were not "fortunate" enough to grow up where she did, at Hailsham. She prefaces several passages with the phrase, "I don't know how it was where you were . . ." before explaining some aspect of Hailsham: medical exams, "collections," the guardians' behavior, or attitudes toward sex. As something akin to eavesdroppers, we, the book's readers, become even more implicated in her fate than if she were addressing us directly. Readers of the novel often experience feelings of uneasiness yet cannot necessarily point to their source, and in unpacking this scene of address we can locate the uncanny and unsettling nature of our involvement with the characters and the text. It can be a revelatory process to locate a name for a formerly inchoate reaction, to cultivate analytical tools to better understand our affective responses.

Furthermore, such "scenes of address" are, as Butler explains, critical to offering an account of self: "I come into being as a reflexive subject in the context of establishing a narrative account of myself when I am spoken to by someone and prompted to address myself to the one who addresses me."[38] Drawing upon Levinas, Foucault, Adriana Cavarero, and others, Butler poses the question: What is the nature of this "structure of address," and how does this encounter ground ethics? This scene of address with Kathy—in its uncanny fictional form—causes us to interrogate our ethical responsibility to the speaker in new and often disquieting ways. And in comparing such scenes of address in literature we become newly attuned to their form and import.

IDENTIFICATION AND REFUSAL

If we are in some sense figured as voyeurs in these opening passages, we also gradually share in the experience of the clones and their terrifying plight. Early on, Kathy cares for a dying "donor" who asks her to share her memories of Hailsham: "What he wanted was not just to hear about Hailsham, but to *remember* Hailsham, just like it had been his own childhood. He knew he was close to completing"—the term for a clone's death at their final donation—"and so that's what he was doing: getting me to describe things to him, so they'd really sink in, so that maybe during those sleepless nights, with the drugs and the pain and the exhaustion, the line would blur between what were my memories and what were his."[39] Though we might resist any comparison with this particular listener, we share in something like this experience as readers—we enter Kathy's recollections, and they are vivid with much that we would recognize and value in our own lives: the vagaries of memory, in all its rich imperfection and contingency; friendship and discord; contentment, confusion, desire, sex, relationships; poetry, painting, imagination; longing, loss. As Kath's tale progresses, our understanding of this world evolves with the maturing students, and our knowledge (and perhaps disavowal as well) grows alongside theirs.

Yet the central question of their childhood remains unanswered: Why was their best artwork taken from them at Hailsham for Madame's "gallery"? These mysteries of the past seem, for Kath, to hold the key to understanding herself and those she loves. Toward the end of the novel she and her dear childhood friend Tommy seek an answer to these questions, violating the rules to visit Madame and Miss Emily, the authority figures at Hailsham, to enquire about a rumored 3-year deferral in "donations" for a couple that can prove they are truly in love. Tommy offers his drawings in hopes of demonstrating his and Kath's inner selves, the integrity of their love for one another. They come, really, in search of their origin story, for they believe that it will determine their fate; understanding themselves, they imagine, will allow them to offer a "complete" account of self and to win a form of liberation, albeit temporary. And they finally do bear witness to their own origin story, in a sense—but it comes at the expense of their humanity. Miss Emily tells them that the 3-year reprieve is nothing more than "a little fantasy." They sense that there is more, and ask the primary question of their childhood: Why did Madame take their best creative work? "We took away your art because we thought it would reveal your souls. Or to put it more finely, we did it to prove you had souls at all," explains Miss Emily.[40] Yet the notion that they were considered *not* to possess souls crashes as a shocking revelation, and every layer of knowledge arrives at further expense to their assumed humanity. Miss Emily continues, explaining that at one time "clones—or students, as we preferred to call you—existed only to supply medical science. In the early days, after the war, that's largely all you were to most people. Shadowy objects in test tubes."[41] This is in fact only the second of two instances of the term "clone" in the text, and Miss Emily reveals it as their primary designation, "students" being an alternate appellation favored by the reformers. And so Kathy cannot complete her account of self, for she has emerged from her story a soul-less clone, just as, in Butler's formulation, "The 'I' can tell neither the story of its own emergence nor the conditions of its own possibility without bearing witness to a state of affairs to which one could not have been present, which are prior to one's own emergence as a subject who can know, and so constitute a set of origins that one can narrate only at the expense of authoritative knowledge." Having unveiled her own foundational narrative, Kathy cannot hold on to her past nor her future; she cannot author her own complete account of self without sacrificing the self she holds most dear. Yet she *does* offer an account, and in its recognition of its own impossibility, in a sense, we find humanity in all of its tragic dimensions.

And what of the "scene of address" here? While Madame and Miss Emily are reaffirming Kath and Tommy's fearsome fate, there is tenderness, too. Kathy and Madame appear to have a moment of recognition; they both recollect the scene of young Kathy dancing to the song "Never Let Me Go" and Madame weeping as she watched from the doorway. "You're a mind-reader," Madame tells Kathy, when Kathy recalls this scene from long ago and describes Madame's sadness. But she cannot read Kathy's mind: "I saw a little girl, her eyes tightly closed, holding to her breast the old kind world, one that she knew in her heart could not remain, and she was holding it and pleading, never to let her go. That is what I saw. It wasn't really you, what you were doing, I know that. But I saw you and it broke my heart. And I've never forgotten."[42] There is a misrecognition here, for Kath was in fact imagining herself holding a child. Yet in a sense there was truth to the misrecognition—for Kathy, in yearning for something she could never have, was also mourning the coming loss of her own innocence. Despite her revulsion for the *unheimlich* clone, Madame was moved to tears and recalls the episode in vivid detail—and in this misrecognition there is, as Felski might suggest, a crucial form of recognition. Similarly, readers may struggle with a sense of recognition with Kath and her friends, shuddering at the horror of their fates yet seeing in their fears and loves something of our own.

Readers respond very forcefully to *Never Let Me Go*, and they are often surprised to find that others respond in powerfully *different* ways. When asked if Kath and her friends experience human emotion, some respond "Of course!"— while others answer, "Of course not—they're not human!" Responding to the register and texture of Kathy's voice, some readers feel that her calm, her introspection and self-management, are commendable signs of her strength, empathy, and adaptability, while others hear intense dissociation in her oddly low affect; they see in it a failure to react emotionally to the horrors in her life, or a willed refusal to make contact with her reality. Still other readers hear in Kath's tone her unthinking compliance—or worse, her complicity in the repressive regulatory system that keeps the clones docile. Is Kathy implicated by her adaptation to a death-dealing entity, or is she a lone voice seeking kinship and understanding—or both? Why the clones don't rebel or run away is a question that often puzzles readers, and this topic leads invariably to a discussion of how the normalization by society of many horrific inequities keeps us from rebelling against things in our world that we find monstrous. We may criticize the clones for their placidity, yet we too are inscribed in punishing systems, in means of social control so vast that we may not even recognize them. We are docile bodies, policing one another just as the "students" in the novel watch each other. This topic can lead students—especially medical students—to consider the ways in which *they* are regulated and limited in thought and action. Is it more ethical, they wonder together, to bluntly expose the Hailsham students to their fate, as their guardian Miss Lucy does, or to leave them in ignorance, as Miss Emily elects, to preserve for them some form of childhood? What responsibilities does knowledge bring? And, in a medical context, how does it moor or unsettle relationships?

Conclusion

It is not because I can't explain that you won't understand; it's because you won't understand that I can't explain.
—Elie Wiesel[43]

In these pages we have sought to give you a glimpse into one narrative medicine course. This ever-evolving syllabus contains many other texts by theorists we haven't room here to expound upon, including bell hooks, Jerome
Bruner, Elaine Scarry, Arthur Frank, Dori Laub, Paul Ricoeur, Jonathan Shay,
and Donnel Stern, all of whom broaden our thinking about the dynamic relationships between people, and between people and narrative. From the work
of philosophers and psychoanalysts, we recognize a conceptual shift from a
model of autonomy to one of relationality. In the clinical encounter this trans-
lates to a shift from the model of seer and seen to a bidirectional interaction
where clinicians recognize themselves and their patients as subjective agents.
Describing such a shift in his domain, Stephen Mitchell writes, "For most of
its history, psychoanalytic technique was based on the premise that the patient's psyche and mental processes could be 'analyzed' independently of their
interactions with the analyst's feelings and behaviors. The latter, it was pre-
sumed, could be factored out or held constant through proper technique . . .
In traditional analytic technique, rigor was maintained by efforts to avoid
interaction . . ."[44] Relational theory registers a fundamental shift away from
this model. Just as relational psychoanalysis has largely shed this notion of
the analyst as a neutral receiver and replaced it with a model of the analyst as
co-constructor of the clinician–patient relationship, so too can the practice
of medicine.

We have found that reading literary texts with a focus on relational dynamics
awakens us to the social, structural, professional, and personal relationships in
our lives. Thinking and writing about the co-constructed and dialogic nature
of human exchanges as represented in literary texts brings readers into a more
finely grained awareness of their own effect on others. In the clinical context
the results of such reflection can be vivid and immediate as, without spending an extra minute, the clinician establishes a deeper rapport, opens herself
to the experience of another despite—or perhaps because of—the limitations
of language. Just as literature enriches and deepens stories, doctors, patients,
nurses, family members—all who work together in caring for the sick—can
thicken the telling and listening, can learn to sit comfortably with ambiguity
and multiple perspectives.

Notes

1. Mitchell, "Attachment Theory," 180.
2. See Kidd and Castano, "Reading Literary Fiction." See also Zunshine, *Why We Read Fiction*.
3. Kidd and Castano, "Reading Literary Fiction," 377.
4. Tóibín, "One Minus One," 273–74.
5. Tóibín, "One Minus One," 274.
6. Tóibín, "One Minus One," 274.
7. Tóibín, "One Minus One," 281.
8. Tóibín, "One Minus One," 278, 282.
9. See Chapter 4, "Dualism and its Discontents II: Philosophical Tinctures" for discussion of phenomenology and healthcare, including the work of Edmund Pellegrino, Richard Zaner, and Fredrik Svenaeus on the reciprocity of the clinical encounter.
10. Dostoevksy, *Notes from Underground*, 3.
11. Dostoevksy, *Notes from Underground*, 4.
12. See Alvan Ikoku's discussion of the theme of refusal in Melville's "Bartleby, the Scrivener." Drawing upon the tools of literary scholarship and bioethics, he explores the notion of the dialogic in a clinical context. As Ikoku demonstrates, a close reading of Melville's story expands our understanding of "the ethical texture of refusal," as he terms it—its disruptive power, which prompts different types of reflection and understanding by the other characters as well as by the reader ("Refusal in 'Bartleby, the Scrivener'," 252).
13. Dostoevksy, *Notes from Underground*, 5.
14. Bakhtin, *Problems of Dostoevsky's Poetics*, 207.
15. Bakhtin, *Problems of Dostoevsky's Poetics*, 236.
16. Bakhtin, *Problems of Dostoevsky's Poetics*, 229.
17. MacIntyre, *Against the Self-Images*, 242.
18. In an interview Bechdel recalls the process of painting the wallpaper, invoking the theme of verisimilitude so critical to *Fun Home*: "God, recreating that wallpaper was insane. I felt like I was serving out some sort of penance. It's William Morris's 'Chrysanthemums', a famous pattern, so I was able to find it online and print it out and slap it on my light box and basically trace it. For an entire weekend. One thing my mother did say about the book was that I didn't get the wallpaper pattern right. And she's right, I didn't get enough contrast in it. I've since learned that there are eleven shades of green in the original—and I was only using five different shades" (Chute and Bechdel, "An Interview," 1008).
19. Michael White, "Narrative Practice and Exotic Lives," 121.
20. Geertz, "Thick Description," 8.
21. Geertz, "Thick Description," 7.
22. Broyard, "The Patient Examines," 39.
23. Bechdel, *Fun Home*, 220–21.
24. Bechdel, *Fun Home*, 219.
25. Felski, *Uses of Literature*, 23.
26. Felski, *Uses of Literature*, 27.
27. Felski, *Uses of Literature*, 28. Felski delicately skirts a thorny issue in these debates, as critiquing the Subject does not in fact amount to a nihilistic denial of the "reality of persons." The notion of an "essential reality of persons"—Felski's phrase quoted above—points toward a notion of autonomous essentialism, a Romantic conception of the subject who is not bound by language, culture, or society. Yet social constructivism places the individual in a broader context but does not negate her existence. Felski's charge that misrecognition and alterity do not offer ground for critical insight—"If we are barred from achieving insight or self-understanding, how could we know that an act of misrecognition had taken place?" (28)—risks eliding the complexity of this body

of 20th-century criticism. Indeed, Michel Foucault's exploration of "archaeologies of knowledge" reveals ways in which the subject is indeed inscribed within structures of knowledge and power yet retains personal agency and can gain empowerment through awareness of such forces (see Foucault, *Archaeology of Knowledge*).

28. Felski, *Uses of Literature*, 49.
29. Bechdel, *Fun Home*, 3.
30. Bechdel, *Fun Home*, 4.
31. Felski, *Uses of Literature*, 36.
32. Felski, *Uses of Literature*, 43.
33. Bechdel, *Fun Home*, 20.
34. The young narrator's self-doubt is reflected in the degradation of writing her own journal, testimony crumbling under the weight of subjectivity, as she inscribes "I think" over every sentence—a Derridean skepticism, effectively putting every line *sous rature*.
35. Broyard, "The Patient Examines," 38.
36. Bechdel, *Fun Home*, 232.
37. The conception of "relational autonomy," grounded in feminist critique, offers a variety of perspectives which share the premise "that persons are socially embedded and that agents' identities are formed within the context of social relationships and shaped by a complex of intersecting social determinants, such as race, class, gender, and ethnicity. Thus the focus of relational approaches is to analyze the implications of the intersubjective and social dimensions of selfhood and identity for conceptions of individual autonomy and moral and political agency" (Mackenzie and Stoljar, "Introduction," 4). Yet the term "autonomy"—often employed without such relational emphasis—is still quite prevalent in bioethics discourse.
38. Butler, *Giving an Account*, 15.
39. Ishiguro, *Never Let Me Go*, 3–4.
40. Ishiguro, *Never Let Me Go*, 260.
41. Ishiguro, *Never Let Me Go*, 239.
42. Ishiguro, *Never Let Me Go*, 249.
43. Academy of Achievement, "Elie Wiesel—Interview."
44. Mitchell, *From Attachment to Intersubjectivity*, 69–70.

CHAPTER 2

This Is What We Do, and These Things Happen: Literature, Experience, Emotion, and Relationality in the Classroom

Maura Spiegel and Danielle Spencer

... we have much less control over our own affective experience than is generally comfortable for us. Our emotions and our behaviors have, to some degree, a messy life of their own, in the gaps, the spaces, between oneself and others.
—Stephen A. Mitchell, *"An Interactional Hierarchy"*[1]

How can it be described? How can any of it be described? The trip and the story of the trip are always two different things. The narrator is the one who has stayed home, but then, afterward, presses her mouth upon the traveler's mouth, in order to make the mouth work, to make the mouth say, say, say. One cannot go to a place and speak of it; one cannot both see and say, not really. One can go, and upon returning make a lot of hand motions and indications with the arms. The mouth itself; working at the speed of light, at the eye's instructions, is necessarily struck still; so fast, so much to report, it hangs open and dumb as a gutted bell. All that unsayable life! That's where the narrator comes in. The narrator comes with her kisses and mimicry and tidying up. The narrator comes and makes a slow, fake song of the mouth's eager devastation.
—Lorrie Moore, *"People like that are the only people here"*[2]

At six-thirty in the morning of July the first, I was swallowed by the House of God and found myself walking down an endless bile-colored corridor on the sixth floor. This was ward 6-South, where I was to begin. A nurse with magnificently hairy forearms pointed me to the House Officer's On-Call Room, where rounds were in progress. I opened the door and went in. I felt pure terror. As Freud had said via Berry, my terror was "a straight shot from the id."
—Samuel Shem, *House of God*[3]

Socio-relational Dynamics and Medical Education

First-year medical students often wonder whether it is "right or wrong" to really feel for the patients they are just beginning to encounter in clinical settings. In narrative medicine electives at the Columbia University College of Physicians and Surgeons, the question is reliably voiced in one way or another: Do we *need* to/should we *feel* sympathy for a patient—or can appropriate concern and gestures serve as well? Strong feelings of inadequacy can surface if students find themselves unable to achieve the depth of emotion they would feel "if that were my grandmother" while contending with the tremendous stresses and challenges of medical education.

Most clinicians agree that regulating the expression of emotions is a necessary and important feature of professionalism. A colleague recalled that after the birth of her son, her obstetrician burst into tears breaking the news to her that her baby had Down Syndrome: "It made me so mad that she cried. Doctors are supposed to make you feel that everything is going to be alright." Another person described feeling comforted and less alone when he saw a trace of a tear in the corner of his physician's eye when he was delivering a cancer diagnosis. Perhaps, then, it is not surprising that mixed messages about what to feel and how to express it are common in medical education. Such contradictions may account in part for the paucity of attention to emotion in medical education. As educator Joanna Shapiro writes, "The formal [medical school] curriculum rarely considers trainee emotions directly, although it periodically enumerates officially desirable attitudes and values of respect, altruism and caring."[4] She goes on to point out, however, that the informal curriculum can convey the alternate message that "emotional distance and detachment" are the appropriate professional postures. Among physicians, she proposes, the dominant attitude is that emotions are "untrustworthy, having little or no place in the practice of medicine" because they are perceived as either self-indulgent or leading to "compassion fatigue." The overwhelming message received by medical trainees, according to Shapiro, is that inadequate emotional control, or "caring too much," can result in "emotional exhaustion" and "professional failures."[5] Such suspicion of emotion extends to both negative *and* positive feelings.

Educators have long understood that emotions are not a neutral factor in learning. As psychologist Daniel Goleman writes, "Students who are anxious, angry, or depressed don't learn; people who are caught in these states do not take in information efficiently. . . ."[6] Feminists and race theorists recognize both the pedagogical and *political* value of learning to speak about feeling in the classroom. As Derald Wing Sue describes in *Race Talk and the Conspiracy of Silence*, students appreciate instructors who are unafraid to recognize the racial tension that can emerge in class discussion and to name the feelings that can attend it: "The skilled facilitator helps others make sense of these feelings and frees the individual from being controlled by them. As long as feelings remain unnamed and unacknowledged, they represent emotional roadblocks to having a successful dialogue."[7] What's more, as educator Elizabeth Vogel points out:

> Who gets to show emotions and who does not is not politically neutral. The people who get silenced are usually the ones on the margins—people of color, females, etc. Often this silence is a reaction to real pain, and so not an inappropriate reaction. In this way, emotions create a web of influence that is difficult to untangle and analyze.[8]

Such complex dynamics occur on every level of interaction, from the medical school classroom to the clinic. Rhetorician Lynn Worsham argues for making a place for emotion in the classroom, and she offers a definition of emotion that is helpful in this context. Emotions are

> a tight braid of affect and judgment, socially and historically constructed and bodily lived, through which the symbolic takes hold of and binds the individual, in complex and contradictory ways, to the social order and its structure of meaning.[9]

As medical educators and clinicians grow increasingly aware that attention to emotional self-awareness is a crucial missing dimension in classrooms and in healthcare training, the consequences of this neglect are coming into greater clarity. As many have observed, medical students and young physicians are not encouraged to become familiar with their own emotional responses nor those of others. Prominent among these feelings is the understandable need to defend one's emotional investment in the values of the dominant medical culture. What's more, as Shapiro observes, "little effort is exerted to develop emotional honesty in medical students or residents." One consequence is that when trainees experience "confusing, unsafe, and difficult" feelings, "they sometimes decide to adopt a position of emotional detachment and distance."[10]

In *What Doctors Feel: How Emotions Affect the Practice of Medicine*, Dr. Danielle Ofri observes that clinicians, throughout their careers, are plagued by such negative emotions as fear, shame grief and anger. Furthermore, their experience of being emotionally overwhelmed often leads to burnout. Such "primal emotions" understandably follow from the onslaught of sickness and death faced by young doctors training in hospitals, as well as from the anguish of medical error and from the hazard of disillusionment in medicine itself, when ideals

and reality come into conflict.[11] Other educators observe that vulnerable patients, in particular, "can evoke fear, revulsion and pity in medical students"
because, having entered medicine to "'help' patients and 'fix' problems," they
may "feel overwhelmed by the extent and number of problems vulnerable patients present."[12] How are doctors to navigate this difficult professional terrain? What messages are conveyed when students are exposed to emotionally
jarring scenarios of profound suffering, fear, poverty, and health disparities,
and are not provided strategies for integrating these experiences into their
sense of the world or of themselves?

A further challenge to correcting this missing element in medical education
and training is that, as Sarah de Leeuw et al. observe, "Too much emotional-
ity, complexity, or critical and self-reflective focus is viewed, by some students,
as detracting from what they were meant to learn in medicine, particularly in
the 'practical and applied/clinical' realm."[13] Indeed, asking students to "talk
about their feelings" often leads to embarrassed silences and resentment on the
part of the students toward the well-meaning educators. As sociologist Arthur
Frank observes, "Professional culture has little space for *personal becoming*.
Young doctors are not trained to think of the careers ahead of them as trajec-
tories of their own moral development."[14] Recognizing that medical culture
can become a training ground for the silencing of emotion, literary scholar and
teacher Suzanne Poirier encourages emotional honesty in medical learners,
with the goal of recognizing and acknowledging one's own feelings and those
of others, and their implications.[15]

These are exemplary goals, but the question remains: how exactly does one
teach "emotional honesty"? While the right questions regarding emotion in
medical training have been raised, the "solutions" remain scant. Some medical educators have invoked the model of "emotional intelligence" (Shapiro) or
"emotional skill" or "labour" (McNaughton) or training in emotional regulation, but the strategies for achieving these goals are not clear.[16] We have found,
in narrative medicine, that close reading of works of creative representation
provides the distance that allows students to speak about feelings, to enter
into experiences that are meaningful to them. Reading a compelling story or
looking at a scene from a film can bring feelings forward, and, through such
mediation and the pleasurable act of making connections, students find themselves drawn to consider the ways their own stories interface with those under
discussion. As we proceed to describe "what we do and what happens," we will
endeavor to explore some of the philosophical and psychological ground on
which we base our work.

Among our propositions is the notion that it is better to know something
about your affective responses, to explore them honestly, than to

1. Extend energy trying to make your feelings conform to an idealized model of bottomless compassion
2. Bring to your encounter with a patient a confused or defended affective state
3. Push down or away your unwelcome feelings, be they "too much" or an absence of emotion

And our premises include the following:

1. Narrative medicine does not seek to judge, correct, or educate affective responses. Rather, it aims to reduce fear of them and to find words to name—or other modes of expression to convey—emotions in order to develop a greater capacity to be present to self and other
2. People are uncannily sensitive to what others feel toward them; there is really no hiding your emotions
3. It is not possible to shut out the suffering of others. It will find its way into your mental life, or keeping it at bay will be psychically costly and contribute to burnout
4. As we continue to locate the many ways in which narrative medicine can be put at the service of social justice, we are attentive to the role emotions play in the nature and structure of bias and racism
5. Narrative medicine seeks to create an environment where aesthetic experience can unlock affective responses, where trust and collaboration replace competition, and where the nature of engagement allows for recognition of self and other

In medicine, one affective term has dominated in recent years and has generated an enormous bibliography: *empathy* is commonly proposed as the most important if not the only relevant feeling in the medical context. We do not have room here to explore the ongoing discussions and disputes surrounding this term except to note that some are critical of this concept, finding in it a misguided assumption that one can enter into or know another's experience. Some wonder whether empathy is "teachable," while others are offended by the suggestion that practitioners and students need to be taught what to feel. We have not found empathy to be a useful term in our work for some of these reasons, and also because there are so many dimensions to any human interaction that to focus on one idealized relational affect or dynamic is simply inadequate. After describing "what happens" in the classroom, we will turn below to philosopher-educator John Dewey to assist us in understanding and articulating the complex interactions between aesthetic, affective, and learning experiences as they relate to our classroom and workshop methods. For Dewey, the arts and aesthetic experiences must never be segregated from everyday life; there is "no such thing in perception as seeing or hearing plus emotion. The perceived object or scene is emotionally pervaded throughout."[17]

The classroom is a complicated, rich combination of information process-ing and emotional responding. In narrative medicine we seek to establish that feelings are part and parcel of our intellectual work and to allow and invite them into the room, recognizing the role emotion plays in relationships and relatedness. This chapter explores some of the affective and experiential di-mensions of the methods we employ in narrative medicine workshops and classrooms toward addressing the relational dimension of healthcare—what we might call its *socio-relational dynamics*. In the previous chapter we ex-plored the theme of relationality in literature; here we will investigate the role of emotions and relationality through group discussion of a literary work and prompted writing.

A Narrative Medicine Classroom / Workshop

There is a range of different contexts for this work. A narrative medicine semi-nar in a university program (undergraduate or graduate, in a healthcare pro-fessions school or in another context) typically has a recognizable "academic" form involving assigned readings, analytic papers, and formal assessment of student work. The academic classroom serves many goals, including training students to practice and teach narrative medicine, either within their own clinical practice or working with clinicians, patients, families and others in-volved in healthcare as well as fields such as social work, law, and chaplaincy. The workshop is a much more flexible entity: it may be a single or recurring meeting or an intensive immersion; it may take place in a hospital conference room with pagers arrayed on the table, or in a nursing home, with caregivers, patients, or families; as part of an international gathering of chaplains or social workers; with a group of public school teachers; or with a team of colleagues in a high-stress environment. Workshop participants may be offered supple-mental readings, but the emphasis is typically on short works of prose, poetry, spoken-word pieces, or other creative media that can be read, seen, or heard together during the session and then discussed.

Within these different spaces our methods vary, but there are common themes and practices. Close reading—of literary texts, film, visual art, dance, music—is integral, as is short prompted writing and discussion. In all con-texts we call upon our analytic skills while remaining attentive to our affec-tive responses to the texts and to one another. We encourage participants to listen to their own observations, to what they can find in themselves that is informative and useful to them. In the workshop setting we see ourselves more as facilitators, while in the "classroom" our roles may shift between teacher and facilitator with the goal of creating a collaborative learning environment in which all play an active role. Here we will explore some of the ways in which we approach this work in different contexts, including specific work with a text and the exercises we may utilize.

We have found the story "Floating Bridge" by Alice Munro to be an inviting and evocative text in the academic classroom as well as in workshops and other contexts where participants are able to read longer texts in advance of the meeting. This is the story of a woman, Jinny, undergoing treatment for advanced cancer. As noted in the previous chapter and elsewhere in this volume, we often choose texts that do not address themes of healthcare directly; here we are not focused *primarily* on the protagonist's experience as a person undergoing an experience of illness, but rather on the rich complexity and relational dynamics of the story. Jinny's cancer, her medical treatment, and mortality are all elements of the narrative, but part of the strength of Munro's storytelling is that it challenges a reductive pathologizing lens. And while some workshops and classrooms will take as the starting point of discussion the particular circumstances of a work's production—its historical, racial, cultural, socioeconomic context—some, like the example offered here, focus on the text with relatively little attention to such context. Particularly in a workshop setting, participants may interpret the biographical details of a work's author as authoritative—*Oh, his wife died of cancer; that's what this work is "about"*—and while such understandings are certainly valid, they may foreclose the kind of open and generative discussion we seek to engender. We are keenly aware that there is no neutral pedagogical stance, and we are not arguing that expediency obviates consideration of social and cultural context—quite the contrary. This is a particular choice—one of a great range of narrative medicine strategies—which often serves to open readers to different interpretations and perspectives, including considerations of ideology, race, gender, ethnicity, and other aspects of personal and cultural identity.

"Floating Bridge" takes place over the course of a hot summer afternoon. Jinny's husband Neal is picking her up after she has been to see her oncologist, where she received some news about her prognosis. In the van with them is a young woman, Helen, whom Neal has employed to look after Jinny in what they anticipate will be her final months. Neal is preoccupied with his excitement and delight at Helen's presence, and so Jinny decides not to inform him (or the reader) of the news the doctor has just delivered. Neal insists on making a detour to pick up Helen's shoes, though Jinny is feeling depleted by the heat. The three ultimately drive some way out of town to the trailer home of Matt and June, Helen's foster parents, where Neal accepts an invitation to stop for a beer. Jinny remains outside despite the others' appeals for her to join them, inciting Neal's irritation at what he interprets as her coolness toward their hosts. Jinny walks into a cornfield, urinates, nearly becomes lost, and then makes her way back to the car. Matt and June's son Ricky—a young man, 17 or 18—arrives on his bicycle and, adeptly perceiving Jinny's state of physical exhaustion, asks if she would like him to drive her home. She surprises herself by accepting the offer and they leave without telling the others. As the evening darkens, Ricky takes an unexpected route, excitedly promising to show her something she has never seen before. "If this was happening back in her old, normal life," Jinny thinks to herself, "it was possible that she might now begin to be frightened."[18] They step out of the car and he urges her onto a floating bridge of wooden planks. The experience stirs her imagination unexpectedly as they observe the reflection of the stars in the water; the young man then surprises her with a kiss, which she accepts with a sense of wonder and even gratitude, and the story ends with her thoughts returning to Neal.

When we read this story in an academic setting we may ask students to write responses online, before class, to one of several different discussion prompts. In replying, readers must gather and articulate their thoughts, making the critical move from passive to active engagement with the text. The responses offer a valuable glimpse of readers' initial reactions to the story which can aid the instructor/facilitator in orienting the classroom discussion. The replies also come into conversation with one another, which helps foster dialogue; class discussion, then, may draw upon points made in the posts, including examples of different reactions to the text. The topics of these prompts and of class discussion often highlight themes that are particularly relevant to healthcare, such as relationality, memory, judgment, and so forth. They range from the analytic—we often pair the text with a particular theorist also on the syllabus—to more creative prompts. It is quite purposeful that we mix these modes together, as analytical thinking is also creative, and creativity can, of course, be highly analytical. One example of a discussion prompt for "Floating Bridge" engaging with a critical text begins with a quotation: *Elaine Scarry writes in the Introduction to* The Body in Pain *that her book "is about the way other persons become visible to us, or cease to be visible to us."*[19] *Discuss the idea of people becoming visible or invisible in the story.* Another productive prompt emphasizing the theme of relationality asks students to *Provide a close reading of one interaction or exchange (spoken or unspoken) between two or more characters.*

The diversity of responses to these questions demonstrates the myriad ways of interacting with and responding to a text. When asked to point to a particular passage or aspect of a literary work which a reader finds compelling, the response can also become a form of personal expression. Some readers focus on Neal's behavior and castigate him for his apparent callousness toward his wife, expressing unbridled moral censure and disgust. One writes of Neal and Jinny's "monotonous and trying marriage," describing Jinny's unwanted ride in her "deadbeat husband's hippie van in search of some missing shoes of a nubile young girl hired to step into Jinny's own figurative shoes as she is leaving this earthly world." Another criticizes Neal for his flirtation with Helen, asserting that he is attentive to his wife's comfort only out of obligation, as she has, in fact—invoking Scarry—"become invisible" to him. Some are quite surprised—dismayed or intrigued—when others do not share these reactions. Neal's character tends to evoke memories of reviled ex-partners, of failed relationships, perhaps of experiences of illness and caregiving, and when other readers respond differently they may become proxies for such figures and trials from one's own past.

In any setting we remain hypervigilant about privacy and do not probe into personal experiences, nor do we set any expectation for self-disclosure. With such safeguards in place, the relational space of the classroom or workshop may become suffused with powerful feelings. The potent life experiences of participants hover in the air and are expressed through close reading and reflection on the piece under discussion. The text creates the opportunity for a productive projection, allowing readers to locate their own feelings and to discuss and examine their judgments and responses. Through such shared close reading we are challenged to open ourselves to different interpretations beyond an initial reflexive distaste at a character's behavior. For example, some might point toward passages in "Floating Bridge" that complicate a neat judgmental interpretation, such as Neal's expressions of tenderness, the ways in which Jinny's death remains, in some way, unthinkable to him. When Jinny jokes about her death, warning Neal not to "let the Grief Counselors in," he responds "in a voice of rare anger": "Don't harrow me."[20] Drawing on such nuanced moments in the text, we might discuss the ways in which the seeming heedlessness of Neal's actions in the story is evidence of a reciprocity characteristic of long-term relationships; by not behaving in an overly solicitous manner toward his sick wife he is also refusing to reduce her to the status of "sick wife." By making jokes about the cemetery as they drive past he asserts their continued humor and humanity. Some readers note that he is dedicated to looking after her, picking her up from appointments, and preparing the home for her care down to the smallest detail.

Remaining close to the text, we might also reconsider Neal's flirtatious behavior toward Helen in light of Jinny's interior reflections: "When Neal was around other people, even one person other than Jinny, his behavior changed, becoming more animated, enthusiastic, ingratiating. Jinny was not bothered by that anymore—they had been together for twenty-one years. And she herself changed—as a reaction, she used to think—becoming more reserved and slightly ironic."[21] Perhaps these behavioral "transgressions" are a testament to Neal and Jinny's foundational presence to one another, to their compact that he will never leave her and will continue to bring a messy vitality to their shared lives, whatever the circumstances. We may see Neal fulfilling his role as the one doing the imperfect and sometimes inappropriate *expressing*—connecting Jinny to herself and the world—while Jinny remains reserved and impassive. For example, the story begins, "One time she had left him"—and what follows is Jinny's recollection of her anger at Neal after a perceived slight. Contemplating her departure and her future solitude, she reads the graffiti on the walls of the bus shelter:

> She felt herself connected at present with the way people felt when they had to write certain things down—she was connected by her feelings of anger, of petty outrage (perhaps it was petty?), and her excitement at what she was doing to Neal, to pay him back. But the life she was carrying herself into might not give her anybody to be angry at, or anybody who owed her anything, anybody who could possibly be rewarded or punished or truly affected by what she might do. Her feelings might become of no importance to anybody but herself, and yet they would be bulging up inside her, squeezing her heart and breath.[22]

To be connected by anger is perhaps a counterintuitive notion. But as we read attentively, we begin to respect the specific forms that intimacy takes between these two people in Munro's complex, subtle portrait. We begin to glimpse, too, the specter of aloneness for Jinny—interestingly, the suffocation of solitude in this passage evokes the apparition of cancer, "bulging up inside her, squeezing her heart and breath." Each of these characters is a relational self, as we all are, and our understanding of them is embedded in their complex connections with one another as Munro depicts them in such a rich and intricate fashion.

By attending to the particularity of these characters and these relationships in a dynamic discussion, participants begin to step outside of their own identifications and projections; together we can listen to a voice which is not our own, and can better see where we stop and something else begins. Moreover, we can observe our own initial responses to the story, and perhaps marvel at how our experiences can always find their way into our relationships—including relationships with characters in a story. In a conventional literature class such emotional readerly responses may be of little or no interest, while in our practice they become a vehicle to acknowledge and recognize our own judgments, how they often operate without our conscious awareness.

Becoming alert to those times when we are projecting our own emotions and values onto others is of critical importance in healthcare, and discussion of a fictional text can be especially helpful in this context. For example, many years ago a medical student began a response to the prompt, "Write about the suffering of someone that moved you" with the following: "I felt sorry for Mrs. T. because she was the only person in the ER that night who hadn't brought her problems upon herself." This was a challenging moment. How to open a discussion of such a sentiment without shaming the student—without placing a judgment on the student's judgment? On another occasion a similar feeling was expressed by a medical student, but this time the blame was directed toward a fictional character—in fact a quite sympathetic character, Sister Rosa, played by Penelope Cruz, who contracts AIDS in Almodovar's film *All About My Mother*: "I feel no sympathy for her because she brought her disease upon herself," he wrote. In contrast to the prior example, it was a simple matter to ask the class how they felt about the character, one they all had encountered on an even footing. A fruitful discussion ensued regarding the complex contingencies of sympathy. Asked to respond to the prompt, "Write about a time you wanted to feel sympathy for someone but couldn't," the students opened up and explored their own judgments—including those they regretted. Because it is particularly challenging to find ways to effectively address people's assessments and feelings, the mediating function of a creative work becomes especially apparent.

In discussing "Floating Bridge" we are interested in what provokes our own reactions, and also in how the story itself is working to explore the question of judgment. Part of the attraction of castigating a literary character is that it can serve to "solve" the story and put it to rest; in this case criticism of Neal may ascribe Jinny's plight to his failings—a more accessible demon than illness and mortality. Static closure, however, is precisely what we seek to challenge. The judgment of Neal's behavior is not at all *wrong*, but it is not *enough*, and close reading demonstrates that reductivism does not do justice to the enormous complexity of relationships and human experience—just as perceiving Jinny solely through the lens of her disease does not do justice to her experience and character. The discussion may not eradicate people's assessments of or hostility towards Neal—nor need it—but the point is to open ourselves to recognize how much room there is for interpretation in even a brief exchange. Hearing classmates' perspectives can enlarge or alter our own and can help us observe the shape of our own response.

Returning to the story, we attend not just to its events but also to its structure. Within the text are the happenings which occurred—what literary critic Gerard Genette terms *histoire*, or story—but of course there is also the particular way that events unfold—what Genette calls *récit*, or narrative.[23] The summary of "Floating Bridge" we offered above is mostly an account of the "story" in this sense, of the events in chronological order. Yet a focus on plot can be quite reductive; in taking up questions of temporality, point of view, narrative structure, and figurative language in class discussion, we become aware of the story's many layers and nuances. For example, "Floating Bridge" begins not with Neal picking up Jinny from her appointment but with Jinny's recollection of the time she had "left" her husband, followed by her recollection of the oncologist's "priestly demeanor" during their appointment; we only enter the oppressively hot van with Neal and Helen on the third page.[24] Jinny's memories are woven into the narration throughout the story, such as her vivid memory of a woman calling her a *"nice nellie"* years in the past, and her outrage at "having to sit there and listen to people's opinions of her."[25] She revisits these moments in her past, and our understanding of the story is further shaped by these narrative choices. In addition to discussing sequence and temporality, we may ask the group to consider the type of narrator. Indeed, the story is told largely from Jinny's perspective with a "third person limited" narration; we hear many of her interior thoughts and recollections but none from the other characters in the story, and our understanding (and perhaps our sympathies) are necessarily informed by this type of narration. As we discuss the role of perspective in the story we are made aware of our own and other readers' particular perspectives.

Finally, we discuss the floating bridge, both its literal function and its symbolic role within the story. What does it mean for Jinny, whose future is now less certain? For we have learned, late in the story, shortly before we travel to the floating bridge, that the medical news she has been carrying from her visit to the oncologist is in fact cautiously optimistic. As she is ostensibly listening to Helen's foster father Matt tell a joke, she is replaying her doctor's voice: *"I do not wish to give the wrong impression. We must not get carried away with optimism. But it looks as if we have some unexpected results here."*[26] The delay of this revelation and its awkward insertion during the conversation with Matt may reflect a fear of acknowledging the news. Hope can be dangerous, and she is in some sense newly afraid: "A dull, protecting membrane that she had not even known was there had been pulled away and left her raw."[27] And so the floating bridge is also a bridge toward an uncertain future for Jinny—and for Neal, too, though he is not physically present—a passage over dark waters that cannot be seen, can only be felt. It also mirrors the structure of the story itself, as we do not know where we are headed, do not know what is a beginning and what is an end. It is an unexpected and perhaps bewildering plot twist, yet as we rest on the floating bridge we must sit quietly with what is around us, with the uncertainty and doubt that subtends human experience. The tone of the narration shifts as well, and we are bathed in rich figurative language, a new and unexpected lyricism and poeticism:

> The slight movement of the bridge made her imagine that all the trees and the reed beds were set on saucers of earth and the road was a floating ribbon of earth and underneath all was water. And the water seemed so still, but it could not really be still because if you tried to keep your eye on one reflected star, you saw how it winked and changed shape and slid from sight. Then it was back again—but maybe not the same one.[28]

In class we spend time reading aloud these luminous descriptive passages and discussing the scene. We then offer a writing prompt. The guidelines for this exercise have been explained thoroughly to the group: participants have a short amount of time to write, typically around 5 minutes. Those who wish to share what they have written may do so, sometimes with a partner but more often with the entire group. The facilitator/instructor writes to the prompt as well, and often shares what she has written with the group. No one is required to read, and in an academic setting a student is not graded on willingness to share the writing, nor do we attempt to assess the creativity of the response. Every context is different and must be approached with great sensitivity. For example, prompts that tend to elicit more personal stories may become appropriate only after a group has met several times and the facilitator has gauged the level of trust and willingness. Regardless of the setting, a prompt should certainly not aim to directly elicit painful experiences; it must be open-ended enough to allow the writer to decide how to calibrate her response. In some settings, particularly those with strong institutional hierarchy (such as a group of clinical fellows, residents, medical students, and their supervising attending physician) we may specify that participants have the option to write from their own voices or from the imagined perspective of another. Discussion leaders *must* be attentive to the dynamics of a particular setting and the needs of each individual. At the same time, emotions play a valuable role in the classroom or workshop setting—a theme to which we will return later in this chapter.

The writing prompt relates to the discussion of the story which has just taken place and invites readers to articulate their individual personal relationship to the text, including associations that are often brought into awareness through the writing exercise. Crafting a narrative medicine prompt is a delicate balance. It must not be too specific, such as *Write about a time you were driven around in a hot car for hours looking for someone's shoes and then were kissed by a teenager on a floating bridge*—nor too pointedly personal, such as *Write about a time you cared for someone with a terminal diagnosis*—nor too vague, such as *Write about a time something unexpected happened*. With "Floating Bridge" we often ask participants to *Write about a time you were on a floating bridge.* The prompt evokes the physical description of standing on a floating bridge in the story as well as its metaphoric associations while relating them to the writer's own experiences. While there is no set amount of writing expected or required, respondents are aware that time is limited so they tend to begin fairly swiftly. Within the span of 5 minutes one can write quite a bit, typically ranging from one to several paragraphs.

The short pieces which emerge from this process are often fresh and surprising. The format allows people to discover and articulate what the story elicits in them and gives them an opportunity to elaborate on what they found most meaningful. Sometimes they observe that they had no idea what they were going to write when they started, but that the exercise helped them achieve a new angle on a feature of their own experience. They are often amazed at the voice that emerges and the complexity of what they have written, and reflecting those qualities back to the writer is an important and gratifying element of the discussion. Here are some examples of responses to the *Write about a time you were on a floating bridge* prompt from students in a master's program class in narrative medicine:

> I have never been on a floating bridge, although I have driven on a swinging bridge, known as the largest suspension bridge in the world—the Mackinaw Bridge, which connects the Upper and Lower Peninsula of Michigan. But when I think of a floating bridge, I am drawn to the metaphorical meaning. I think of how my relationships are floating bridges that sometimes have broken apart and sometimes hold together in an uneasy fashion. Take my brother. We once had more a solid bridge—or at least that's how I saw it. Then he was my older brother, a hero, a role model and I was the younger brother. Used to be I thought if I had one phone call to make before I'd die, I'd call him. It seemed that this relationship was rock solid. But then things changed and sometimes I wonder if the relationship we could have is still out there in the swamp, waiting to connect us, but we can't connect because we cannot forget the old stationary bridge.

* * *

> I interviewed a friend of mine for our oral history class because of her work in advocacy, or so I thought. But yesterday when I was writing my final essay for the class and listening again to our interviews, I realized that I really interviewed her for the story we share. Our fathers both died suddenly when we were young—and we both have spent our lives caring for our mothers. Listening to the interviews I could hear in my friend the story I tell myself about resilience and responsibility. A story that makes me at once sad and in a certain sense proud. The bridge my friend and I are on is the

shifting waters of our mothers' needs and the work we do to keep our balance—to keep ourselves afloat.

* * *

There is a space back home, a 4x4' spot of leveled roofing material on the pinnacle of a sloping roof—the rest of the roof's shingles reaching both for the heavens and earth at a sharp 30°.

The surface of this small patch of lofted architecture is black—dirtied with the wash of rainy winters and gusty dry summers.

But this is my spot. In the summer, during the late sunsets, I often lie curled up on this 4x4' expanse—warmed by the sun-soaked material.

I watch the grapefruit sunsets fall to indigo until the light of the cosmos reveals itself to me. Here . . . in the countryside, the stars are clear and infinite. And it is here that I both begin to think and cease thought—as I become infinite under the late summer's sky.

* * *

Passage

With six months left

hovering, early January

75 degree Southern California winter boasting through

fresh roses parading in the streets

football on everyone else's mind

and our small house on Mar Vista Avenue

suspended about it all

tubes of morphine, swabs of saline

stains of blood, shit, scraps of hair

looking out we'd see

signs of life

brown squirrels budgeting

blue jays jousting

ivy climbing the gazebo

she wouldn't sit beneath

* * *

Yesterday I came home to my 13 year-old sister wearing my boots when she did not ask me and it was the last straw. My dad says "Well, you weren't here to ask." I can't bring it up because I know I must respect the unwritten rules of the house and God knows I've "borrowed" shoes before, but just fucking ask. I'll say yes, just let me say yes.

I was late for my MRI appointment because the shoe debacle delayed my dad from going grocery shopping and I had to wait for a ride in the one-car-for-seven-people system. My dad offered to wait and go in with me but I knew Sarah (the 13 year old) had basketball practice and it would throw off the one-car-for-seven-people system. So I went up alone.

I took off my clothes and all metal jewelry and got strapped into the stretcher and thought how this pain is probably all mental anyway and I probably just wasted an hour and $20 copay. They turned the machine on and drew me into the huge loud whirring structure and told me not to move even though it was uncomfortable. They moved me in further to the machine than I expected and I couldn't breathe but I couldn't move because I had to get the picture of my pounding hip. I sat and prayed and listened to the bad pop music and felt my muscles spasming from my control until I heard, "good job, you were very still."

I let my parents take care of my sister first, and still didn't mention the shoes. It was over.

As these pieces demonstrate, good narrative medicine prompts do not ask for an answer or an analysis but rather ask readers to look inward, to find a resonance with the text's ambitions and allow them to co-mingle with one's own memories and experiences. It is often striking and intriguing to note the ways in which the literary work that has just been discussed is literally and/or figuratively echoed in the pieces' tone and subject matter, frequently to the surprise of the writer. Such mediation is helpful as it reframes, re-infuses, reinterprets, readjudicates a moment which was important to the writer, perhaps an experience she needed to tell herself. For example, the piece which is set on a square of roofing material reflects a feeling of pleasurable solitude akin to Jinny's experience in Munro's story; it evokes a sense of timelessness and an enigmatic yet powerful sense of melting into the cosmos which characterizes the scene of the floating bridge. As the prompted piece concludes, "the stars are clear and infinite. And it is here that I both begin to think and cease thought—as I become infinite under the late summer's sky." In contrast, another response may begin by stating a *lack* of literal connection with the prompt: "I have never been on a floating bridge . . ." Yet more often than not such an assertion serves to spark a series of associations. Beginning with a negative—a lack of connection—also reflects the theme of uncertainty in the story, and we may ask this author if he knew where he was headed when he began. Indeed, this response can be read as a floating bridge into uncertainty, with the painful recognition of loss: "I wonder if the relationship [my brother and I] could have is still out there in the swamp, waiting to connect us, but we can't connect because we cannot forget the old stationary bridge." This piece reflects, too, the importance of relationality, a theme we see again and again, as in the piece about the oral history interview: *How do we tell our own stories through one another?*—is the question the author poses. This is one of the fundamental objectives in our work, to explore the ways in which we express ourselves *through* other texts and selves—through our response to a short story, to a discussion question, to a writing prompt, and to one another's writing. Indeed, the richness of participants' writing arises directly from the relational space of the group and the combinations of these different factors.

These are just a few examples of possible responses to the prompted writing—ideally arising in discussion, with dynamic engagement from the participants—and of course it will vary in different contexts. In addition, depending upon the composition of the group, it can be revelatory to note the ways in which writing styles reflect the ways people are trained and expected to write and think professionally. For example, clinicians will often break a narrative down into discrete sequential steps, employing short sentences: *First this happened. Then this happened*—echoing the highly structured form of a clinic note or a patient history. In addition, it is interesting to note whether or not people write directly in the first person—how much they write themselves into the story, *finding* themselves in the experience—something clinicians and scientists are trained *not* to do, in fields where the passive voice is greatly encouraged and deployed. When we highlight such stylistic trends it may prompt a conversation about the ways in which participants have been influenced by their training and by the rubrics governing their professional thinking and writing. In such discussions clinicians frequently note the length of time since they last had the opportunity to write in a more "creative" or open-ended format; sadly, it is often quite a long time.

As facilitators we typically write and share what we have written as well, with the goal of forging mutual trust. We encourage all who share to read what they have written without prefacing or commentary. The premise is similar to that of a writing workshop, with an emphasis on what is written. Participants may have varying skill levels in writing and fluency, and it is understood that they are not evaluated on such abilities. Central to our work is the fact that people articulate things in writing quite differently than they do in speech, and reading what one has written expresses a different type of commitment and, again, creates a different kind of rapport in the room. Readers sometimes wish to qualify what they have written or to offer modest disparagement (*It's no good, I didn't get to finish . . .*) yet they are frequently pleasantly surprised by the work's positive reception—indeed, these short pieces often feel complete within themselves, without offering a sense of forced closure. Sometimes the writer is tempted to elaborate verbally on the story she has just read, though we try to forestall such extemporaneous storytelling. Likewise, there can be an inclination for others to respond to a written account with concerned questions about the writer's predicament. Such expressions of kind sympathy can be quite natural, but in this context they effect a change of register, shift the emphasis away from *forms* of expression, when in fact it is the mediation of the exercise that has, in many cases, allowed the person to share that particular experience and the feelings that accompany it. Moreover, we preface these exercises with—and reinforce as needed—a caution about privacy, that even if an individual has chosen to share a personal experience in a workshop, others must respect each participant's confidentiality. In this context, writing about a topic is not an invitation to others to offer opinions or to have a conversation about the experience outside the parameters of what the writer has chosen to share. Two students in our master's program addressed this issue in a workshop they were co-facilitating; they described the episode as follows:

> One participant wrote about memories—and the wish to alter these memories—of hardship facing cancer. The writing was clear, imaginative, and powerful. However, other students, two in particular, began to ask questions about this personal experience, unrelated to the writing exercise. The questions felt prying and invasive: "How long have you had this cancer? Has it affected your schoolwork?" The participant was brave and willing to answer these questions, but this discussion was clearly too much for the workshop setting. We (the facilitators) turned the conversation back to his writing, and thanked him for sharing. Then [my co-facilitator] stated, stretching his hand out to the center of the table, "I would like to jump in, and point out . . ." He discussed the importance of commenting only on participants' writing during the workshop, and acknowledging the writing as a means of giving respect to people's stories and to their personal choices of sharing.

This incident exemplifies the risks of this work and the importance of proper training for facilitators who must frame the exercise with great care and model the response to participants' written work, emphasizing the structure and style of the text, practicing close reading with attentiveness and rigor, just as with the Munro story.

Conclusion

> Meaningful learning underlies the constructive integration of thinking, feeling, and acting leading to empowerment for commitment . . .
>
> Joseph D. Novak[29]

In medical training and practice there are few opportunities for attending to the emotional content of a difficult experience or encounter, or for deploying strategies to help one's patients or colleagues grapple with what discomforts or troubles them. Those strategies that are offered are frequently inept or inapt. One such ineffective strategy was recently parodied by two Columbia

University medical students in a screenplay they co-wrote about third-year rotations, a project they developed as part of a fourth-year project in narrative medicine. Here they depict a non–narrative-medicine curricular activity designed—with the help of a clown—to sensitize third-year students to be more observant and mindful of their patients' unvoiced emotions. The student, Elizabeth, is waiting outside the classroom to be summoned back to guess which emotion her classmates are expressing by miming gestures and facial expressions:

INT. HALLWAY OUTSIDE GENERIC CLASSROOM – DAY

ELIZABETH is waiting in the hallway and walks aimlessly for a moment before fixing her hair in the semi-reflective glass surface of a portrait in the hallway. She glances at her watch and then knocks on the door to the classroom. The clown opens the door and ELIZABETH walks into a silent room. Some students are sitting, some are standing, and they all exhibit empathetic posturing and facial expressions.

One walks up to ELIZABETH and briefly places her hand on her shoulder. ELIZABETH looks confused and concentrates as she looks from student to student.

ELIZABETH
Pity?

The students continue to look at her.

CLOWN
Close … empathy. So you see, we can convey a lot through
body language alone. Humor can be equally important.
So remember, you always have a red nose in your pocket!

JAMIE takes an actual foam red nose out of her pocket, puts it on her nose, and sternly whispers to ELIZABETH.

JAMIE
You have cancer.

ELIZABETH looks at her with confusion and disdain.

In this scene, the exercise (exaggerated here but not by much) does not have its intended effect; it takes the students, Elizabeth and Jamie, in the wrong direction, arousing their contempt. Elizabeth reads "pity" in the expressions of her classmates who intend to simulate empathy. Pity is no one's idea of a desirable emotion, so the scenario wittily undercuts the discursive distinction drawn in medical school argot between empathy—the approved affect—and pity. One looks just like the other, as far as Elizabeth is concerned, so what are we playing at? The clown's reminder that humor serves as an additional affective resource also backfires. Forced humor (in the form of a red nose) does not correspond with Jamie's state of mind, and instead the two students share a moment of *black* humor—a reliable, if defensive, fallback for medical students. Throughout their screenplay these medical students employ humor to explore the charged emotional dimensions of medical training, beautifully illustrating such bundled feelings as eagerness and fear; inadequacy and self-importance; competitiveness and remorse for feeling competitive; loss of identity; and loss of free time (one medical student recently began to cry when reading a piece she'd written about taking half a day off from studying to take a walk in the woods). Along with these stressful emotions, the screenplay also depicts feelings of satisfaction and pride in accomplishments, joy in learning, admiration for colleagues and teachers, and a warm sense of comradery.

Similar to the possibilities opened by the screenplay-writing exercise, one of the unexpected consequences of the work we do with close reading and prompted writing is that participants often observe that they feel less afraid to approach difficult topics, experiences, or emotions. They command an increased confidence in their capacity to examine and metabolize what in the past they might have held at bay or fended off—including in consultations with patients. We don't know exactly how to account for this effect. Are we seeing an increase in affective agility? A greater creative and critical capacity to contextualize a moment or circumstance? A burnished trust that difficult situations and feelings can be explored without disastrous results? A greater confidence in others' ability to take in what one has to say, and a faith that one can communicate with greater nuance? Unlike in the clown exercise portrayed above, our work focuses on connecting with others from where you are in a specific moment in time. Checking in with and working on yourself are part and parcel of the job for healthcare providers—for healers. A professional demeanor, like a red nose in your pocket, can come in handy but only goes so far.

In this chapter we have described some of what happens in a narrative medicine classroom or workshop. More than a sum of its parts, these procedures involve participants in a rigorous aesthetic experience, a collaborative and creative unpacking of a literary text or work of art, an opportunity to speak and/or write about something of importance, and the surprise and delight of commissioning language in a fresh way. When a group member shares an insight or experience in a candid fashion, the level of trust accelerates dramatically in the room. Participants find the activity of making sense of their internal experience—their responses to a work of art or to a recent professional encounter—deeply satisfying and *interesting*. As John Dewey might put it, they are engaged in an act of *integration*, of bringing together their professional, intellectual, and existential selves. Competition and mistrust, two enormous factors in the erosion of collegiality, are banished from the experience. Each person is engaged in asking questions and in allowing for the limits of their own certainty.

As discussed, we do not ask participants to speak about their emotions or make the sharing of feelings an objective for the session. In a well-guided discussion of a story, a poem or any work of creative expression, feelings—with all their ideational and social complexities—surface organically and not according to an assigned agenda. In the examples of prompted writings quoted above, we detect the presence of many different feelings; students, however, do not articulate them directly, as in "this story reminded me of my feelings of guilt toward my sibling" or "this poem evoked the sensation of peaceful self-forgetting which I sometimes miss." Generally, we find that explicit or categorical expressions of this latter kind are less gratifying for the writer and listener both, whereas a more oblique or indirect delivery, by way of an image or as part of a storied memory, allows an emotion state to find more authentic expression.[30] To simply give a label to an experience does not necessarily bring us into contact with it or enliven it, nor does it express the complexity of our inner lives.

These many pedagogical elements produce a distinct atmosphere, one that is singular and experiential and belongs, in a sense, to the people in the room. John Dewey's theory of what he terms *an experience* offers one way to account for this rare alchemy in at least some of its aspects. In his book *Art and Experience*, Dewey emphasizes that *aesthetic perceiving* is a commonplace experience; it is ubiquitous in everyday life and does not belong only to a trained or privileged few. The creative work of the artist, in its broad outline, belongs to all intelligent human activity. Like the making of art, the imaginative use of intelligence draws upon emotion, as does the aesthetic experience. Creative thought calls upon our many faculties. When we concentrate on a work of art, we approximate the activity of the maker; we become interested in noticing details and the connections between parts, we select and gather specific elements into a whole. This kind of aesthetic attentiveness draws us into a work of art, and, Dewey observes, it can draw us closer to aspects of our daily lives. Dewey is proposing that we can perceive aesthetically (in our terms, *close read*) events in our lives. Such activity can lift us out of our daily "non-experience" wherein we drift, evade, and compromise. "In much of our intercourse with our surroundings we withdraw," Dewey writes, "sometimes from fear, if only of expending unduly our store of energy; sometimes from preoccupation with other matters . . ."[31] When we bring to our own experience the kind of pleasurable attentiveness we give to a work of art, then we have *undergone* something. In narrative medicine this *undergoing* allows people to meet one another in a different way. In such moments, aesthetic experience is not a solitary but a collective activity. For Dewey, such experiences help us to achieve greater aliveness.

Perception, Dewey writes, "involves surrender. But adequate yielding of the self is possible only through a controlled activity that may well be intense"—such as, we contend, close reading and prompted writing.[32] Inchoate happenings can, through aesthetic relatedness, find form and shape—and sometimes meaning. Addressing the role of aesthetic form in our mental lives, Dewey notes that "the aesthetic is no intruder in experience from without, whether by way of idle luxury or transcendent ideality, but . . . it is the clarified and intensified development of traits that belong to every normally complete experience."[33]

One of the formative figures in early twentieth-century progressive education, Dewey concerned himself with the subjective quality of a student's experience, focusing as much on process as on content, on *how* children learn as well as what they learn. By promoting a classroom culture where collaborative skills are honed toward developing creative solutions and where learning is understood to be a creative act that stimulates emotion and imagination along with thought, Dewey sought to create a classroom where learners and teachers are able to integrate elements of the self. Bringing one's whole (integrated) self to the task of teaching and learning is and should be a creative act—indeed, one on which responsible and active citizenship in democracy depends. In these and other ways, he offers a pedagogical model that informs our work in narrative medicine. Teaching is also a relationship of care.

In narrative medicine the attention to character actions, nuances, how the story is told, perspective, temporal unfolding, tone, images, and the rest is in the service of having an experience as Dewey describes it, and, as he implies, of creating habits of mind to become more noticing (via aesthetic engagement) of the dynamics of one's own experiences—with patients, colleagues, and institutional structures. This necessarily involves attending to crucial affective responses of bias, of making judgments, of uncertainty and impatience. Recognition that what one hears in someone else's story can depend on one's own experiences and state of mind can change everything—can be culture change. "Where am I in this patient's story?" and "Where am I in the story of healthcare today?" are questions that, if asked consistently and honestly, can change the face of healthcare.

Notes

1. Mitchell, *Relationality*, 67.
2. Moore, "People Like That," 237.
3. Shem, *House of God*, 26.
4. Shapiro, "Feeling Physician," 310.
5. Shapiro, "Feeling Physician," 310–11.
6. Goleman, *Emotional Intelligence*, 76.
7. Derald Wing Sue, *Race Talk*, 237.
8. Vogel, "What We Talk About," 12.
9. Worsham, "Coming to Terms," 105.
10. Shapiro, Movies Help us Explore," 22–23.
11. See Ofri, *What Doctors Feel*.
12. Shapiro, "Feeling Physician," 311.
13. De Leeuw, Parkes, and Thien, 6.
14. Frank, *Wounded Storyteller*, 159.
15. Poirier, *Doctors in the Making*.
16. See Shapiro, "Feeling Physician," and McNaughton, "Discourse(s) of Emotion."
17. Dewey, *Art as Experience*, 51.
18. Munro, "Floating Bridge," 82.
19. Scarry, *Body in Pain*, 22.
20. Munro, "Floating Bridge," 60.
21. Munro, "Floating Bridge," 57.
22. Munro, "Floating Bridge," 56.
23. Genette, *Narrative Discourse*, 27.
24. Munro, "Floating Bridge," 55–57.
25. Munro, "Floating Bridge," 74.
26. Munro, "Floating Bridge," 76.
27. Munro, "Floating Bridge," 77.
28. Munro, "Floating Bridge," 84.
29. Novak, "Theory of Education," 1.
30. See Kuiken, "Locating Self-Modifying Feelings."
31. Dewey, *Art as Experience*, 55.
32. Dewey, *Art as Experience*, 55.
33. Dewey, *Art as Experience*, 48.

PART

II

DUALISM, PERSONHOOD, AND EMBODIMENT

CHAPTER **3**

Dualism and Its Discontents I: Philosophy, Literature, and Medicine

Craig Irvine and Danielle Spencer

I might regard man's body as a kind of mechanism that is outfitted with and composed of bones, nerves, muscles, veins, blood and skin in such a way that, even if no mind existed in it, the man's body would still exhibit all the same motions that are in it now except for those motions that proceed either from a command of the will or, consequently, from the mind.
—René Descartes, *Sixth Meditation*[1]

This is Descartes' error: the abyssal separation between body and mind, between the sizable, dimensioned, mechanically operated, infinitely divisible body stuff, on the one hand, and the unsizable, undimensioned, un-pushpullable, nondivisible mind stuff; the suggestion that reasoning, and moral judgment, and the suffering that comes from physical pain or emotional upheaval might exist separately from the body. Specifically, the separation of the most refined operations of mind from the structure and operations of a biological organism.
—Antonio Damasio, *Descartes' Error: Emotion, Reason, and the Human Brain*[2]

That the best physician is also a philosopher.
—Galen of Pergamon, A.D. *129–199*[3]

"Hi. How are you feeling today?"—Tales of Alienation in Healthcare

In the opening of "A Burst of Light: Living with Cancer," Audre Lorde writes about her visit to an oncologist after a large mass is discovered in the right lobe of her liver. The highly regarded specialist considers it very likely that the

tumor is malignant and suggests immediate surgery. Lorde, who has undergone a mastectomy and treatment for breast cancer in the past, responds that
she needs time to "feel this thing out and see what's going on inside" herself
first.[4] She does not want to act out of panic, she explains. The oncologist, however, will brook no delay. As Lorde describes:

> What the doctor could have said to me that I would have heard was, "You have a serious
> condition going on in your body and whatever you do about it you must not ignore it or
> delay deciding how you are going to deal with it because it will not go away no matter
> what you think it is." Acknowledging my responsibility for my own body. Instead,
> what he said to me was, "If you do not do exactly what I tell you to do right now without
> questions you are going to die a horrible death." In exactly those words.
>   I felt the battle lines being drawn up within my own body.[5]

In vivid detail, Lorde describes the pernicious confluence of medical paternalism and bias in this painful scene:

> From the moment I was ushered into the doctor's office and he saw my x-rays, he pro-
> ceeded to infantilize me with an obviously well-practiced technique. When I told him
> I was having second thoughts about a liver biopsy, he glanced at my chart. Racism and
> Sexism joined hands across his table as he saw I taught at a university. "Well, you look
> like an *intelligent girl*", he said, staring at my one breast all the time he was speaking.
> "Not to have this biopsy immediately is like sticking your head in the sand." Then he
> went on to say that he would not be responsible when I wound up one day screaming in
> agony in the corner of his office![6]

The alienation in this tale is acute. As clinician-philosopher Edmund
Pellegrino explains, "To care, comfort, be present, help with coping, and to al-
leviate pain and suffering are healing acts as well as cure. In this sense, healing
can occur when the patient is dying even when cure is impossible . . . Cure may
be futile but care is never futile."[7] The absence of such comfort and presence in
the scene Lorde describes is itself a material form of injury.

Sadly, experiences of this type are a familiar trope in Western healthcare
and are thematized in many works of memoir, literary fiction, film, and theater about illness. Offering an imagined perspective of an historical encounter, Sara Maitland's short story "Forceps Delivery" is the tale of Dr. Hugh
Chamberlen's seventeenth-century demonstration of the forceps—which his
family had invented and kept secret for a century—for Dr. Francois Mariceau,
who was recognized as the leading obstetrician in Europe at the time. In the
story's introduction the date, place, and cast of the drama are listed, including
a description of the story's circumstances. Unwilling to pay the proposed price
for Dr. Chamberlen's unspecified product, Dr. Mariceau proposed a test case:

"He had in his care a *severely deformed rachitic dwarf primipara* aged twenty-eight and nameless. After examining her [Dr. Mariceau] concluded that the case was impossible; if Dr Chamberlen could deliver her the secret would be worth paying for."[8] Following the introduction, Maitland's story shifts into first-person narration from the imagined perspective of the "test case", and we hear the voice of the person who has been described in such reductive clinical terms as she recounts her story:

> The baby has its face pressed to my belly . . . I wonder if the effects of the senna repelled it, made it turn around. There are things you do not ask doctors. Clearly, they agreed, the case was impossible. Let Dr Chamberlen try his secret; if it works on me it's worth the price.
>
> You see their rhythm imposes itself on mine. I too become rational, worldly, slightly jaundiced, hearing them. I cannot fly back into my silence and my weighted waiting. Not in their presence.
>
> They like each other, these two. I realize that. It is a game they are playing, a game with some pride and some money invested, but a game nonetheless and played between friends who respect each other. I would like to play too, I would. I think I could hold a strong hand in this game, but then it would not be between friends. It does not matter who wins this expensive game. It will not be me. It will not be me.[9]

The "expensive game" is one of technology and craft, of research and distance. The sense of isolation is palpable here, echoing the estrangement in Lorde's account. We hear, too, the yearning for affinity between patient and doctor, the desire to play the "game" between friends rather than to play the objectified victim.

In a more contemporary setting, Margaret Edson's celebrated 1995 play *W;t* offers a brutal portrait of such disaffection and technological dominance in healthcare. The opening scene begins with Professor Vivian Bearing—scholar of seventeenth-century poetry—newly diagnosed with cancer, speaking directly to the audience from her hospital room:

> VIVIAN: (In false familiarity, waving and nodding to the audience) Hi. How are you feeling today? Great. That's just great.[10]

Here we are immediately implicated, addressed by the protagonist who is play-acting the role of doctor or nurse to emphasize the insincere intimacy of this salutation. The "you" is an abstracted idealized patient, perfectly compliant and infantilized; it is also the body, estranged from context and history. For recognition of Vivian's personhood in the hospital is cursory at best. When her oncologist, Dr. Kelekian, brings a gaggle of fellows to her bedside on rounds, they palpate and scrutinize her body and compete with one another to impress Kelekian with their medical knowledge. They barely acknowledge Vivian, for only her corporeal signs and symptoms are of interest. Jason, the clinical fellow, presents "the patient," employing the characteristic passive voice: "At the time of first-look surgery, a significant part of the tumor was debulked, mostly in this area—*here. (He points to each organ, poking her abdomen.)* Left, right ovaries. Fallopian tubes. Uterus. All out." Simultaneously, Vivian offers her commentary to the audience, noting that the ritual resembles a graduate literature seminar, except that "in Grand Rounds, *they* read *me* like a book."[11] When the doctors conclude, Kelekian stops Jason as the team is about to leave the bedside, prompting him with the reminder: "Clinical." "Oh, right," replies Jason, and turns to Vivian, saying, "Thank you, Professor Bearing. You've been very cooperative"—whereupon they leave her, with her torso still undraped. "Clinical" attention to—or in this case, perfunctory acknowledgement of— the individual patient is here opposed to research, a stark divide in *W;t's* somewhat heavy-handed portrayal. As Jason explains to Vivian later in the play, this obligatory fellowship is an impediment on his path to research; clinicians are "troglodytes" and bedside manner is "a colossal waste of time for researchers."[12]

Playwright Margaret Edson's experiences as a unit clerk on a cancer and AIDS inpatient ward of a research hospital informs the depiction of medical care in *W;t*,[13] and such scenes offer a fictional patient's perspective of the hospital's myriad aggressions—both micro and macro—against an individual's personhood. Yet the play also draws many parallels between Vivian's character as an uncompromising scholar and the research-oriented physicians operating within the rigid hierarchy of academic medicine. The opening scene of diagnosis establishes a mutual identification between doctor and patient: Kelekian begins by addressing Vivian as "Miss Bearing" and shifts to "Dr. Bearing" as they discuss their shared professorial despair at the perceived inadequacies of their students. In describing the harsh regimen of chemotherapy he is recommending, Kelekian invokes their mutual pursuit of knowledge, a commonality which Vivian embraces. We learn that Vivian exhibits unapologetic pride and even arrogance in her academic achievements —as she states, "I can say with confidence, no one is quite as good as I."[14] A glimpse of her student days shows her choosing the library over socializing, and we learn that she has been a strict and ruthless professor. At the age of 50 she does not have a partner nor children, and she is not currently sexually active. Thus we are given to understand that Vivian has eschewed her own body, selfhood, and personal relationships in favor of a life of the mind. As the end draws near, her nurse, Susie, brings up the issue of a DNR, suggesting that doctors prolong life for the sake of research: ". . . [T]hey always . . . want to know more things," she explains. "I always want to know more things," replies Vivian. "I'm a scholar. Or I was when I had shoes, when I had eyebrows." No longer in possession of shoes nor eyebrows, she chooses the DNR with Susie's encouragement—manifestly the right decision, given her abject suffering, the futility of further treatment, and the violence of such resuscitation—yet in so doing she must repudiate her identity as a thinker, for it has been stripped away:

> VIVIAN: (Quickly) Now is not the time for verbal swordplay, for unlikely flights of imagination and wildly shifting perspectives, for metaphysical conceit, for wit.
>
> And nothing would be worse than a detailed scholarly analysis. Erudition. Interpretation. Complication.
>
> (Slowly) Now is a time for simplicity. Now is a time for, dare I say it, kindness.[15]

Why must Vivian slow her speech and disavow her love of knowledge in order to embrace kindness? As Jacqueline Vanhoutte argues, *W;t* can be read as a tragedy in which Vivian's cancer is punishment for the hubris of neglecting her humanity, an arrogance that mirrors coldhearted modern medicine in the play's reductive portrait: "*W;t*'s doctors are all monsters of insensitivity, devoted to knowledge and to intellectual one-upmanship. Only when she rejects their values can Vivian be saved."[16] That she falls victim to the arrogance and inhumanity of the hospital is just retribution for her proud valorization of the mind and abnegation of the body and spirit, and her final redemption and ascension—with her soul rising from her body on her deathbed—reinforces this division. Thus *W;t* offers a trenchant critique of the separation between mind and body in the healthcare space, as medical research and technology are opposed to the patient's body and spirit—and the play further reinforces this divide by inflicting great pain and suffering on Vivian, who has privileged intellect over emotion.

Whether or not one agrees with this particular interpretation of the play or the realism of its depictions, readers and spectators *experience* the dramatic transformation of its protagonist, faced not just with the cruelties of a fatal disease but the dissociation and alienation of modern medicine. Indeed, common to these three examples—"A Burst of Light: Living with Cancer," "Forceps Delivery," and *W;t*,—is the elaboration of an individual patient's perspective in contrast to that of clinicians/researchers. Reflecting the genres of memoir, historical fiction, and dramaturgy, these works convey each narrator's personal experience of *illness* as Arthur Kleinman describes it: "the innately human experience of symptoms and suffering . . . how the sick person and the members of the family or wider social network perceive, live with, and respond to symptoms and disability."[17] Their stories also depict the diminution or outright elision of such experience subject to a clinical gaze focusing exclusively on what Kleinman terms *disease*: "In the narrow biological terms of the biomedical model . . . disease is reconfigured *only* as an alteration in biological structure or functioning."[18] It is no accident that these selected passages give voice to the illness experiences of female patients—Lorde as an African-American lesbian woman, and the narrator of Maitland's story bearing a body type that differs significantly from the norm—for power imbalances amplify the alienation of a clinical encounter of this type. Prevalent prejudice and silencing of the voices and experiences of persons of color, the disabled, trans* patients, those with mental illness, and many others is endemic in our society and thus in healthcare, accentuating the vulnerability of illness and attenuating trust between clinician and patient.

Yet one need not have faced a diagnosis of cancer or an impossible pregnancy to feel some recognition—though not to say full understanding—of these characters' stories. One experiences this type of objectification all too frequently upon entering a doctor's office or hospital, learning to identify by ID numbers or doctor's last name, as Vivian Bearing quickly does. One hears the odd rhythms of an unfamiliar language reducing patients to injury or pathology, mapped to a disease entity,[19] and becoming "the knee in room 3"—an assemblage of seemingly fungible organs and body parts, each treated by a different service of the hospital. One becomes, too, a virtual body of electronic medical records and digital scans, with the scope of human experience relegated to "social history" in the medical chart. There are, to be sure, many works of autobiography and fiction that reflect tremendous compassion and effectiveness in the clinical setting, just as our experiences of healthcare are complex and varied. However, the discontent reflected in these passages is indeed pervasive.

Clinicians increasingly feel diminished and disempowered as well, caught in the maw of bureaucratic documentation and burdensome regulation, estranged from the call to care and the intimacy of the doctor–patient relationship. From Doctor X to Samuel Shem to Danielle Ofri, memoirs by physicians—often focusing on the years of medical school and residency— invariably recount experiences of profound bewilderment, humiliation, fatigue, brutality, and a loss of empathy and idealism.[20] Illustrating the prevalent theme of desensitization in this genre, Salvatore Iaquinta's 2012 memoir *The Year THEY Tried to Kill Me: Surviving a Surgical Internship . . . Even if the Patients Don't* includes an orientation lecture from his Chief Resident offering the following advice to incoming interns:

> "If a surgeon tries to break you, don't. Remember that they are trying to break you. Let their insults roll off you like a bead of water. If you snap back once, it will haunt you. Nobody here forgets anything. You will be paid back every day if you bite once. Do not cry. Even at home, do not cry. Remind yourself that it is only one year and that you just

got through one more day. I have seen some great people leave this program because they couldn't take it. [. . .] They are ruthless here," Bradford said without a smile. He delivered this information with the same flat affect he would use to describe a patient's vitals. These weren't opinions, these were the facts.[21]

This dramatic passage reflects the often harsh nature of medical education and its parallels to military indoctrination. And here the junior clinician experiences a dissociation that runs parallel to the patient's: One must learn to separate from oneself—to disregard the needs of one's own body and spirit—to successfully withstand the crucible of medical training.

Such examples paint a necessarily reductive portrait, one that certainly does not include the breadth of experience of patients and clinicians both. Yet they illuminate a woefully familiar lament about contemporary healthcare, and although there is widespread recognition of these concerns and substantive efforts to address them, it is important to investigate the roots of these issues.

Biomedicine in Recent History

The evolution of healthcare toward its present state of alienation, institutionalization, and specialization is a complex tale.[22] It has occupied and bedeviled many patients, social scientists, cultural critics, writers, and clinicians, and we may well ask how we have arrived at our current state. A watershed moment within the scope of this history in the United States is Abraham Flexner's 1910 Carnegie Foundation report on medical education.[23] Flexner described a chaotic and unregulated state of affairs in healthcare curricula, arguing for standardization and a strong foundation in the biological sciences. He stressed that medical school admission must depend on an applicant's knowledge of chemistry, biology, and physics—still largely the case today—and that "every departure from this basis is at the expense of medical training itself."[24] Flexner's report instantiates the pervasiveness of the biomedical model in medical education and practice, a scientism that has brought truly revolutionary advances in healthcare and medical science. Yet, as physician Charles Odegaard wrote in *Dear doctor: A personal letter to a physician* (1986), the weakness of Flexner's model "lies not in the kinds of knowledge it includes, but in the kinds of knowledge it ignores." As Odegaard explains:

Man belongs not only to the animal world observed by the biologist. He is, as the philosopher has observed, a social animal, and as the novelist has described, a creature of affect. The physician who is educated to see his patient as only a collection of interrelated tissues and organs is not seeing his patient whole; and, except as he may be aided fortuitously by untutored intuition, he will not be able to deal with his patient's health in all its aspects.[25]

In fact, a lesser-known aspect of Flexner's report is his acknowledgment that the biomedical sciences are merely the minimal qualification for medical practice, which also demands "requisite insight and sympathy on a varied and enlarging cultural experience" and entails a broader social and moral responsibility.[26] Significantly, however, Flexner does *not* suggest specific training in ethics, social sciences, or humanities; we are left to ponder whether and how we might preserve and inculcate such "insight and sympathy." Many studies have demonstrated that medical education succeeds in *blunting* empathy, and so we are still struggling to prevent such erosion of compassion and understanding.[27] Certainly such accounts as Iaquinta's indicate that we face a formidable challenge in changing the culture of medical training. Similarly, Samuel Shem's legendary 1978 *House of God*—a satirical fictionalized account of internship at an academic medical center based closely upon the author's own experiences[28]— offers a scathing tale in which a young physician imagines patients as grotesque creatures of this animal world during his first day on the wards:

> I started to panic. And then finally the cries coming from the various rooms saved me. All of a sudden I thought "zoo," that this was a zoo and that these patients were the animals. A little old man with a tuft of white hair, standing on one leg with a crutch and making sharp worried chirps, was an egret; and a huge Polish woman of the peasant variety with sledgehammer hands and two lower molars protruding from her cavernous mouth became a hippo. Many different species of monkey appeared, and sows were represented in force. In my zoo, however, neither were there any majestic lions, nor any cuddly koalas, or bunnies, or swans.[29]

This question of how to protect and nurture clinicians' insight and sympathy is one that many voices have raised throughout the twentieth century and up to the present, and periodic clarion calls alert the medical community to restore its humanistic calling. In 1926, physician (and Flexner critic) Francis Peabody delivered a speech to Harvard Medical School students in which he warned about the depersonalization of the practice of medicine and the degradation of the doctor–patient relationship. As he famously cautioned:

> Disease in man is never exactly the same as disease in an experimental animal, for in man the disease at once affects and is affected by what we call the emotional life. Thus, the physician who attempts to take care of a patient while he neglects this factor is as unscientific as the investigator who neglects to control all the conditions that may affect his experiment. The good physician knows his patients through and through,

and his knowledge is bought dearly. Time, sympathy and understanding must be lav-
ishly dispensed, but the reward is to be found in that personal bond which forms the
greatest satisfaction of the practice of medicine. One of the essential qualities of the
clinician is interest in humanity, for the secret of the care of the patient is in caring for
the patient.[30]

The seeming tautology of Peabody's dictum invites us to consider the
scope of care itself beyond laboratory science, disease processes, and an objectification of the body, a question that has continued to arise throughout the
twentieth century and into the new millennium. In Eric Cassell's influential
1982 article in *The New England Journal of Medicine*, "The Nature of Suffering
and the Goals of Medicine," he addresses *suffering* as the experience of illness or injury that is not limited to physical pain but includes threats to one's
personhood—threats often including medical intervention itself. Referencing
the objectification of patients' physical bodies still so pervasive in medicine,
Cassell argues that

> . . . so long as the mind-body dichotomy is accepted, suffering is either subjective and
> thus not truly "real"—not within medicine's domain—or identified exclusively with
> bodily pain. Not only is such an identification misleading and distorting, for it deper-
> sonalizes the sick patient, but it is itself a source of suffering. It is not possible to treat
> sickness as something that happens solely to the body without thereby risking damage
> to the person.[31]

As Cassell describes, the dissociation of illness from personhood is itself
a form of injury, a harm that we should endeavor to avoid. Such dissociation
can also be understood in narrative terms, as in the work of sociologist Arthur
Frank, who identifies a set of narrative typologies characterizing accounts of illness. As Frank describes, the "restitution narrative"—"Yesterday I was healthy,
today I'm sick, but tomorrow I'll be healthy again"—predominates in our culture to a prescriptive extent.[32] This story promises the return of a body that is
"as good as new" after it is given over to medical science. As Frank explains:

> The temporarily broken-down body becomes "it" to be cured. Thus the self is dissoci-
> ated from the body. [. . .] The body is a kind of car driven around by the person inside;
> "it" breaks down and has to be repaired. The restitution story seems to say "I'm fine but
> my body is sick, and it will be fixed soon." This story is a practice that supports and is
> supported by the modernist deconstruction of mortality: mortality is made a condition
> of the body, the body is broken down into discrete parts, any part can be fixed, and thus
> mortality is forestalled. Sickness as an intimation that my whole being is mortal is ruled
> out of consideration."[33]

Frank challenges us to consider the potentially coercive effects of the restitution narrative: How might it elide the experience of *being* ill, of feeling one's
body and experiencing change? Such an understanding helps us to identify the
underlying attitudes toward mind and body within a given story and to recognize the prevalence and effects of restitution narratives in our culture.

Such criticisms of the dissociative effects of healthcare are hardly novel. In
his study of the mutability of diagnosis and the historical contingency of the
notion of a discrete disease entity, historian of science Charles Rosenberg laments the "antireductionist critique" of biomedicine as a hackneyed refrain.
Rosenberg readily acknowledges the alienating aspects of contemporary healthcare, yet argues in Foucauldian terms that the individual's abstraction into the
institutional space of diagnostic categories is in some sense inevitable and also
creates meaning; such a "simulacrum thriving in a nurturing environment of
aggregated data, software, bureaucratic procedures, and seemingly objective
treatment plans" is also productive and quite real.[34] Citing Arthur Kleinman's
distinction between illness as a person's experience and disease as the biomedical construction of that process, Rosenberg argues that it is a false dichotomy:

> [I]n practice, sickness is, of course, a mutually constitutive and interactive merging of
> the two; we are not simply victimized, alienated, and objectified in the act of diagnosis.
> Disease categories provide both meaning and a tool for managing the elusive relation-
> ships that link the individual and the collective, for assimilating the incoherence and
> arbitrariness of human experience to the larger system of institutions, relationships,
> and meanings in which we all exist as social beings.[35]

In order to understand this nuanced relationship between the individual
and the space of medical care, we must explore its underpinnings. We must
try to understand how care has become a commodity to be "delivered" by
"healthcare providers," reducible to a matrix of CPT and ICD-10 codes,
Relative Value Units, and Quality-Adjusted Life Years—and, heeding
Rosenberg, investigate the ways in which we, too, are constituted by these categories, designations, and divisions, for we ignore or discount them as unreal
at our own peril. And in order to find our way, we must first tell a story—one
possible narrative among many, to be sure—of how we arrived here. As philosopher Alisdair MacIntyre writes, "I can only answer the question 'What
am I to do?' if I can answer the prior question 'Of what story or stories do I
find myself a part?' "[36]

While there are many stories of which medicine finds itself a part, one
that is particularly important to tell is the story of the evolution of dualism in
Western philosophy. As Drew Leder notes, "it is by now a cliché that modern
medicine often neglects the import of psychosocial factors in the etiology and

treatment of disease. Not as widely recognized are the metaphysical roots of this neglect."[37] Indeed, this philosophical story has profoundly shaped medicine's understanding of *embodiment*—the relation between body and self—and *intersubjectivity*—the relation between one embodied subject and another. Through better understanding the philosophical roots of medicine's dualistic frame we will better appreciate, draw upon, and advance the work of those seeking to move beyond it, as we explore further in the following chapter.

The Cave and the Machine: Philosophical Roots of Dualism

We begin in a prison, deep beneath the surface of the earth, where a group of men has been chained since childhood, unable to look from side to side. On the wall before them they watch a play of shadows—of cows, deer, people and all else—and this, for them, is the only reality. Behind them, unseen, puppets dance in front of a flame, casting the shadows to which the prisoners attend. One day, one of the men's chains are loosed. Rising, he turns around, sees the puppets, and realizes that he has been deluded all his life—that the puppets are what is real, the shadows merely images. This realization is only the beginning of the prisoner's enlightenment. He will eventually ascend to the world's surface, where he will discover the real cows, deer, people and all else on which the puppets are modeled. When he is ready, he will look at last to the Sun, without which nothing would appear.

The allegory of the cave in book VII of Plato's *Republic* represents a journey through higher and higher levels of abstraction. Socrates—Plato's teacher, and a character in the *Republic*—asks that we "liken the domain revealed through sight to the prison home, and the light of the fire in it to the sun's power; and, in applying the going up and the seeing of what's above to the soul's journey up to the intelligible place, you'll not mistake my expectation."[38] In other words, the cave represents the world we live in—the concrete, physical world of bodies, in which we must rely on our senses to smell, hear, taste, touch, and, most importantly for Plato, *see* all that we know. In this world our senses frequently deceive us, leading us to accept mere shadows, or illusions, as reality. The prisoners' chains represent our bondage to our senses and to our bodies—to their pleasures and pains.

Pleasure and pain alike prevent us from ascending the path to the universality of Wisdom by keeping us bound to the particular—to *this* delicious flavor, *this* raging fever, *this* pleasing sound, *this* piercing injury. For instance, I might take pleasure in the chair in which I now sit: the way it curves to support my back, the color and texture of its fine-grained oak frame, its pleasing, well-balanced form. But if I never rise above the contemplation of this particular chair, I will never know what makes a chair a chair—will never know the nature of "chairness" itself. Based only on my experience of *this* chair, I might convince myself that it is the essential nature of a chair that it *must* be made of oak, or that it *must* have arms of a specific height or a back that curves in just this particular way. Limited to my experience of this particular chair, I might never realize that all chairs have "accidental" qualities (arms, oak, a back that curves just so) that are not essential to the nature of chairness itself. In order to know that essential nature I must therefore abstract from those nonessential qualities, and that is only possible if I am released from the chains that bind me to the particularity of my embodied experience. If this is true for the nature of chairness, how much truer must it be for the nature of Beauty itself, or of Justice, or Goodness. I must therefore rise above my body, from which I can see only the particular (represented by the shadows cast on the wall of the cave), through disciplined training of my mind, for it is the mind alone that can see the universal (metaphorically represented by the Sun, which brings to light the True nature of all things). For Plato, only the universal is truly *real*. The allegory of the cave represents the movement of the mind out of the darkness and bondage of the world of particular, concrete, physical bodies—shadows of the real—to the light and freedom of the universal, *meta*-physical Ideas.

After narrating the allegory, Socrates offers a proposal for the education of the guardians of the ideal city-state designed to free them from the cave, from bondage to their bodies. The most gifted among them will become philosopher kings, ruling in the light of the Wisdom granted only to those capable of contemplating the Sun. The first subject the guardians must master, Socrates insists, is gymnastics: the effort to free one's soul from the shackles of embodiment begins, paradoxically, with focused training of the body: "[O]ne of their tests, and that not the least, is what each will show himself to be in gymnastic."[39] Only those with the most fit bodies, enjoying ideal health, are strong enough, *disciplined* enough, to undergo the rigors of an education that will allow them to *transcend* their bodies. For Plato, there is no room for the chronically ill nor the incurably infirm among those who rule, for there is no wisdom in illness and disability, which only trap us, bind us yet more firmly to the body. Medicine, in fact, should be reserved, Socrates insists, for those who can be restored to health as quickly as possible, so that they might go about their business. Those with lingering diseases, disabilities, chronic illnesses—all those who cannot be restored to "productive" health—should not be treated but left to die.[40] Most importantly, the excessive care of the body necessitated by chronic illness "makes any kind of learning, thought, or meditation by oneself hard; it is always on the lookout for tensions and spinning in the head . . ."[41] Thought proceeds from health—the highest thought from the most perfect health. Socrates insists that, in choosing those who should pursue the education that might produce the philosopher kings, "[t]he steadiest and most courageous must be preferred and, insofar as possible, the best looking."[42] The philosopher kings' education thus begins in the body—an ideal, white, *male* body, that is—*so that they might transcend it.*

Already here, over two thousand years in the past, we find the theoretical roots of the estrangement of the ill, the infirm, and the disabled, to say nothing of women and persons of color. In *W;t*, no one on the team in charge of "caring" for Vivian need trouble themselves with what her cancer or chemotherapy *means* to her, as this particular embodied subject, because that meaning is irrelevant to the essentializing higher operations of mind, for which Vivian is just an *instance*, a data-point—patient number XXXX—in their study of a disease that is, for all intents and purposes, abstracted from the particulars of the life of the one who suffers from it.

This ascent of abstraction, from the body to the Ideas, is reinforced in Plato's *Symposium*. Here, Socrates recollects a dialogue in which the character of Diotima, a woman from whom he claims to have learned the nature of love, describes the ascent from the cave as an *erotic* journey. Early in their dialogue, Diotima convinces Socrates that the goal of all eros, or desire, is the possession of good things. This is true, she tells him, "because the happy are happy by the acquisition of good things," and happiness is *the* end-in-itself of all desire.[43] One's desire to possess good things is, Diotima adds, necessarily the desire to possess them forever, for who can be happy knowing that the good they possess might be snatched from them at any moment? To possess good things forever, Diotima argues, we must give birth, "both in terms of the body and in terms of the soul," to something that will outlast our mortality.[44] Diotima therefore weds happiness—the goal of desire—to immortality. We may be temporal, mortal beings, but the goal of our desire is the transcendence of time, a transcendence accomplished only through generation.

It is beauty, Diotima argues, that makes generation—and thus immortality—possible, for it is our desire for what is beautiful that inspires us to give birth, whether to actual children or to poetry, laws, sciences, or philosophy: "It is impossible for [pregnancy and bringing to birth] to happen in the unfitting; and the ugly is unfitting with everything divine, but the beautiful is fitting."[45] The student of eros must ascend the ladder of love one rung at a time, giving birth first in the lowest form of beauty before moving to the next, higher level, then on to the next, and the next, until finally reaching the summit. The lowest form of beauty is that of the body, so it is here that the student must begin. As in the Republic, therefore, we begin the journey to transcendence with a focus on a healthy, beautiful body: "He who is to move correctly in this matter must begin while young to go to beautiful bodies. And first of all, if the guide is guiding correctly, he must love one body and there generate beautiful speeches."[46] Loving this one, beautiful body, and giving birth to the poetry (and hence the share of immortality this poetry grants) inspired by this beauty, the student, if guided aright, soon realizes "that the beauty that is in any body whatsoever is related to that in another body; and if he must pursue the beauty of looks, it is great folly not to believe that the beauty of all bodies is one and the same."[47] Having recognized that beauty does not inhere in one beautiful body only, the student is eventually able to abstract beauty from embodiment itself and thus consider a higher form of beauty: "After this he must believe that the beauty in souls is more honorable than that in the body. So that even if someone who is decent in his soul has only a slight youthful charm, the lover must be content with it, and love and cherish him, and engender and seek such speeches as will make the young better; in order that [the lover] . . . may come to believe that the beauty of the body is something trivial."[48] Note that the student of erotics must, at this point, himself become a teacher ("engender and seek such speeches as will make the young better") if he is to ascend to the next, higher level of abstraction: from the love of the beauty common to all beautiful bodies to the love of the beauty of the soul.

This pedagogical force driving the ascent is further reinforced at the next level:

> And after these pursuits, he must lead [the beloved] on to the sciences, so that he [himself, the lover] may see the beauty of sciences, and in looking at the beautiful, which is now so vast, no longer be content like a lackey with the beauty in one, of a boy, of some human being, or of one practice, nor be a sorry sort of slave and petty calculator; but with a permanent turn to the vast open sea of the beautiful, behold it and give birth—in ungrudging philosophy—to many beautiful and magnificent speeches and thoughts; until, there strengthened and increased, he may discern a certain single philosophical science.[49]

The lover must therefore teach the beloved the sciences—through which are revealed how all beauty (of bodies and souls) is "akin to itself"—if he is himself to give birth to knowledge inspired by the beauty of the sciences and thus ascend to the very highest level of abstraction: the Idea of Beauty that unites all sciences, which only philosophy can behold.

Before describing this final, highest form of knowledge—the revelation of the Beauty that is philosophy's true object—Diotima instructs Socrates (and thus Plato instructs us) to "pay as close attention as you can." We are still paying close attention today, for Diotima's description of the goal of all intellectual labor—the very highest form of knowing, at the highest level of abstraction from the mundane, the earthly, the bodily—has remained a powerful ideal of knowledge in the West since Diotima instructed Socrates almost two-and-a-half millennia ago. The highest form of knowledge—the Beauty of which generates the greatest share of immortality—is knowledge, Diotima tells Socrates, that is *Eternal* ("always being and neither coming to be nor perishing"), *Unchanging* ("nor increasing nor passing away"), *Objective* ("not beautiful in one respect and ugly in another"), *Universal* ("nor at one time so, and at another time not—either with respect to the beautiful or the ugly—nor here beautiful and there ugly, as being beautiful to some and ugly to others"), *Noncorporeal* ("nor in turn will the beautiful be imagined by him as a kind of face or hands or anything else in which body shares"), and *One* ("and not as being somewhere in something else . . . but as it is alone by itself and with itself, always being of a single form").[50] In other words, Truth is Truth for all time, in all places, from all perspectives, for all peoples. The highest form of knowing, then, is one that abstracts most radically from the *temporal* (from knowledge bound to that which changes, coming to be and passing away), from the *subjective* (from knowledge bound to that which is particular to an individual perspective, bound to a particular place and time), from the *many* (from knowledge scattered across many particulars without a unifying, totalizing view).

Given Plato's view that the ideal objects of knowledge—Beauty and all the rest of the Ideas—exist in a hyperuranion realm transcendent to the earthly, the mortal, it is not surprising he contends that those who hope to contemplate the Ideas must work to free their souls from the prison of their own bodies. The body is a hindrance to contemplation, distracting us, dragging us back to earth with its importunate needs, pleasures, and pains. As we saw in the *Republic*, where only those who excel at gymnastics are deemed worthy to become guardian/rulers, and as was reinforced in the *Symposium*, the erotic drive to transcendence begins with the ideal of healthy, male embodiment. All others, presumably, are doomed to exist in the cave, and the best we can do for them is to make sure the shadows they view are salutary ones. This drive to free the soul from the body, with body/emotion/disease/mortality on one side and soul/rationality/purity/immortality on the other—proved instrumental in the development of thought in the West, including Christian, Jewish, and Muslim theology,[51] for more than 2000 years, reaching a kind of apotheosis in the middle of the seventeenth century when Descartes published his *Discourse on Method*.

It is impossible to understand the central role of dualism in contemporary medicine without considering how Descartes influenced its development. It was the *Discourse on Method*'s radicalization of Platonic dualism that placed the split between mind and body at the very foundation of the scientific revolution. Descartes begins his *Discourse* with an assertion of the universality of reason: "[T]he power of judging well and of distinguishing the true from the false (which is, properly speaking, what people call 'good sense' or 'reason') is naturally equal in all men. . . . [I]t exists whole and entire in each of us."[52] It is this conviction that reason is universal, that it is *One*, that grounds Descartes' confidence that he can establish a single, unified science. Because there is one reason, the same for all "men" of all times, there should be one Truth for all "men" of all times. Plato may have established the unity, universality, and atemporality of True Wisdom more than 2000 years before Descartes but, Descartes laments, even though philosophy (literally, "the love of wisdom") had been "cultivated for many centuries by the most excellent minds that have ever lived . . . nevertheless, there is still nothing in it about which there is not some dispute, and consequently nothing that is not doubtful."[53] If this is true of philosophy and all the sciences, then *a fortiori* it is true of poetry, plays, and all other imaginative representations of reality, whether fictional or nonfictional: "[F]ables make one imagine many events to be possible which are not so at all. And even the most accurate histories, if they neither alter nor exaggerate the significance of things in order to render them worthy of being read, almost always at least omit the baser and less noteworthy details."[54] To establish science on a firmer foundation, Descartes resolves to "reject as absolutely false everything in which [he] could imagine the least doubt, in order to see whether, after this process, something in [his] beliefs remained that was entirely indubitable."[55] Since reason is universal, Descartes contends, whatever he establishes as indubitable through this thoroughgoing process of doubt should serve as an incontestable foundation on which finally to build the One, True Science.

The first, most obvious thing Descartes rejects as a source of indubitable knowledge is the evidence of the senses: "[B]ecause our senses sometimes deceive us, I wanted to suppose that nothing was exactly as they led us to imagine."[56] Whatever the foundation for Wisdom might prove to be, the body will most assuredly not be its source. Until Descartes has established an irrefutable foundation for reason, from which he might firmly judge the truth of anything we sense, he must set aside all that our bodily senses provide. Yet Descartes' next move is even more radical: "And because there are men who make mistakes in reasoning, . . . I rejected as false all the reasonings that I had previously taken for demonstrations."[57] Even mathematical deductions, which seem the most sound of all possible reasonings, must be set aside as false until Descartes has established an absolutely unassailable ground on which he might then establish the certainty of all that he reasons. After thus setting aside all former reasonings, however, Descartes is still not satisfied: "[C]onsidering the fact that all the same thoughts we have when we are awake can also come to us when we are asleep, without any of them being true, I resolved to pretend that all the things that had ever entered my mind were no more true than the illusions of my dreams."[58] With this, Descartes casts aside the contents of everything he has ever thought, felt, or experienced as candidates for the first principle of science. What, then, is left? "But immediately afterward I noticed that, while I wanted thus to think that everything was false, it necessarily had to be the case that I, who was thinking this, was something. And noticing that this truth—*I think, therefore I am*—was so firm and so assured that all the most extravagant suppositions of the skeptics are incapable of shaking it, I judged that I could accept it without scruple as the first principle of the philosophy I was seeking."[59] Though he can doubt all other things, Descartes reasons, he cannot doubt his own existence, so long as he is doubting. The entire system of science must therefore be built on the certainty of his own existence that follows necessarily from his own thinking. As Merleau-Ponty writes in the *Phenomenology of Perception*, "Descartes . . . *freed* the subject or consciousness by establishing that I could not grasp anything as existing if I did not first experience myself as existing in the act of grasping . . ."[60]

Having established the Cogito (from *cogito ergo sum*, the Latin form of "I think, therefore I am," which appears in his *Principles of First Philosophy*) as the first principle of the philosophy that will ground the One, True, Eternal, Unified Science (the development of which would finally achieve Diotima's ideal), Descartes writes this:

> Then, examining with attention what I was, and seeing that I could pretend that I had no body and that there was no world nor any place where I was, I could not pretend, on that account, that I did not exist at all, and that, on the contrary, from the very fact that I thought of doubting the truth of other things, it followed very evidently and very certainly that I existed; whereas, on the other hand, had I simply stopped thinking, even if all the rest of what I had ever imagined had been true, I would have had no reason to believe that I had existed. From this I knew that I was a substance the whole essence or nature of which is simply to think, and which, in order to exist, has no need of any place nor depends on any material thing. Thus this "I," that is to say, the soul through which I am what I am, is entirely distinct from the body and is even easier to know than the body, and even if there were no body at all, it would not cease to be all that it is.[61]

With this, Descartes radicalizes Plato's separation of soul from body into a separation, as Elizabeth Grosz writes, of "soul from nature."[62] Following Descartes, Grosz argues, the body becomes "a self-moving machine, a mechanical device, functioning according to causal laws and the laws of nature. The mind, the thinking substance, the soul, or consciousness, has no place in the natural world. This exclusion of the soul from nature . . . is the prerequisite for founding a knowledge, or better, a science, of the governing principles of nature, a science which excludes and is indifferent to considerations of the subject. . . . Descartes, in short, succeeded in linking the mind/body opposition to the foundations of knowledge itself."[63] The body is on the side of nature—part of the "external" world; it is not essential to consciousness/soul/mind/*self*, which exists outside nature. I am *not* my body. I am *essentially* a rational being, a being not subject to the laws of nature, a being that does not even exist in space—in the *res extensa* that is the substance of all material bodies. The body is thus *acted upon*, subjected to nature, independently of the mind.

Descartes therefore grounds science in an oppositional dualism; it has unquestionably flourished there, and medical science can be said to be the fulfillment of Descartes' fondest dream. In Part Six of his *Discourse* Descartes writes that the purpose of rendering ourselves "masters and possessors of nature" through science is "not only for the invention of an infinity of devices that would enable one to enjoy trouble-free the fruits of the earth and all the goods found there, but also principally for the maintenance of health, which unquestionably is the first good and the foundation of all other goods of this life."[64] Health is the *greatest good*—the good from which all other goods follow—so the development of effective medical science is Descartes' highest goal. Indeed, in his final paragraph, Descartes assures us that he has "resolved to spend the rest of my life on nothing but trying to acquire some knowledge of nature which is such that one could draw from it rules for medicine that are more reliable than those we have had to the present."[65]

It is easy to imagine how proud Descartes might be if he were witness to the marvels of contemporary medicine, from antibiotics and anesthesia to MRI technology, genomics, and beyond. Perhaps ironically, however, advances in neuroscientific research belie the separation of thought and emotion that are often considered so integral to Descartes' philosophy. For example, in *Descartes' Error: Emotion, reason and the human brain*, neurologist Antonio Damasio marshals neurobiological evidence to support the claim that the automatic emotional system is the basis for—and remains an integral component of—logical reasoning and cognition. As he explains, the effects of Cartesianism remain problematic both in terms of scientific insight and healthcare: "For the past three centuries, the aim of biological studies and of medicine has been the understanding of the physiology and pathology of the body proper. The mind was out, largely left as a concern for religion and philosophy . . . The result of all this has been an amputation of the concept of humanity with which medicine does its job."[66] Damasio's pathological metaphor is apt, for humanity is integral to healthcare, and its excision imperils our very body of knowledge and duty of care.

Descartes' role must also be understood within the broad changes of the Renaissance and Enlightenment—a story that includes such pivotal figures as Leonardo da Vinci, Santorio Santorio, Julian Offray de la Mettrie, Francis Bacon, Galileo, and Isaac Newton, whose materialism had a profound influence on the evolution of Western thought, including the development of "iatromechanism" in medical practice. For example, Archibald Pitcairn, a physician and follower of Newton, argued that "Physicians ought to propose the method of Astronomers as a pattern for their Imitation."[67] Depending upon one's view of history, the emergence of mechanism may be understood as a "spontaneous movement" that is not attributable to any one figure.[68] Regardless, the influence of thought articulated by Descartes, among others, has been truly profound. For medicine still lives in this dualistic world. As philosopher S. Kay Toombs writes, "The traditional biomedical paradigm focuses exclusively along 'Cartesian' lines on the body-as-machine, with a concurrent de-emphasis on the personhood of the patient and the reality and importance of the human experience of illness ... Indeed, the prevailing model so effectively separates the biological physical body from the person whose body it is that medical education deems it necessary explicitly to remind students that patients are persons."[69] We see this divide reflected in the pervasive refrain about surgeons who lack humanistic qualities such as communication skills: "Well I would rather have a technically adept surgeon than one with 'good bedside manner'!" Accepting the premise that skill and compassion are incompatible speaks to the age-old split between the mechanistic body and the human spirit.

In another sense the body-as-machine is perpetuated by the focus on the corpse and dissection in medical science and education. As Drew Leder describes, dissection preoccupied Descartes for many years, including "almost daily visits to butcher shops, collecting material for this purpose."[70] Citing Foucault and Engelhardt, Leder describes the eighteenth-century shift in clinical orientation from symptoms to that which can be discerned in dissection; the "epistemological primacy of the corpse" is thus one of the critical roots of contemporary abnegation of individual subjective experience, for the lifeless body/machine does not possess a life-world. Indeed, the central importance of clinical gross anatomy in contemporary medical education speaks to this perspective. In a study of a US medical school anatomy lab in the 1980s, Peter Finkelstein describes a focus on acquiring an immense body of knowledge and adopting an appropriate "clinical attitude" while students routinely internalize and conceal their emotions. As Finkelstein observes, the students' use of such terms as "hacking and whacking" and their behavior "reveals an inclination towards treating the body as material."[71] In addition, humor serves to reduce "the status of the cadaver to one that is less human, or at times even UNhuman. Dehumanization is a useful response. It lessens the impact of the experience."[72] Several decades later, Christine Montross, writing of her experience on the first day in the anatomy lab, describes the presentation of the cadaver:

> Her hands, feet, and head are wrapped in a translucent, cheeseclothlike material and then enclosed by tightly tied plastic bags. This elaborate wrapping, [the instructor] explains, is to protect those parts of the body from desiccation until we begin our study of them. He adds that their coverage also helps depersonalize the body. The hands, feet, and head are parts of the body that are instilled with character. They can most quickly conjure up an individual life.[73]

Montross also describes the ways in which "the humanity of the body emerges in unexpected moments," such as the presence of nail polish—yet, as she explains, the labors of dissection require the students "to turn off, in a sense, our connection with this humanity."[74] Attitudes and practices have evolved considerably, and Montross' thoughtful and respectful reflections upon the experience are evidence of such a shift. Many medical schools now hold ceremonies for the cadavers, and students may write letters to the families of those who donated their bodies for this purpose. Regardless, the dramatic initiation into formal medical education beginning with dissecting a corpse can be said to reflect the pervasive model of the body-as-machine, as nature stripped of its animating force.

The scope of this Cartesian schema extends well beyond medicine. As Grosz writes, "The Cartesian tradition has been more influential than any other tradition in establishing the agenda for philosophical reflection and in defining the terrain, either negatively or positively, for later concepts of subjectivity and knowledge."[75] In detailing the means by which this epistemological terrain has been defined by Descartes, Grosz highlights the other dichotomies correlated with his dualism:

> The mind/body relation is frequently correlated with the distinctions between reason and passion, sense and sensibility, outside and inside, self and other, depth and surface, reality and appearance, mechanism and vitalism, transcendence and immanence, temporality and spatiality, psychology and physiology, form and matter, and so on. These terms function implicitly to define the body in nonhistorical, naturalistic, organicist, passive, inert terms, seeing it as an intrusion on or interference with the operation of mind, a brute givenness which requires overcoming, a connection with animality and nature that needs transcendence.[76]

Grosz goes on to posit that dualism is, at least indirectly, also responsible for myriad distinctions: the historical division of different disciplines, the separation of quantitative and qualitative analysis, and the hierarchy within the sciences elevating mathematics and physics as paragons of knowledge.[77]

The very prevalence of this philosophical lineage sometimes makes its applicability difficult to discern. Reading philosophy demands careful attention and thought, and the relevance of such study is not always immediately apparent to our students. Yet after reading Descartes for the first time for the philosophy core seminar of our narrative medicine Master of Science program, Barbara, an endocrinologist in practice for over 30 years, suddenly bolted upright in her seat, threw up her hand, and exclaimed, "I *get* it now! Medicine is *Cartesian*! It's the way we treat the body, as if it's completely separate from the person." It wasn't until she read Descartes that she understood the centuries-old origins of medicine's objectifying view. Now, several years after her revelation, Barbara reports that her epiphany has reaffirmed her commitment to the treatment of the whole patient: "The patient with diabetes' feeling about having a chronic illness must be explored. The patient can no longer be seen as a 'diabetic' but rather as the 'person with diabetes'." (Indeed, such attentiveness represents a widespread semantic shift in the field of endocrinology and more broadly within healthcare.[78]) As Barbara explains, "I have always been committed to this form of practice. The discussion in class reaffirmed my strong belief. Understanding the Cartesian paradigm offered new tools for helping to challenge this paradigm in medical education."

What Barbara came to realize is that one can welcome the advances of biomedical science and recognize their debt to Descartes' Enlightenment ethos while also identifying the less-than-salubrious sequelae of dualism in contemporary healthcare. For while such a mechanistic view has arguably helped to foster a tremendous growth in scientific knowledge and skill, its very dominance has revealed a paucity of humanism. As Pellegrino and Thomasma described in 1981: "Today, medicine's temptation to technicism is greatly enhanced by its obvious technological abilities . . . Paradoxically, the very triumphs of technicism have revealed how urgently medicine needs understanding and wisdom . . ."[79] And so we turn again to philosophy, among other disciplines and practices, seeking such understanding and wisdom. In the following chapter we will explore philosophical responses to this dualistic heritage.

Notes

1. Descartes, *Discourse on Method*, 100.
2. Damasio, *Descartes' Error*, 250.
3. Galen, *Claudii Galeni Opera Omnia*, vol. 1. Cited in *Brain*, "Galen on the Ideal."
4. Lorde, "A Burst of Light," 149.

5. Lorde, "A Burst of Light," 149.
6. Lorde, "A Burst of Light," 150.
7. Pellegrino, *Philosophy of Medicine Reborn*, 72.
8. Maitland, "Forceps Delivery," 166.
9. Maitland, "Forceps Delivery," 169.
10. Edson, *W;t*, 5.
11. Edson, *W;t*, 37.
12. Edson, *W;t*, 57, 55.
13. "Love and Knowledge."
14. Edson, *W;t*, 20.
15. Edson, *W;t*, 69.
16. Vanhoutte, "Cancer and the Common Woman," 406.
17. Kleinman, *Illness Narratives*, 3.
18. Kleinman, *Illness Narratives*, 3, 5.
19. See Charles Rosenberg for discussion of disease entities: "Diagnosis has always played a pivotal role in medical practice, but in the past two centuries, that role has been reconfigured and has become more central as medicine—like Western society in general—has become increasingly technical, specialized, and bureaucratized. Disease explanations and clinical practices have incorporated, paralleled, and, in some measure, constituted these larger structural changes. This modern history of diagnosis is inextricably related to disease specificity, to the notion that diseases can and should be thought of as entities existing outside the unique manifestations of illness in particular men and women" ("Tyranny of Diagnosis," 237).
20. For scholarship on clinician memoirs, see: Aull and Lewis, "Medical Intellectuals"; Kathryn Montgomery Hunter, *Doctors' Stories*; Koski, *Autobiography of Medical Education*; Poirier, *Doctors in the Making*; Wear and Jones, "Bless Me Reader."
21. Iaquinta, *The Year They Tried to Kill Me*, 11.
22. See Lewis, "Narrative Medicine." For further reading about trends toward "biomedicalization" see Riska et al., *Biomedicalization: Technoscience, Health, and Illness*.
23. Flexner, *Medical Education in the United States and Canada*.
24. Flexner, *Medical Education*, 25.
25. Odegaard, *Dear Doctor*, 16.
26. Flexner, *Medical Education*, 26.
27. There is a rich body of scholarship in this area. See Hojat et al., "The Devil Is in the Third Year," for a representative qualitative study, and Marcus, "Medical Student Dreams," for a fascinating psychoanalytic study.
28. See Shem, "Fiction as Resistance."
29. Shem, *House of God*, 32.
30. Peabody, "Care of the Patient," 882.
31. Cassell, "Nature of Suffering," 640.
32. Frank, *Wounded Storyteller*, 77.
33. Frank, *Wounded Storyteller*, 85–86.
34. Rosenberg, "Tyranny of Diagnosis," 257.
35. Rosenberg, "Tyranny of Diagnosis," 257.
36. MacIntyre, *After Virtue*, 216.
37. Leder, "Tale of Two Bodies," 23.
38. Plato, *Republic* 517b1–5.
39. Plato, *Republic* 537b6–7.
40. Plato, *Republic* 406c3–407e1.
41. Plato, *Republic* 407b8–c1.
42. Plato, *Republic* 535a10–b1.
43. Plato, *Symposium* 205A1–2.

44. Plato, *Symposium* 206b8.
45. Plato, *Symposium* 206c7–9.
46. Plato, *Symposium* 210A4–7.
47. Plato, *Symposium* 210B1–3.
48. Plato, *Symposium* 210B5–C6.
49. Plato, *Symposium* 210C6–D7.
50. Plato, *Symposium* 210E1–211B3.
51. Cross and Livingstone, eds., *Oxford Dictionary of the Christian Church*; Louth, *Origins of the Christian Mystical Tradition*; Ahbel-Rappe, "Plato's Influence"; Walzer, *Greek into Arabic*.
52. Descartes, *Discourse on Method*, 1–2.
53. Descartes, *Discourse on Method*, 5.
54. Descartes, *Discourse on Method*, 4.
55. Descartes, *Discourse on Method*, 18.
56. Descartes, *Discourse on Method*, 18.
57. Descartes, *Discourse on Method*, 18.
58. Descartes, *Discourse on Method*, 18.
59. Descartes, *Discourse on Method*, 18.
60. Merleau-Ponty, *Phenomenology of Perception*, lxxii.
61. Descartes, *Discourse on Method*, 18–19.
62. Grosz, *Volatile Bodies*, 6.
63. Grosz, *Volatile Bodies*, 6.
64. Descartes, *Discourse on Method*, 35.
65. Descartes, *Discourse on Method*, 44.
66. Damasio, *Descartes' Error*, 255.
67. Brown, *Mechanical Philosophy*, 216. Cited in Marcum, *Introductory Philosophy of Medicine*, 50.
68. "No one man created the mechanical philosophy. Throughout the scientific circles of western Europe during the first half of the seventeenth century we can observe what appears to be a spontaneous movement towards a mechanical conception of nature in reaction against Renaissance Naturalism" (Westfall, *Construction of Modern Science*, 30–31; cited in Lee, *Philosophical Foundations*, 29).
69. Toombs, "Illness and the Paradigm," 201–2.
70. Leder, "Tale of Two Bodies," 19.
71. Finkelstein, "Studies in the Anatomy Laboratory," 41.
72. Finkelstein, "Studies in the Anatomy Laboratory," 41.
73. Montross, *Body of Work*, 20.
74. Montross, *Body of Work*, 24–25.
75. Grosz, *Volatile Bodies*, 10.
76. Grosz, *Volatile Bodies*, 3–4.
77. Grosz, *Volatile Bodies*, 7.
78. As endocrinologist Kyle Peters has asserted, the use of the term *diabetic* objectifies persons with diabetes; Peters argues persuasively against its use, as well as terms such as *noncompliant*: "I believe that, by focusing on the individual instead of the disease, health care professionals will allow patients to reach their treatment goals and will, ourselves, find greater joy in managing our patients with diabetes. Calling someone noncompliant is not just rude; it is amazingly inaccurate and vague, and it leads to obvious treatment interventions that are just wrong and worthless. If we continue to refer to patients as diabetics or noncompliant diabetics, no change will occur, and patients with diabetes will not reach their treatment goals" (Peters, "'Diabetic' and 'Noncompliant Diabetic,'" 90).
    Such usage has indeed evolved, as evidenced by the UK journal *Diabetic Medicine*'s Style Guide, which specifies that the journal "does not recognise the term 'diabetic' as

a noun. Preferred style is 'people (or person) with diabetes'" (n.p.). In a 2011 position statement, the advocacy/support organization Diabetes Australia advocated several semantic shifts, including avoidance of the term *diabetic*: "The term 'diabetic' defines the individual as their health condition. It is better to emphasise the person's ability to live with diabetes. Labelling someone as 'diabetic' positions diabetes as the defining factor of their life" ("A New Language").

Similarly, the use of such disease terms as *epileptic* and *asthmatic* as nouns are increasingly discouraged, as they reflect and may indeed perpetuate the reduction of personhood to the scope of a disease category.

79. Pellegrino and Thomasma, *Philosophical Basis of Medical Practice*, 13.

CHAPTER 4

Dualism and Its Discontents II: Philosophical Tinctures

Craig Irvine and Danielle Spencer

Phenomenology and Narrative Hermeneutics

In the previous chapter we told a story about the evolution of dualism in Western philosophy, framed by Alisdair MacIntyre's famous dictum: "I can only answer the question 'What am I to do?' if I can answer the prior question 'Of what story or stories do I find myself a part?' "[1] Understanding the philosophical roots of medicine's dualistic frame, we argued, allows us to better appreciate, draw upon, and advance the work of those seeking to move beyond it. Yet we are not yet through telling our philosophical story. Western philosophy, after all, did not end with Descartes. Since the mid-seventeenth century, many philosophers have challenged Descartes' dualistic ontology. Narrative medicine joins anthropology, women's studies, sociology, disability studies, LGBTQ studies, and many more disciplines in drawing on these philosophers to establish a theoretical foundation for rethinking medicine's alienation of the self from the body—for moving past its dualistic frame. We begin this chapter of our story with a thinker who has inspired scholars across all of these disciplines: Maurice Merleau-Ponty. His philosophy offers one of the most radical challenges to Descartes' conclusion that "the whole essence or nature" of the self "is simply to think." Merleau-Ponty proposes a philosophical method—phenomenology—that makes embodied experience *primary*, overthrowing Plato's hierarchization of the Ideas. This overthrow reorients our relation to the abstractions of science, making them secondary to our primary experience, which is *fundamentally* embodied. As we will see, phenomenology provides a rich foundation for contemporary perspectives in philosophy of medicine.

In the preface to his *Phenomenology of Perception*, Merleau-Ponty describes the project of phenomenology as founded by his teacher Edmund Husserl. It is a philosophy, he writes,

> for which the world is always 'already there' prior to reflection—like an inalienable presence—and whose entire effort is to rediscover this naïve contact with the world in order to finally raise it to a philosophical status. It is the goal of a philosophy that aspires to be an 'exact science,' but it is also an account of 'lived' space, 'lived' time, and the 'lived' world. It is the attempt to provide a direct description of our experience such as it is, and without any consideration of its psychological genesis or of the causal explanations that the scientist, historian, or sociologist might offer of that experience.[2]

Merleau-Ponty challenges empiricism, or what he calls the "naturalistic attitude," for which the world exists independently of consciousness. For empiricism the body is just one thing among others, essentially external to consciousness, which functions as a passive receptor of sensory experience. Merleau-Ponty's challenge to empiricism calls us back to *experience*. He argues that consciousness is *essentially* embodied, *essentially, actively* embedded in its environment. The body is not a mere object among other objects in the world, separate from our minds. The body *is* consciousness, is the very *self*. He encourages us to examine our embodied relation to the world, not as abstracted from the self but as the life of consciousness—to learn to *describe* rather than *explain* our conscious experience. In this way Merleau-Ponty advances phenomenology's commitment to describing *primary*, pre-reflective, prescientific experience:

> Everything that I know about the world, even through science, I know from a perspective that is my own or from an experience of the world without which scientific symbols would be meaningless. The entire universe of science is constructed upon that lived world, and if we wish to think science rigorously, to appreciate precisely its sense and its scope, we must first awaken that experience of the world of which science is the second-order expression.[3]

As Merleau-Ponty writes, the dis-embodied abstractions of science are *dependent* on our embodied, lived experience of the world—on our *being-in-the-world*—"just like geography with regard to the landscape where we first learned what a forest, a meadow, or a river is."[4]

Given a phenomenological perspective, mental states and activities that we ordinarily consider disembodied knowledges are actually constituted in and through our bodily engagement with the world. Indeed, Merleau-Ponty describes the ways in which our bodily interactions with the world constitute *all* our states of consciousness—our very thinking itself. Even, or perhaps most especially, *language*, for Merleau-Ponty, is a *bodily* expression, and it is here that narrative medicine finds one of its strongest philosophical supports.

All speech is a bodily gesture—an elaboration of our embodied being-in-the-world. Speech is, in fact, as gestural as raising one's hand to hail, scowling in displeasure, or pointing to direct. I do not need to call to mind a word, to represent it to myself, before speaking; rather, "It is enough that I possess its articulatory and sonorous essence as one of the modulations or one of the possible uses of my body."[5] Speech is a sonorous articulation of our bodies that *signifies the world* toward which it gestures:

> According to Darwin . . . the knitting of the eyebrows destined to protect the eye from the sun, and the convergence of the eyes destined to permit clear vision become components of the human act of meditation and signify this act for the spectator. Language, in turn, poses no other problem: the contraction of the throat, the sibilant emission of air between the tongue and the teeth, a certain manner of playing with our body suddenly allows itself to be invested with a *figurative sense* and signifies this externally. This is no more and no less miraculous than the emergence of love from desire . . ."[6]

"[W]ords, vowels, and phonemes," Merleau-Ponty writes, "are so many ways of singing the world," each language a unique style "for the human body to celebrate the world and to finally live it. This is why the *full* sense of a language is never translatable into another."[7] In speaking, performing its sonorous gesture, the body becomes "the thought or the intention that it signifies to us. It is the body that shows, that speaks . . ."[8] Thought does not exist prior to this gesture, this showing, this speaking. It is, then, the body that articulates our shared world and thus *brings thought into being*.

Such an understanding of the embodiment and relationality of language stands in contrast to a Cartesian subject, isolated in his disembodied rationality. It interrogates a view of thought as an essentially internal, intra-subjective process, with speech as an extrinsic representation of ideas, just as our bodies, in the Cartesian cosmos, are accidental to our essential selves. Our understanding of thought as embedded in language is reflected in many discourses, such as the Sapir-Whorf hypothesis and variants in cognitive linguistics; it is also one of the common threads in the corpus of poststructuralist thought. Returning to Merleau-Ponty's conception, we find many compelling arguments for the ways in which thought inheres in the embodied gesture of language:

> If speech presupposed thought . . . then we could not understand why thought tends toward expression as if toward its completion, why the most familiar object appears indeterminate so long as we have not remembered its name, and why the thinking subject himself is in a sort of ignorance of his thoughts so long as he has not formulated them for himself, or even spoken or written them, as is shown through the example of so many writers who begin a book without knowing just what they are going to include. . . . For the speaker, then, speech does not translate a ready-made thought; rather, speech accomplishes thought.[9]

Thought, then, is not, as it was conceived by Descartes, an essentially inner function of the mind. In Merleau-Ponty's description, thought does not exist "outside the world and outside of words."[10] We come to believe that thought exists inwardly, independently of its expression in language, because of the already constituted thoughts that we can recall to ourselves at any time. Merleau-Ponty calls these already formulated thoughts "second-order" speech, or "secondary expression," as they are secondary to the primary activity in which they originate. Mundane speech is a kind of sedimentation of thinking—expressing thoughts that are already ready-to-hand, thoughts that "require no genuine effort of expression from us, and that will demand no effort of comprehension from our listeners"; these "banal words" form the basis for most of our everyday use of language, whether silently recalled to ourselves or spoken aloud to others.

> Thus, language and the comprehension of language seem self-evident. The linguistic and intersubjective world no longer causes us any wonder, we no longer distinguish it from the world itself, and we reflect within a world already spoken and speaking. We become unaware of what is contingent in expression and communication, either for the child who learns to speak, or for the writer who says and thinks of something for the first time, in short, for those who transform silence into speech. It is, however, clear that constituted speech, such as it plays out in everyday life, assumes that the decisive step of expression has been accomplished. Our view of man will remain superficial so long as we do not return to its origin, so long as we do not rediscover the primordial silence beneath the noise of words, and so long as we do not describe the gesture that breaks this silence. Speech is a gesture, and its signification a world."[11]

"Authentic speech," in contrast to mundane speech, "formulates [thought] for the first time."[12] Authentic speech is *creative*—an originating gesture— bringing into being a thought that did not previously exist:

For the miracle to happen, the phonetic gesticulation must make use of an alphabet of already acquired significations, and the verbal gesture must be performed in a certain panorama that is shared by the interlocutors, just as the comprehension of other gestures presupposes a perceived world shared by everyone in which the sense of the gesture unfolds and is displayed. But this is not a sufficient condition. If authentic, speech gives rise to a new sense, just as the gesture—if it is an initiating gesture—gives a human sense to the object for the first time. Moreover, significations now acquired must surely have been new significations.[13]

The process of formulating a new thought begins, Merleau-Ponty writes, as "a certain emptiness of consciousness" and "an instantaneous desire"—a "certain lack that seeks to be fulfilled," as if a vacuum had suddenly opened at the center of one's being.[14] Nature abhors a vacuum, and consciousness is no exception: words ("the available significations") rush in to fill the void, intertwining "according to an unknown law, and once and for all a new cultural being has begun to exist. Thought and expression are thus constituted simultaneously when our cultural assets are mobilized in service of this unknown law."[15] Creative speech is the expression, the realization of new thought. Unlike the sedimentation of "ordinary" speech,[16] "The operation of expression, when successful, does not simply leave to the reader or the writer himself a reminder; it makes the signification exist as a thing at the very heart of the text, it brings it to life in an organism of words, it installs this signification in the writer or the reader like a new sense organ, it opens a new field or a new dimension to our experience."[17]

The implications for communication are profound: "For the speaker, then, speech does not translate a ready-made thought; rather, speech accomplishes thought. Even more so, it must be acknowledged that the person listening receives the thoughts from the speech itself."[18] In listening to or reading the speech of others, we are not receiving words external to (mere representations of) their thinking; rather, we are receiving their thought itself, directly, in their speech. My thinking, while listening or reading, *is* the thought of the other: "Through speech, then, there is a taking up of the other person's thought, a reflection in others, a power of thinking *according to others*, which enriches our own thoughts."[19] My relationship to the other is not *mediated* by her language, as if her essential, thinking selfhood were "over there" in some inner, inaccessible realm; rather, her language is the *immediate* presence of her subjectivity. When listening to or reading the other,

I do not primarily communicate with 'representations' or with a thought, but rather with a speaking subject with a certain style of being, and with the 'world' that he aims at. Just as the significative intention that initiated the other person's speech is not an explicit thought, but rather a certain lack that seeks to be fulfilled, so too is my taking up of this intention not an operation of my thought, but rather a synchronic modulation of my own existence, a transformation of my being.[20]

To receive the creative speech of the other is to synchronize one's very existence with theirs: what a challenge this offers to the notion of the clinician as disembodied mind, treating a body dissociated from the personhood of the patient. To recognize the embodiedness of speech is to reaffirm the particularity of the clinical encounter, of any account of self. In narrative medicine we explore the implications of attending to speech as an essentially creative act, investigating the ways in which our work opens the possibilities of creative speech, providing opportunities to break through the sedimentations of "ordinary" speech so that we might think, create, express, and therefore *know* the meaning of our own experience, while attending to the meaning of the other's. We remain mindful of the different forms that speech can take and of the presence and significance of silence— the echoing cries of those who do not have the opportunity to speak or be meaningfully heard.

To heighten our mindfulness to the creative possibilities of language, we turn to literature. Literature, like all creative speech, is an elaboration of our embodied being-in-the-world, each new work of literature a new way of "singing the world." Narrative medicine attends to the style, voice, rhythm, metaphors, perspectives, temporalities, silences, and genres of this singing, through which is expressed the meaning of our own and others' embodied experience. A great work of literature, Merleau-Ponty suggests, "contributes to modifying [the] common meaning" of words, conferring "an existence in itself upon what it expresses" and thus installing it "in nature as a perceived thing accessible to everyone."[21] After reading Ralph Ellison for the first time, I no longer live in the same world. Ellison's speech, as the expression of his being-in-the world, *directly* installs in me a new way of being—a new sense organ through which I perceive a previously unknown world.

Returning to the literary examples with which we began the previous chapter—Audre Lorde's account, the narrator of "Forceps Delivery," and Vivian Bearing in *W;t*—each of these voices articulates, in unique ways, the frequently alienating effects of illness and healthcare. As we investigate the roots of the pervasive dualism subtending Western medicine, we deepen our understanding and perception of the dissociative experiences expressed by these creative works. We also encounter philosophical responses to this legacy offering a phenomenological balm or tincture that may have aided our three protagonists and those who sought to care for them. Elaboration of our embodied lived experience gives rise to a different understanding of illness and, potentially, a more promising model for medical training and practice.

In *Illness: The Cry of the Flesh* philosopher Havi Carel offers an account of her own experience of health and illness interwoven with discussion of Merleau-Ponty and other thinkers. As both protagonist of her own memoir and a scholar, Carel combines "the first- and third-person points of view, the subjective and the objective, the personal and the philosophical," thus enacting the interconnectedness of embodied and intellectual elements of her story.[22] She describes in vivid detail the shock of her diagnosis with an extremely rare and serious lung disease at the age of 35; the effects of the changes in her body on her daily life; the ways in which family members, friends, and colleagues responded to the news; and her experience of the medical care she received. Many of her portrayals of diagnosis and treatment evince a recognizable depiction of depersonalized clinical practice and objectification of the body, virtually indistinguishable from a scene in *W;t*:

> I quickly learned that when doctors ask 'How are you?' they mean 'How is your body?';
> that when an X-ray of my lungs is upon the screen and several doctors stand around
> it discussing my 'case', they will not include me in the discussion. That they will not
> want to know how my life has changed because of my illness, how they could make it
> easier for me.[23]

As Carel explains, such behavior reflects the biomedical model's naturalistic understanding of disease, reducing the body to a material object in good Cartesian form. By contrast, normativism—or social constructivism—points toward cultural understandings of health and illness as determinative of such definitions and categories. Yet both perspectives, Carel argues, minimize or elide the lived experience of a person with an illness or disability. This experience can be understood as a disruption of the seeming congruence between the biological body and the lived body, effecting a rift in the warp and woof of habitual experience. Here phenomenology affords a means of acknowledging the significance of this rent. S. Kay Toombs, a philosopher who has also written about her own experience of living with chronic illness and disability, describes the way in which phenomenology "allows us to recognize that *illness-as-lived* is a disruption of *lived body*. As such, it . . . strikes at the very heart of 'I am'"—for the self is constituted in and through my bodily being-in-the-world.[24] Moreover, a phenomenological perspective offers a means of mending this rupture. According to Carel, it does not bracket or abstract the experience

of illness but rather sees it "as a way of living, experiencing the world and interacting with other people. Instead of viewing illness as a local disruption of
a particular function, phenomenology turns to the lived experience of this
dysfunction. It attends to the global disruption of the habits, capacities and
actions of the ill person."[25] Such an approach also offers a structure for integrating illness into "the good life" by acknowledging and exploring the ways in
which one's world has evolved and by reuniting the ill body with lived experience. Indeed, while injury or illness may bring about swift change, the evolution of the relationship between an individual, the physical world, and society
is part of the natural aging process, and so foregrounding a phenomenological
understanding offers a productive toolkit for all, whether or not one is facing a
precipitously altered somatic experience.

Alongside such rich philosopher-patient perspectives, a number of
philosopher-clinicians have explored the intersection of phenomenology
and medical practice with particular emphasis on the clinical encounter.
For example, internist Richard Baron cites the frequent occurrence of a
patient beginning to speak as he is listening to his chest through a stetho-
scope: "Quiet," he instructs his patient—"I can't hear you while I'm listening."[26] As Baron explains, this exchange is illustrative of the divide between
doctors and patients in the face of objectified disease entities and the dominance of anatomicopathology and technology. Citing Husserl's conception
of *epoché*, or phenomenological reduction—a meditative suspension of pre-
conceptions and beliefs in order to "understand the world as it is given in
consciousness rather than as we think about it scientifically"—Baron imagines a clinician engaging in this practice and thus investigating the experience of illness in a radically different and productive fashion.[27] Such an
approach would, Baron maintains, open the physician's understanding of
the lifeworld-disrupting aspects of illness and forge a bridge to better understanding his patient's experiences.

As a physician writing extensively about bioethics and philosophy, Edmund
Pellegrino occupies a particularly significant role in the development of
twentieth-century philosophy and medicine and medical ethics in the United
States. Pellegrino describes himself as a "medical truant," though he maintains, invoking philosopher-psychiatrist Karl Jaspers, that "we must have two
commitments—to a scientific attitude and to philosophical reflection on the
meaning of that science."[28] He joins the critique of a too-narrow focus of biomedicine, explaining that "[t]echno-medical good does not exhaust the good
the physician is obliged to do. It is an essential but not a sufficient component
of good medicine."[29] In formulating an ethics of good medicine, Pellegrino
argues that it must be grounded in the very nature of clinical practice:

My approach has been to derive a philosophy of medicine from the phenomena of the clinical encounter, the confrontation of doctors and patients whose lived worlds intersect in the moment of clinical truth. This is the omega point upon which the actions of individual doctors as well as the whole health care system converge—that moment when some human being in distress seeks help from a physician within the context of a system of care.[30]

What is the nature of this meeting? In Pellegrino's description the physician is not omniscient, nor is a medical encounter an exchange of fungible commodities between two agents in equal possession of knowledge and authority.[31] The encounter is a highly individual one, a dialogical healing relationship, and is the foundation for Pellegrino's philosophy of medicine and medical ethics.

Moreover, Pellegrino invokes the *telos*—the end or purpose—of health, and its role in Hippocratic, Aristotelian, and Platonic thought. Lamenting the dissolution of such purpose-guided hierarchy from the Middle Ages to the present,[32] Pellegrino argues for a conception of the good of the patient of which the "medical good" is but one element, focusing rather on the patient's values, experiences, and agency.[33] Thus an awareness of the phenomenology of illness is an ethical imperative for the physician. Again citing Plato, Aristotle, and the Stoics, Pellegrino articulates a need for a conception of virtue ethics applicable to the healing professions, including a responsibility for "fidelity to trust and promise," benevolence, effacement of self-interest, compassion and caring, intellectual honesty, justice, and prudence.[34] There is reciprocity in the clinician-patient relationship, to be sure, and the negotiation of different values and ethics becomes a focus of Pellegrino's work in clinical ethics. Philosophically, however, Pellegrino argues for a restoration of a conception of the Good and its intrinsic role in healthcare, and a continued attentiveness to the many dimensions of illness and caregiving in lived experience.

Clinical ethicist Richard Zaner, too, points toward the clinical encounter as the ethical foundation of medicine, drawing our attention to the phenomenological complexity of the "lifeworld" in this "living context." As Zaner describes, "To focus on a clinical encounter, then, is to focus on a complex context characterized by presenting multiple points of view, hence, points for reflective entrance . . . and is thus to come into the responsibility for respecting that context: its constituents, their mutually constituted and multiple interrelationships, and the always changing, temporally and socially variable situation . . ."[35] In exploring this encounter, Zaner emphasizes its dialogical character and draws upon such phenomenological concepts as Hegel's *ecstasia* and Husserl's *epoché*, as well as Husserl's fundamental transcendental method of "free-fantasy variation" in understanding concepts and essences.[36] Zaner describes the mutual process of the clinical encounter as a particular example of the human encounter, in which neither patient nor clinician can be dispossessed nor emptied of himself: "Rather, I believe, it is *precisely* by being myself, including all I value, before and with the other (who must similarly be encouraged to be himself with all he values, before and with me), that dialogue is at all possible in the first place."[37] In this encounter, critically, both presences are corporeal—they are embodied selves.

Discussing Zaner's work in light of her own experience as an internist, Rita Charon emphasizes the incarnate aspects of the clinical encounter, describing "the ways in which the clinician/listener's body becomes the transducer of knowledge that bypasses words altogether and is registered on the sensate soma."[38] Recounting a visit from a patient with a serious decubitus ulcer on her back, Charon describes her own anxiety and irritation at her uncertainty concerning how to treat the wound properly. As she explains, it was only after she sought advice from a specialist and her worry abated that she could be fully present with her patient: "It was a very odd feeling—as if my clinical brain had been traveling outside of my body, seeking answers to these vexing questions, humiliated that I didn't know what to do, and therefore rendering me unavailable to my patient. But once I found the answers I needed, the brain came back home with a start, reconstituting my entire self within my body."[39] Charon describes her own position and posture in relation to her patient in vivid detail, as well as the way in which her receptiveness created a space for her patient to share her own life-world more fully, including her fears and anxieties. Thus we see how the ideas of phenomenologist philosophers find their way into a clinical ethicist's writings about medicine, and take on new form and life with a physician-scholar who is attentive to this tradition and to the delicate nuance of her own practice and is able to convey these revelations to others in rich, particular detail.

In discussing the role of the body, Zaner describes, too, the dislocation of illness. I and my body are one, in a sense—yet my body can also be, as in illness, beyond my control, offering an experience of alienation and uncanniness:

> If there is a sense in which my own body is intimately mine, there is, furthermore, an
> equally decisive sense in which I belong to it—in which I am at its disposal or mercy,
> if you will. My body, like the world in which I live, has its own nature, functions,
> structures, and biological conditions; since it embodies me, I thus experience myself
> as implicated by my body and these various conditions, functions, etc. I am exposed
> to whatever can influence, threaten, inhibit, alter, or benefit my biological organism.

Under certain conditions, it can fail me (more or less), not be capable of fulfilling my wants or desires, or even thoughts, forcing me to turn away from what I may want to do and attend to my own body: because of fatigue, hunger, thirst, disease, injury, pain, or even itches, I am forced at times to tend and attend to it, regardless, it may be, of what may well seem more urgent at the moment. Hence despite its evident 'intimacy', my own-body is as well the experiential ground for frustration, anguish, pain, fear, dread, as well as joy, satiation, pleasure, well-being ('health' as Kass says), and ultimately of death, my own ceasing-to-be.[40]

Acknowledging the uncanniness of the illness experience, then, becomes a critical element of clinical practice and of understanding experiences of illness—a theme to which we will return below in discussing the work of Fredrik Svenaeus. Alongside Baron, Pellegrino, and Zaner, there are many other important voices in phenomenology and medicine—including a critical branch of feminism and phenomenology—and it is not possible to do justice to these thinkers and to the breadth of this discussion in such truncated form; yet these brief snapshots offer a window into this rich realm of scholarship and practice.[41]

Another contemporary philosophical perspective on illness and identity closely aligned with phenomenology arises from narrative hermeneutics, which emphasizes the dynamic interpretive process of meaning-making and its narrative structure. As Brockmeier and Meretoja explain, "the project of narrative hermeneutics is to explore how and to what degree acts of meaning are realized by narrative practices and how individuals, through these practices, bind themselves into their cultural worlds while binding the cultural world into their minds."[42] Drawing upon thinkers such as Hans Gadamer, Paul Ricoeur, and Martin Heidegger, this understanding of narrative identity is one in which stories play an active interpretive role; they do not simply reflect experience, but they form it in a process of continual reciprocal exchange. We are always already inscribed within multiple stories, and our process of understanding the world through narrative also constructs our identities and the world. Recalling Havi Carel's account of her diagnosis, we see that illness can bring a radical change in the story that one tells of oneself—*I am an active person, I ride my bicycle to work, I expect to have children and live for many decades more*—and can effect a dramatic shift in the story that one receives from others about oneself, either tacitly or explicitly. In this sense illness experiences offer us particular insight into the ways in which we construct our identity and relationships within and through narrative, well beyond the context of health and medicine.

Narrative hermeneutics shares an interest in the particularity and materiality of our being-in-the-world with phenomenology, as we experience stories in singular, specific, and often profoundly corporeal ways. As Anna Donald describes, the process of creating narratives is one that is often unconscious and also deeply physical:

> [T]he symbolic/story-making process is not an abstract one that goes on somewhere in the intellect, or solely in the white and grey matter of the cortex. Rather ... in relay with the brain, narratives are processed and programmed into the rest of the body: the musculature and autonomic nervous system; that whole domain of feelings: of rage, of pain, of joy, the felt responses to information that we carelessly call emotions.[43]

Donald investigates the ways in which differences within healthcare—such as the often discordant perspectives of clinicians and patients, or practitioners of different types and traditions of medicine—may be understood not simply or solely as an argument about who has the correct naturalistic interpretation but also as a skirmish over which is the dominant narrative.[44] Recall Audre Lorde's description of her diagnosis and the competing narratives of a paternalistic medical authority, of racism and sexism, of Lorde's knowledge of her own body and mind and experience. Similarly, in Havi Carel's experience, the alienation from clinicians she describes is also a form of narrative injury, as physicians largely ignored her experience in its singular embodied complexity. In this sense narrative hermeneutics (and narrative ethics—see Chapter 5) offers additional tools to understand rupture and difference between different stories and to hone our awareness of the operation of power and authority in narrative framing. For example, Hilde Lindemann Nelson points toward the role of narratives in constructing identity, and their capacity to limit or expand one's moral agency; in the face of a "master narrative" perpetuating an oppressive identity for a particular group, she describes the operation of *counterstory* effecting a "narrative repair," thus altering others' perception of an oppressed group as well as the self-perceptions of those within the group.[45] Finally, as a perspective that privileges interpretation in an ongoing, dynamic process, narrative hermeneutics resists objectifying closure, encouraging us to remain attentive to the significance of the stories we live and tell one another.

Drawing upon both phenomenology and hermeneutics, contemporary philosopher Fredrik Svenaeus offers a particular understanding of medical practice. Acknowledging Descartes' pervasive influence in healthcare, Svenaeus argues that "phenomenology and hermeneutics provide better tools than dualism for thinking about the ill as something more than molecules, tissues and organs."[46] In the face of a narrow biostatistical orientation in contemporary medicine and the objectification of the patient under a reductive pathological lens, he seeks a means of explicating "what is medicine" and "what is medical knowledge"—an articulation of healthcare as it is *experienced* by clinicians and patients.[47] Integral to the ontology of medicine, as Svenaeus describes, is the *meeting* and *practice* occurring between doctor and patient, an emphasis shared by medical phenomenologists such as Pellegrino and Zaner, as we have seen. This meeting is not understood as an isolated dyad; "doctor" is shorthand for any number of professional roles within the clinical context, and Svenaeus describes the patient's experience as embedded within a complex social and relational web. In offering a history of medicine, however, Svenaeus describes features common to different eras, theories, and modes of practice:

> [M]edicine is an interpretive meeting, which takes place between two persons (the doctor or some other clinical professional and the patient) with the aim of understanding and healing the one who is ill and seeks help. Clinical medicine . . . is thus first and foremost a practice and not a science. Medical science must be viewed as an integrated part within the clinical interpretive meeting and not as its true substance; that is, not as the core mode of clinical practice, which is here merely 'applied' in contrast to the pure science of the laboratory.[48]

The scientific knowledge so privileged by physicians in Edson's *W;t*, then, is understood as a critically valuable tool of medicine but not its primary end. Such an ethic surely would have been beneficial to *W;t*'s protagonist; as Vivian is dying, clinical fellow Jason and nurse Susie physically tussle over whether or not to resuscitate—Susie grabs Jason and cries, "She's DNR!"—to which Jason shouts, "She's Research!"[49] As Svenaeus insists, however, the clinician's drive toward truth and knowledge may *not* subsume the care of the patient: "This attunement of curiosity and wonder must . . . clearly be wedded to the attunement of helping if it shall not lead to perverted behaviour in the clinic. The patient is always first and foremost a person to help and not a research object."[50]

Here Svaneaeus draws upon the phenomenological tradition, particularly Heidegger (in an admittedly unorthodox reading) and others, including Gadamer, Straus, and Merleau-Ponty, to offer a conception of health and illness.[51] The "attunement" of curiosity and of helping invoked above is understood in the Heideggerian sense as "a being delivered to the world, a finding oneself in the meaning-structure of the world as an understanding existence."[52] As a being-in-the-world I move outside of myself and *into* the world and its structures of meaning and intersubjectivity in a process of attunement as well as transcendence. Svenaeus invokes the concept of *homelikeness* (*heimlichkeit*), a being-at-home in the world, as well as *unhomelikeness*, both of which I experience: "[T]he world I live in is certainly first and foremost my world (and not the 'objective' world of atoms and molecules), but to this very 'mine-ness' also belongs otherness in the sense of the meaning of the world belonging to other people. The otherness of the world, however, is not only due to my sharing it with other people, but also to nature (as opposed to culture) as something resisting my understanding."[53] Thus the familiarity and "alien nature" of the world both permeate our existence. Building upon the work of Richard Zaner, Svaneaeus explains that in a state of health being-at-home eclipses not-being-at-home, whereas illness allows "homelessness" to come to the fore, affecting our attunement and transcendence into the world. Svenaeus is not referring to a transitory discomfort but illness that has a lasting character and ruptures one's meaning-structure, as embodied experience is central to selfhood.[54] As Svenaeus describes, "The unhomelikeness of illness is consequently a certain form of senselessness, an attunement of, for instance, disorientedness, helplessness, resistance, and despair."[55]

Svenaeus offers the example of a patient, Peter, who visits Dr. X with a persistent sore throat and fatigue; the doctor prescribes antibiotics and rest, but the illness remains. Peter returns, and after an extensive workup, including visits to specialists, he is diagnosed with chronic fatigue syndrome, a poorly understood (and somewhat contested) disease at the present time. The illness affects Peter's ability to work, his relationship with his family members, and his emotional state. Such is the experience of homelessness, a profound and unwelcome breach in Peter's "lifeworld." Dr. X and Peter continue to discuss therapeutic options, his job, his situation with his family, and various approaches to his new embodied experience. As Svenaeus describes, biomedicine is but one aspect of these meetings; even if Dr. X cannot offer a satisfactory scientific understanding of this particular condition, she can recognize the ways in which Peter's being-in-the-world has been altered and can relate it both to biomedicine—such as potential treatments and therapies—and Peter's lifeworld, including his work, social network, and attitudes toward his own life.[56]

Clinical practice, then, seeks the goal of health as a restoration of "homelike being-in-the world," and the clinical encounter as described above is integral to this process.[57] This meeting is understood in a hermeneutic context as, drawing upon Gadamer, Svenaeus emphasizes its dialogic and interpretive nature. The medical meeting is "the gradual fusion of two horizons— the patient's perspective of unhomelikeness, and the doctor's perspective of medical expertise and mission to help. The meeting of the two horizons as the inter-nesting of interpretations means that both parties must come to see things from the other party's point of view in order to reach a new, more

productive understanding."[58] Doctor and patient have different horizons—
notably, the patient is experiencing the unhomelikeness, and the doctor typically possesses greater medical knowledge and is charged with helping the
patient—and the meeting between the two is characterized by a reciprocal
acknowledgement of the other's role and the particularity of each one's experience: "if the goal of the meeting is to be attained it is not only necessary
that the doctor is able to put himself in the patient's situation; the patient too
must come to see things from the medical viewpoint of the doctor."[59] Thus
drawing upon the phenomenological and hermeneutic traditions, Svenaeus'
understanding of the clinical encounter is both descriptive—this *is* the operation and significance of these meetings, though it may not be widely recognized—and normative: this is how it *should* be.[60] Svenaeus' description of
the clinical encounter may appear so remote from Audre Lorde's tale of her
visit with her oncologist ("I felt the battle lines being drawn up within my
own body") as to seem fantastical—and in that context it may serve as an
instructive ideal alongside her powerful account.

Such understanding of our experience as embodied, interpretive, and relational, as we have seen in our all-too-brief survey of certain strands of contemporary philosophy and medicine, is certainly a contrast from the type of essentialism or dualism that we find in the Western philosophical tradition. And it is,
one hopes, a particularly salutary perspective for persons experiencing illness,
injury, and disability. As Havi Carel explains, philosophy can offer pragmatic
and therapeutic benefit; she cites ancient Greek philosopher Epicurus: "Empty
is the argument of the philosopher by which no human suffering is healed;
for just as there is no benefit in medicine that does not drive out bodily diseases, so there is no benefit in philosophy if it does not drive out the suffering
of the soul."[61] Of course, just as medicine is not limited to "driving out bodily
diseases," philosophy need not be confined to practical advice for living—yet
both may inform and enrich one another. As the accounts of Toombs, Carel,
Kleinman, and many others illustrate so richly, philosophy offers us the tools
to guide our own experiences of illness and care. And by deepening our understanding of the legacy of philosophical discourse and its effects, we are better
suited to address the challenges we face in healthcare today.

Philosophical Narratives: Complexity and Multiplicity

In these chapters we have offered portraits of particular philosophers in the
Western tradition and a narrative spanning these ideas and their influence
on contemporary medical practice. One of the great gifts and challenges of
philosophical enquiry, however, is that it never ceases; we find in this dialogue

different narratives altogether, and a complexity that only serves to enrich our understanding.

For example, our reading of Plato emphasizes the hierarchy between soul and body, with the physical realm serving as mere distraction. The *Phaedo* offers another articulation of this order, describing a Pythagorean conception of the soul's immortality and reincarnation and its elevation in contrast to the contingency and deceit of phenomenal experience: "And indeed the soul reasons best when none of these senses troubles it, neither hearing nor sight, nor pain nor pleasure, but when it is most by itself, taking leave of the body and as far as possible having no contact or association with it in its search for reality."[62] Such an understanding of the material and intelligible realms is integral to Platonism and proves to be a foundational schema in Western thought.

However, to what degree did this model influence medical practice of the era? Second-century A.D. physician-philosopher Galen—arguably the most influential figure in the development of early Western medicine through the Middle Ages until the Enlightenment and beyond, particularly in his contributions to anatomy and physiology—articulated a vision of the soul and the body that is to some degree Platonic, yet to some degree not. He follows Plato's tripartite division of the soul with the logical/rational, spirited, and appetitive portions corresponding to the brain, the heart, and the liver—yet also reflects Aristotelian and Stoic thinking in his formulation. As R. J. Hankinson describes, "Galen, in common with Greek thought on the subject, considered there to be no radical distinction of type between the physical and the mental (or more properly, the psychic.)"[63] Furthermore, Galen does *not* impute immortality to the soul, and draws a distinction between the speculative domain of philosophy and the empirical realm of medicine.[64]

Furthermore, the role of health and medicine *within* Platonic thought is quite complex. As Pellegrino and Thomasma describe, philosophy and medicine are often aligned—such as in the *Protagoras* and the *Gorgias*—with medicine adjuring proper care of the body and philosophy the correct cultivation of the soul. Yet the prescription for philosophers' ascension from the material to the intelligible realm is *not* coextensive with the role of the physician, as we see in the *Symposium*. Here the figure of the doctor Eryximachus functions as an example of overweening technism. In Pellegrino and Thomasma's portrayal, he is "promulgating the cultivation of the body as the true end of human life: 'And this is what the physician has to do, and in this the art of medicine consists: for medicine may be regarded as the knowledge of the loves and desires of the body, and how to satisfy them or not . . .' While the physician exalts the body, the philosopher tends to dream of a form of perception which would transcend the body."[65] According to Pellegrino and Thomasma, such "ambiguities and tensions" between medicine and philosophy characterize Plato's works.

One may also find in Plato's corpus a conception of medicine that can be said to presage the humanism we seek in contemporary practice. The goal of medicine is health, as we see in *Lysis* and elsewhere; as Socrates argues in Book I of *The Republic*, the true physician "in the precise sense" is one who treats the sick (rather than being a money-maker), and medicine seeks the ends of its craft—which is the advantage of the body—rather than its own enrichment.[66] And, as we have seen, Pellegrino argues that the teleological ethic of Platonism provides defining *ends* for the practice of medicine—its practice in service of the *Good*—an ethical substrate that Pellegrino seeks to recuperate for contemporary medical practice. Moreover, the relationship between body and soul in Plato's discussion of health is often predicated on the principle of balance—a Hippocratic and Galenic balance within the body as well as a balance between the soul and the body, as in the *Timaeus*:

> Hence we must take it that if a living thing is to be in good condition, it will be well-proportioned. [. . .] In determining health and disease or virtue and vice no proportion or lack of it is more important than that between soul and body—yet we do not think about any of them nor do we realize that when a vigorous and excellent soul is carried about by a too frail and puny frame, or when the two are combined in the opposite way, the living thing as a whole lacks beauty, because it is lacking in the most important proportions.[67]

Thus while the soul is associated with the higher realms of intelligibility in contrast to the material world, it must, critically, remain in balance with the body. Indeed, as William Stempsey describes, Plato's discussion of health and medicine is—in comparison to a narrow medico-scientific conception—in many ways holistic, advocating equilibrium and serving a conception of the good life. As Stempsey explains, in Platonic thought "health cannot be understood reductionistically in purely scientific terms. We need to understand the Form of health in order to understand our experience of being healthy or not."[68] In the *Charmides*, for example, Socrates describes a headache charm that is in fact a treatment of body and soul, quoting a Thracian physician: " 'Let no one persuade you to cure his head, until he has first given you his soul to be cured by the charm. For this,' he said, 'is the great error of our day in the treatment of human beings, that men try to be physicians of health and temperance separately'."[69] Such holism may be said to model the reforms we seek in contemporary healthcare: rather than bracketing a biomedical fix, we must honor and attend to the soul alongside the body.

These perspectives emphasize the importance and complexity of the philosophical questions posed in Platonism, such as the relationship between the soul and the body as it pertains to medicine and health—questions that continue to fascinate and torment us to this day. Similarly, close study of dualism in Cartesian thought reveals great nuance and controversy within philosophy and philosophy of medicine. Richard Zaner, for example, points to Descartes' writings about medicine, particularly his 1645 letter to Princess Elizabeth, as evidence of his conception of the "continuous daily interaction and union of the mind and body":[70] in suggesting that Princess Elizabeth's fevers were due to "the bad temperament of the blood which is caused by sadness," Descartes prescribes taking the waters at the spa, as well as ridding the mind of sad thoughts.[71] Descartes' writings on medicine, Zaner argues, offer a different perspective from the articulation of the *cogito* in the *Meditations*. Zaner cites portions of the *Discourse on Method and Meditations* that speak of the body and soul as functionally united—as Descartes writes:

> nature also teaches me by these sensations of pain, hunger, thirst, etc., that I am not only lodged in my body as a pilot within a vessel, but that I am very closely united to it, and so to speak so intermingled with it that I seem to compose with it one whole.[72]

According to Zaner, then, the conception of Cartesian dualism as it is commonly employed is "almost pure fable, a concoction of subsequent history."[73] Whether or not one agrees with this contention, the *role* of this model of mind–body dualism within history is, as we have seen, extremely potent. It is not our purpose here to adjudicate the matter of dualism in Descartes' corpus (puns intended), but simply to gesture (perhaps maddeningly) toward the many different interpretations and narratives spun between philosophy and medicine and to argue for continued rigorous study of this vital history and these essential quandaries.

Such questions may indeed be universal, may continue to challenge us even as medical science advances beyond our wildest imagination. In Ian McEwan's novel *Saturday*, neurosurgeon Henry Perowne contemplates the inside of his patient's brain, a familiar sight—"a kind of homeland, with its low hills and enfolded valleys of the sulci, each with a name and imputed function, as known to him as his own house."[74] Yet this experience of homelikeness is permeated by the unknown as Perowne ponders the mysteries of mind, body, and spirit:

Just like the digital codes of replicating life held within DNA, the brain's fundamental secret will be laid open one day. But even when it has, the wonder will remain, that mere wet stuff can make this bright inward cinema of thought, of sight and sound and touch bound into a vivid illusion of an instantaneous present, with a self, another brightly wrought illusion, hovering like a ghost at its centre. Could it ever be explained, how matter became conscious?[75]

Soul

Thus we find ourselves returning to the literary arts, now with visions of Cartesian dualism and phenomenology dancing in our heads. Read this poem, aloud if possible. Read it again. If you are near someone, read it aloud to them; have them read it aloud to you.

Soul

What am I doing inside this old man's body?
I feel like I'm the insides of a lobster,
All thought, and all digestion, and pornographic
Inquiry, and getting about, and bewilderment,
And fear, avoidance of trouble, belief in what,
God knows, vague memories of friends, and what
They said last night, and seeing, outside of myself,
From here inside myself, my waving claws
Inconsequential, wavering, and my feelers
Preternatural, trembling, with their amazing
Troubling sensitivity to threat;
And I'm aware of and embarrassed by my ways
Of getting around, and my protective shell.
Where is it that she I loved has gone to, as
This cold sea water's washing over my back?

—David Ferry[76]

"What am I doing inside this old man's body?"

Who is the "I" who speaks here? Perhaps the soul? But what, then, is the relationship between the speaker—or the soul—and his corporeal existence? "I feel like I'm the insides of a lobster," he writes. Not that he *is* a lobster, but that he is the *insides* of a lobster. We picture the flaky white flesh ("packed in like feathers," as Elizabeth Bishop imagines the flesh of the fish), the boiled green innards staining our fingers. The gullet, the guts. In these insides we are trapped, confused, vulnerable, following we know not what for sure, feelings of doubt, of interiority. And then we move, progressively, to observations of the outside world, including ourselves—"seeing, outside of myself, / From here inside of myself . . ."—and then finally to another, to a lost love. We begin with one question, "What am I doing inside this old man's body?" which leads us, inexorably, inevitably to another: "Where is it that she I loved has gone to, as / This cold sea water's washing over my back?" For we are, finally, embodied selves and relational selves. Our insides and our outsides are connected. We cannot tell our stories without telling the tale of our bodies and those who have touched us.

What and who we are in relation to others, to our bodies and our mortality, defines our existence. In Ferry's haunting, luminous voice we may hear the plaintive cry of an older man who is incredulous at the body he inhabits, foreign and unwelcome to him—an unhomelike experience in Svenaeus' conception, a palpable alienation within this carapace. Yet the poem is not simply about aging. When we change—as a result of a stroke, of dementia, of infirmity, or as a result of adolescence, of friends and lovers gained and lost, of the sea currents and crashing waves of life's fortunes—are we the same person? Is the "I" who speaks essential, unchanging? Or is the soul nested in the body, the body nested in the soul, and all of us nested in the fates and fortunes of those surrounding us—those present in body and those now only present in spirit?

The shell is both a home and a figure of unhomelikeness, and as we navigate our way along the cold ocean floor we ponder and *experience* afresh the questions that thinkers have considered for millennia. It is critically important to study and question the philosophical tradition as well as to explore the ways in which the arts express these questions, these barbaric yawps and cries and exultations. This intersection of philosophy and literature and experience— arriving at ideas through different *forms* of knowledge—exerts a powerful influence on our understanding of illness and healthcare and is integral to the principles and practice of narrative medicine.

Notes

1. MacIntyre, *After Virtue*, 216.
2. Merleau-Ponty, *Phenomenology of Perception*, lxx.
3. Merleau-Ponty, *Phenomenology of Perception*, lxxii.
4. Merleau-Ponty, *Phenomenology of Perception*, lxxii.
5. Merleau-Ponty, *Phenomenology of Perception*, 186.
6. Merleau-Ponty, *Phenomenology of Perception*, 200.
7. Merleau-Ponty, *Phenomenology of Perception*, 193.
8. Merleau-Ponty, *Phenomenology of Perception*, 203.
9. Merleau-Ponty, *Phenomenology of Perception*, 182–83.
10. Merleau-Ponty, *Phenomenology of Perception*, 188.

11. Merleau-Ponty, *Phenomenology of Perception*, 189–90.

12. Merleau-Ponty, *Phenomenology of Perception*, 530.

13. Merleau-Ponty, *Phenomenology of Perception*, 200.

14. Merleau-Ponty, *Phenomenology of Perception*, 189.

15. Merleau-Ponty, *Phenomenology of Perception*, 189.

16. See also Paul Ricoeur's description of narrative's "living" nature, dependent upon both sedimentation and innovation. As he explains, "The variations between these poles gives the productive imagination its own historicity and keeps the narrative tradition a living one" (Ricoeur, "Life in Quest," 25).

17. Merleau-Ponty, *Phenomenology of Perception*, 188.

18. Merleau-Ponty, *Phenomenology of Perception*, 183–84.

19. Merleau-Ponty, *Phenomenology of Perception*, 184.

20. Merleau-Ponty, *Phenomenology of Perception*, 189.

21. Merleau-Ponty, *Phenomenology of Perception*, 185, 188.

22. Carel, *Illness*, 13.

23. Carel, *Illness*, 39.

24. Toombs, "Illness and the Paradigm," 207.

25. Carel, *Illness*, 8–9.

26. Baron, "Introduction to Medical Phenomenology," 606.

27. Baron, "Introduction to Medical Phenomenology," 608.

28. Pellegrino, *Philosophy of Medicine Reborn*, xv. See Jaspers's *Philosophy and the World*, 234.

29. Pellegrino, *Philosophy of Medicine Reborn*, 168.

30. Pellegrino, *Philosophy of Medicine Reborn*, 63.

31. Pellegrino, "Toward a Reconstruction," 66–67.

32. "From the late thirteenth and fourteenth centuries to our times, the foundations for a teleological ethic have been seriously eroded. The Nominalists began the process by rejecting the ideas of universals or of essence in the nature of things, thus disarticulating the connections between the ends and the good. This process accelerated in the eighteenth century and has continued to the present" (Pellegrino, *Philosophy of Medicine Reborn*, 71).

33. Pellegrino, *Philosophy of Medicine Reborn*, 72–73.

34. Pellegrino, "Towards a Virtue-Based," 269–270.

35. Zaner, "Phenomenon of Vulnerability," 287.

36. Zaner discusses Husserl's "free-fantasy variation": released from established empirical facts one considers any possible examples, including what might be considered fictions. Indeed, "it is most important for the working philosopher to 'fertilize his phantasies' to the utmost" ("Examples and Possibles," 25)—and here creative works can aid in this nourishment. Any given case in clinical ethics, Zaner explains, must be understood in its own singular terms; yet, considering different cases for philosophical analysis is a form of such free-fantasy variation ("Phenomenon of Vulnerability," 290–91).

37. Zaner, "Medicine and Dialogue," 321.

38. Charon, "Ecstatic Witness," 179.

39. Charon, "Ecstatic Witness," 180.

40. Zaner, *Context of Self*, 52. Cited in Svenaeus, *Hermeneutics of Medicine*, 111.

41. For further reference see Toombs, *Handbook of Phenomenology*.

42. Brockmeier and Meretoja, "Understanding Narrative Hermeneutics," 7.

43. Donald, "The Words We Live in," 19.

44. Donald, "The Words We Live in," 18.

45. Lindemann Nelson, *Damaged Identities*.

46. Svenaeus, *Hermeneutics of Medicine*, 19n.

47. Svenaeus, *Hermeneutics of Medicine*, 5–6.

48. Svenaeus, *Hermeneutics of Medicine*, 11.

49. Edson, *W;t*, 82.

50. Svenaeus, *Hermeneutics of Medicine*, 174.
51. Svenaeus, *Hermeneutics of Medicine*, 92.
52. Svenaeus, *Hermeneutics of Medicine*, 94.
53. Svenaeus, *Hermeneutics of Medicine*, 93.
54. Svenaeus, *Hermeneutics of Medicine*, 117.
55. Svenaeus, *Hermeneutics of Medicine*, 115.
56. Svenaeus, *Hermeneutics of Medicine*, 130.
57. Svenaeus, *Hermeneutics of Medicine*, 100.
58. Svenaeus, *Hermeneutics of Medicine*, 179.
59. Svenaeus, *Hermeneutics of Medicine*, 157.
60. Svenaeus, *Hermeneutics of Medicine*, 166.
61. Inwood and Gerson, *Epicurus Reader*, 99. Cited in Carel, *Illness*, 127.
62. Plato, *Phaedo*, 65c.
63. Hankinson, "Galen's Anatomy," 199. Also see Richard Zaner: "Galen had serious difficulty accommodating his medical ideas to Plato's notion of psyche (soul), and eventually considered it merely a temperament of the body: 'I have not come upon anybody who geometrically demonstrated whether it is altogether incorporeal, or whether any [species] is corporeal, or whether it is completely everlasting, or perishable'. He had 'nowhere dared to state the essence of the soul'" ("Medicine and Dialogue," 322n1).
64. Hankinson, "Galen's Anatomy," 201. Indeed, Galen's influence can be said to have strengthened the dogmatic tradition in ancient Greece, whose opposition with the methodists (also skeptics or empirics) in some sense presaged our current debate over the proper scope and nature of medical practice. Citing Ludwig Edelstein, Richard Zaner points out that "The complex form of reasoning about the patient's experience, history, values, etc., was the main concern of the ancient methodists' method (semeosis) and its form of reasoning (epilogismos): the deliberative weighing of all those factors and facets of a patient's actual life, in order to understand the person and the illness fully, and thus to reach appropriate therapies" ("Medicine and Dialogue," 308). The skeptics' emphasis on interpretation of specific symptoms, the singularity of a given person, and the importance of his holistic context can be said to anticipate Kleinman's understanding of *illness* in contrast to a biomedical focus on *disease*.
65. Pellegrino and Thomasma, *Philosophical Basis of Medical Practice*, 11.
66. Plato, *Republic* 341c–342c.
67. The quote continues: "... That's how we ought to think of that combination of soul and body which we call the living thing. When within it there is a soul more powerful than the body and this soul gets excited, it churns the whole being and fills it from inside with diseases, and when it concentrates on one or another course of study and inquiry, it wears the body out. And again, when the soul engages in public or private teaching sessions or verbal battles, the disputes and contentions that then occur cause the soul to fire the body up and rock it back and forth, so inducing discharges which trick most so-called doctors into making misguided diagnoses. But when, on the other hand, a large body, too much for its soul, is joined with a puny and feeble mind, then, given that human beings have two sets of natural desires—desires of the body for food and desires of the most divine part of us for wisdom—the motions of the stronger part will predominate, and amplify their own interest. They render the functions of the soul dull, stupid, and forgetful, thereby bringing on the gravest disease of all: ignorance" (Plato, "Timaeus" 87c–88b).
68. Stempsey, "Plato and Holistic Medicine," 203.
69. Plato, *Charmides* 157b. Cited in Stempsey, "Plato and Holistic Medicine," 206.
70. Zaner, *Ethics and the Clinical Encounter*, 111.
71. Riese, "Descartes as a Psychotherapist," 243.

72. Descartes, *Philosophical Works*, vol. 1, 192. Cited in Zaner, *Ethics and the Clinical Encounter*, 114.
73. Zaner, *Ethics and the Clinical Encounter*, 119.
74. McEwan, *Saturday*, 262.
75. McEwan, *Saturday*, 262.
76. Ferry, *Bewilderment*, 7.

CHAPTER 5

Deliver Us from Certainty: Training for Narrative Ethics

Craig Irvine and Rita Charon

Neither our understanding of who we are nor our very existence in a
cultural world can be separated from the stories that we and others tell
about ourselves.

—Jens Brockmeier, *Beyond the Archive*[1]

Stories are the primordial means through which we make sense of and convey
the meaning of our lives. It is to this that the philosopher Paul Ricoeur points
when he speaks of "life *as an activity and a passion in search of a narrative.*"[2]
Indeed, for Ricoeur, a life is "the field of a constructive activity, by which we
attempt to discover . . . the narrative identity which constitutes us."[3] Medical
sociologist Arthur Frank continues Ricoeur's thought by proposing that
"[o]ur very selves are perpetually recreated in stories. Stories do not simply
describe the self; they are the self's medium of being."[4] Narrative accounts of
oneself—autobiography, memoir, psychoanalytic transactions, clinical accounts, dreams, that which one tells oneself in secret, or casual tales one tells
to friends—not only report one's narrative identity but, more radically, create
that which is experienced as the "self."

Narrative medicine arises from the awareness of this relation between narrativity and identity. Our principles and practices of intersubjectivity and relationality, our election of close reading as a signature method, our elevation
of creativity in the work of healthcare, our collaborative teaching methods,
and our narrative clinical practices all bear the mark of this centering commitment to comprehend and live in the light of this narrativity/identity reciprocity. Since illness and injury are among the most exposing experiences of the
mortal life, the experiences that lift the veil on the large objects in the room of
one's life, narrative medicine is present when a person urgently comes to face

or question or embrace his or her identity. Who *am* I now suffering, now recovering, now dying? What matters to me now? In the face of this illness or injury, what is the best way forward in my life?

In this chapter we try to articulate the practical consequences of narrative medicine's growing understandings of the possibilities for a narrative identity. Within healthcare, questions of narrative and identity frequently arise in the setting of bioethics, and so we probe here the role of narrative medicine in the practice of bioethics. This probe brings us to concentrate on narrative ethics, that subdiscipline of clinical bioethics that starts with the narrative accounts patients give of their lives and helps patients to envision and then choose among the alternative futures ahead. Sometimes practiced in the face of thorny ethical dilemmas at the end of life and sometimes practiced in the relative calm of everyday healthcare, narrative ethics extends skilled close listening to patients, families, and clinicians so as to midwife a narrative view of a person's situation. Unlike other bioethical approaches that attempt to apply universal laws and principles to solve individual ethical problems, narrative ethics arises from the patient's singular situation to bring unique algebras to the tangle of values, meanings, choices, desires, and loves in this particular life or this particular death. We also acknowledge the contributions of the *literary* field called narrative ethics. Parallel but distinct from bioethics' narrative ethics, it illuminates the fundamental duties of the listener or reader of another's narrative. These duties are incurred both in listening to oral narratives and reading literary written texts. Finally, we propose that narrative ethics *is* narrative medicine as it unfolds in the setting of bioethics, bringing methods of teaching and practice to those who try to help others in their living and their dying.

What Stories Do for Us: Narrative Understanding as Ethics

The primacy of narrative acts in perceiving, experiencing, representing, and interpreting the world is acknowledged across diverse disciplines.[5] Historians,[6] psychologists,[7] social scientists,[8] educators,[9] theologians,[10] philosophers,[11] psychiatrists,[12] and literary critics, as detailed in this chapter, have all come to recognize the central role that narrative plays in our lives.[13] While the interest in narrative theory and practice may be a relatively recent phenomenon in many disciplines, the salience of narratives—and of the narrative capacities that are developed in and called forth by engaging with them, at least for literary texts—have enduringly been recognized as foundational in human learning and thought. Ricoeur argues that ethics first turned to narrative more than

24 centuries ago, when Aristotle wrote his *Poetics*: "Aristotle did not hesitate to say that every well-told story *teaches* something . . . [I]t is certain that tragedy, epic and comedy, to cite only those genres known to Aristotle, develop a sort of understanding that can be termed narrative understanding and which is much closer to the practical wisdom of moral judgment than to science, or, more generally, to the theoretical use of reason."[14] While theoretical understanding can only speak abstractly of the relation between ethical principles and human action, narrative understanding as a form of practical or phronetic understanding offers imaginative thought experiments through which we learn, in Ricoeur's words, "to link together the ethical aspects of human conduct and happiness and misfortune" (p. 23). From this Aristotelian opening, Ricoeur develops his thesis that emplotment, or "the process of composition, of configuration" central to narrative, "is not completed in the text but in the reader and, under this condition, makes possible the reconfiguration of life by narrative. I should say, more precisely: the sense or the significance of a narrative stems from the *intersection of the world of the text and the world of the reader*" (p. 26). The literary text opens before it a world of possible experience, in which it is possible to live. Not something closed in on itself, the text is a projection of a new universe distinct from that in which we live. When we read, therefore, we belong, at the same time, to the world-horizon of the work in imagination and the world-horizon in which the action of our "real life" unfolds, multiplying exponentially that which can properly be called one's lived experience. We will see that listening to the oral narratives heard in clinical bioethics has similar consequences for the listener of widening horizons and enlarging one's actual experience.

The philosopher Hans Gadamer speaks of the "fusion of horizons" essential to the art of understanding a text.[15] Through the actions of this fusion we expand our own vision of reality, our own state of being, indelibly changing us toward the next encounter with a text. Each new narrative work opens new horizons in which we might experience, explore, and try on alternative realities, new ways of being-in-the-world. Visual art, music, drama, and dance each expand horizons in their particular sensory and imaginative ways.[16]

We always already live in imaginative worlds. The very worlds of sense and experience are configured uniquely by each perceiver, for consciousness itself is shaped by narratives we have heard. Thought, fantasy, belief, emotion, attachment, and ultimately action are *in their making* shaped by the stories that have framed each person's individual consciousness. Hence, what we call experience is not a pure blank reality. It rests in some way on prior perceptions, on antecedents and imagined subsequents. This is not to suggest that there is no innovation, for the imagination *creates* the new and the never-seen, yet always from a perceptual foundation inflected by one's individual private experience.[17]

If each person perceives and experiences reality, at least in part, through individual narrative means, reality cannot be treated as replicable or universal fact. Serious engagement with narrative texts—reading them closely, writing them, grappling with what they mean—challenges the belief that we can define and dominate reality through technical mastery. The indeterminacy of stories baffles the mind that seeks concrete, unambiguous conclusions. As one enters the narrative world of a text, one lets go of the conviction that a key to its meaning is to be found anywhere but in the experience itself of encountering it.[18] Cleanth Brooks, one of the American leaders of the New Critical literary movement of the 1940s and 1950s, asserted that the poem is something that cannot be paraphrased:

> Is it not possible to frame a proposition, a statement, which will adequately represent the total meaning of the poem; that is, is it not possible to elaborate a summarizing proposition which will "say" briefly and in the form of a proposition, what the poem "says" as a poem. . . . Could not the poet, if he had chosen, have framed such a proposition? Cannot we as readers and critics frame such a proposition?
>
> The answer must be that the poet himself obviously did not—else he would not have had to write his poem.[19]

In like manner, a story is something whose content cannot be reduced to analyzable data. Meanings, ethical and otherwise, are not extractable from a story as if they exist separate from its form. Instead, a story relinquishes its meaning only to the reader or listener who undergoes all the story's elements—its plot, its genre, its diction, its metaphors, its allusions, its temporal and spatial natures. The reader or listener who enters that story experiences the integrated flow of all these features, none of which is elective to the full measure of the story. The full story is required for the reader to understand its ethical or personal or affective meaning. The reverse is true as well, suggests literary scholar Marshall Gregory in *Shaped by Stories*: "*Not to understand the ethical vision of a story is also not to understand its aesthetic shape.*" (italics in original).[20]

The reader who enters the world of a text recognizes its rules of conduct and is influenced by its moral compass and its shaping power. Narrative ethics as we understand it in narrative medicine reminds writers and readers that narratives of any kind by necessity privilege certain perspectives and positions, that marginalized voices are often silenced, and that commitments to equality require "equal access" to the author/teller position. We can learn to respond to stories that exclude the marginalized with a demand for additional stories—not just any additional stories, but ones in which the point of view shifts to favor how the world looks to the characters previously silenced.

Narrative and Bioethics

How have these concepts about narrativity and identity come to influence the work of bioethics? Novelist Richard Powers, who has placed several of his novels in medical settings, proposes a profound use for serious reading:

> Story is the mind's way of molding a seeming whole from out of the messiness of the distributed, modular brain. At the same time, shared stories are the only way anyone has for escaping the straightjacket of self. Good medicine has always depended on listening to histories. So any attempt to comprehend the injured mind naturally inclines toward all the devices of classic storytelling. . . . Only inhabiting another's story can deliver us from certainty.[21]

Escaping the straightjacket of self: this could be the clarion call of ethical practice. As Powers makes clear, this straightjacket that imprisons us in our selves is fashioned by our own *certainty*. By allowing oneself to enter into an alien narrative world—as glimpsed through a conversation with a friend, an interview with a patient, or a novel by Richard Powers—one can shift the strictures of assumption, prejudice, genealogy, and habit to expand the mind by contact with the world of another. Many of the consequential acts of ordinary life require the capacity to perform acts of envisioning otherness—a capacity, we assert, that is developed in becoming a close reader. Whether the other is an intimate or a stranger, the inhabiting of the other's narrative world requires feats of imagination, self-stilling, empathy, and challenging of assumptions.

Philosopher and novelist Iris Murdoch is among those who have helped us understand the importance to moral life of imagining the other's story. In her novel *The Black Prince*, Murdoch's protagonist Bradley Pearson says, "When we do ill we anaesthetize our imagination. Doubtless this is, for most people, a prerequisite of doing ill, and indeed a part of it."[22] As Martha Nussbaum has written, "Murdoch felt that we would only get to the right choices if we understood better the inner forces militating against goodness. And in her view, the main such force was our inability to see other people correctly."[23]

Consider Powers' escape from certainty in the context of healthcare. Typically, the professional is assumed to know more—and to know with certainty—about the illness situation of the patient than does the patient. The patient's lived experience of having the disease does not automatically count for much in healthcare's proceedings. The power is all on one side. When disagreements between them arise, the power asymmetry privileges the stance of the professional. If a patient consents to medical treatment, the treatment proceeds. If a patient refuses medical treatment, the patient is charged with incompetence.

Such asymmetries of power in healthcare and beyond were challenged in the 1960s by the emerging Civil Rights movement, the women's movement, and the populism that included a commitment to patients' rights. Beginning around the same time, medicine itself was rocked by a series of events that either created new ethical quandaries or amplified existing ones, each of them demonstrating a power asymmetry between patients and clinicians and requiring a response from bioethics. Chief among these events included the redefinition of death as the cessation of brain rather than of cardiac activity (1968), publication of information about the Tuskegee syphilis experiment (1972), the nationwide legalization of abortion (1973), the suit brought by Karen Ann Quinlan's parents requesting that she be removed from a ventilator (1975), and the death of "Baby Doe," a child born with Down syndrome whose parents withheld lifesaving treatment (1982). Biomedical ethics arose as an institutionalized, interdisciplinary academic discipline in response to these and other events, as the nation faced an urgent need for ethics experts to help resolve the escalating number of increasingly complex biomedical ethics cases. When ethical or legal dilemmas in the care of a particular patient arose, clinicians turned to the bioethics consultant for help in deciding what to do.

While there were several competing ethical frameworks governing the development of medical ethics practice, principlism soon emerged as the dominant approach. In 1979, Tom Beauchamp and James Childress published their *Principles of Biomedical Ethics*.[24] Elaborating and expanding on the principles promulgated in the *Belmont Report*,[25] published the year before, Beauchamp and Childress invoked four principles—(1) respect for autonomy, (2) nonmaleficence, (3) beneficence, (4) justice—"to provide frameworks of general guidelines that condensed morality to its central elements and gave people from diverse fields an easily grasped set of moral standards."[26] The ethics expert applies these universal principles to a particular case, determining which among the principles should govern action. Beauchamp and Childress insist that the method principlism employs in resolving ethical dilemmas is not one of simple deduction: "[N]either rules nor judgments can be *deduced* directly from principles, because additional interpretation, specification, and balancing of the principles is needed in order to formulate policies and decide about cases."[27] Principles are understood as *prima facie* duties. When a conflict arises among these principles, Beauchamp writes, "some balance, harmony, or form of equilibrium between two or more norms must be found; or, alternatively, one norm overrides the other."[28] Beauchamp and Childress insist that their principles should be understood only as guidelines. Applying these guidelines in clinical decision making requires, Beauchamp writes, that they be "*interpreted and made specific* . . . [I]nventiveness and imaginativeness in their use is essential and to be encouraged."[29]

We applaud Beauchamp for noting the essential role inventiveness and imaginativeness play in clinical decision making; we believe their use should be more than simply "encouraged." Indeed, to note that inventiveness and imaginativeness are essential without providing the tools for developing and applying them is problematic. The application of universal principals, even only as guidelines, without sufficient attention to the complexity and uniqueness of each particular situation—an attention that *requires* creativity and imagination—fosters a sense that clinicians and ethicists, or clinician ethicists, are "above" the stories of the patients and families facing ethical quandaries. Such detachment reflects an all-too-pervasive attitude in healthcare—the adoption of an ideal of objectivity that rests on the assumption that one must remain outside the story of the other.[30]

During his research on physicians who are genetic counselors, medical sociologist Charles Bosk asked "Bill Smith," a physician caring for patients with severe congenital illnesses, how he "came to grips with all the 'accidents' or 'mistakes'" in human biology that manifest in the genetic illnesses he saw. Following is Smith's response:

> What you have to do is this, Bosk. When you get up in the morning, pretend your car is a spaceship. Tell yourself you are going to visit another planet. You say, "On that planet terrible things happen, but they don't happen on my planet. They only happen on that planet I take my spaceship to each morning.[31]

Arthur Frank recommends that Smith's response "should be read aloud to every medical school class as an example of how professional practice can warp an otherwise decent mind."[32] Assuming this disembodied perspective, Frank continues, physicians, nurses, social workers, chaplains convince themselves that they are shielded from the "terrible things" happening on hospital planet. They practice a "spaceship ethics," taking refuge in principles that place them outside, or above, the complicated, ambiguous, contradictory lives of those others who sicken and die (p. 147). To board the spaceship they must deny their own embodiment, a denial for which they pay dearly.[33]

Since the mid-1980s, several alternative ethical frameworks have challenged principlism's dominance in biomedical ethics. Among the most prominent of these challenges is the common morality framework proposed by K. Danner Clouser and Bernard Gert.[34] Common morality's primary objection to principlism is that there is no comprehensive theory undergirding its principles. Clouser and Gert contrast the principles of Beauchamp and Childress with traditional ethical principles, like those of utilitarianism, that are "shorthand" for comprehensive ethical theories and systems. They suggest that principlism is not supported by such comprehensive theories or systems; on the contrary, it acts only as a reminder to "think about justice" or "think about helping people."[35] By suggesting that a comprehensive theory undergirds their principles, Clouser and Gert argue, principlists mislead us into believing they have provided a firm foundation for our moral decision making when they have not. Instead, they have provided a way to justify our personal, biased, often arbitrary moral reasoning: "Since the principle was not nearly sufficient for determining judgment," Clouser asks, "what idiosyncrasies, what biases, what subjective elements entered into the moral decision or judgment?"[36] In contrast to the superficiality of principlism's principles, Clouser asserts that common morality's approach combines cognitive, aspirational, procedural, and juridical elements in a

> complex system that has four main components: moral rules, moral ideals, the morally relevant features of situations, and a detailed procedure for dealing with conflicts. . . . [Common morality] begin[s] with the moral system that is actually used by thoughtful people in making decisions and judgments about what to do in particular cases . . . [that] impartial, rational persons would find acceptable as a public system that applies to everyone, including themselves and those they care about (pp. 227, 228).

Casuistry is an alternative—or possibly a complement—to principlism that bases its reasoning in cases rather than abstract principles.[37] A centuries-old form of moral reasoning, casuistry reentered the ethical arena in 1988 with the publication of *The Abuse of Casuistry: A History of Moral Reasoning*, by Albert Jonsen and Stephen Toulmin.[38] It was then applied to bioethics in 1992, when Jonsen, Mark Siegler, and William Winslade published the first edition of their *Clinical Ethics*.[39] Cases are concrete because they represent a "congealing" of circumstances. While each case is a unique combination of actors, actions, places, and times, it is also generalizable to other, similar types of cases. Jonsen describes how the ethicist schooled in casuistry sets about describing and evaluating the "circumstances, that is, the particulars" of a case— the "who, what, why, when, and where"—including the "manifold institutions and practices that constitute a social order," which moral philosophers, in their fascination with a universalist rationality that "transcends particular practices of life," have too long ignored.[40] Ethicists who focus on universal forms of reasoning may be very skilled at theorizing, but they have proven themselves inept, casuists contend, in considering the particular circumstances of ethical cases. Yet casuistry is not simply a method for calling attention to the particular circumstances of a case; it is also a way of assessing these circumstances in seeking a resolution for ethical dilemmas. The arguments casuistry makes in seeking resolution are not long chains of reasoning; instead, they are en-thymemes ("No one is obliged to do what is futile") or maxims ("Do no harm") that, Jonsen writes, "are open to challenges of various sorts. . . . In some cases, these challenges can be met within the casuistry itself, as with the question, 'Is resuscitation in this case truly futile', but in others, they require an ascent to a more speculative philosophy, for example, the careful examination of the concepts of efficacy, authority, and probability that underlie the term 'futil-ity'" (pp. 244–45). In the latter cases, casuistry must call on moral philoso-phy, although the need for this arises infrequently. In every instance, however, the final step is to compare cases, "seeking to identify cases similar to the one under scrutiny and to discern whether the changed circumstances justify a dif-ferent judgment in the new case than they did in the former" (p. 245).

Virtue-based ethics, also an ancient form of moral reasoning, offers another alternative to principlism. The primary focus of virtue ethics is not on prin-ciples, a comprehensive ethical system, or cases, but, as Edmund Pellegrino asserts, on "the agent; on his or her intentions, dispositions, and motives; and on the kind of person the moral agent becomes, wishes to become, or ought to become as a result of his or her habitual disposition to act in certain ways."[41] Of course, this standard—the model of the virtuous person—varies from culture to culture and era to era. As Alisdair MacIntyre argued in his seminal work, *After Virtue*, the dominance of virtue ethics declined, post-Enlightenment, with the gradual decrease of consensus on philosophical and theological norms of moral judgment.[42] Pellegrino emphasizes that the revival of virtue ethics, which he bases on the Classical-Medieval conception of virtue, focuses on "professional ethics," or the "realm of the ethics of physician- or nurse-patient relationship," not on "the growing body of other ethical issues commonly sub-sumed under the rubric of 'bioethics'—i.e., the issues of withholding or with-drawing life-support, euthanasia and assisted suicide, embryo research, organ and tissue transplantation, managed care and the like; the whole panorama of new issues growing out of medical technological advances."[43] There is little hope for recovering a normative role for virtue in resolving these dilemmas, Pellegrino insists, because there is no agreement about the foundations for the virtues that apply to them, whereas in professional ethics, agreement on the nature of the end, or *telos*, of the healing relationship is possible (p. 267). For Pellegrino, the virtues that most facilitate healing in the clinical relationship are (1) fidelity to trust and promise, (2) benevolence, (3) effacement of self-interest, (4) compassion and caring, (5) intellectual honesty, (6) justice, and (7) prudence (*phronesis*, or practical wisdom) (pp. 269–70).

In the dynamism of contemporary bioethics, principlism and the chal-lenges to principlism continue to help practitioners and patients choose fit-ting approaches to individual ethical concerns. The alternatives to principlism considered above have arisen in efforts to rectify the impersonality, detachment, or superficiality of principlism. Other ethical frameworks—feminist bioethics, collective ethics, and perspectives from social justice— raise overarching concerns about autonomy, structural justice, and institutional morality that challenge all mainstream bioethical approaches' concentration on personal as compared to public morality.[44] We turn now to discuss narrative ethics, an ethical practice that centers on the contributions of narrative knowledge to moral lives. We will propose that a narrative approach answers the shortcomings of principlism while recognizing feminist and structural justice frameworks as means to move forward in facing both the personal and global ethical concerns within healthcare.

Narrative Ethics

Narrative ethics emerged from within mainstream clinical bioethics in the 1980s as a means to perform a "ground-up" ethics that would start with the situation of the singular patient and move toward fitting ways of thinking about a particular patient's situation instead of trying to fit sanctioned theories or rules to the individual case. As we will see below, its emergence coincided with the development of a conceptual narrative ethics from within literary studies, separate from but supportive of the narrative ethics of healthcare. A community of clinicians and scholars dedicated to the practice of bioethics who were trained in literary theory, narratology, philosophy, and religious studies came to realize the importance of narrative approaches to the concerns of patients and their families. Unlike principlism and its accompanying alternative modes of bioethical practice summarized above, which arose to adjudicate medical wrongdoings or to resolve technology-driven biomedical problems, narrative ethics emerged from broad intellectual movements within literary and interpretive thought. Influenced by and convened in such movements as the medical humanities, human values in medicine, and patient-centered healthcare, narrative ethics merged the perspectives of humanities scholars with the viewpoints of clinicians facing ethical situations in patient care. Together, they sought ways to bring ethical decision making closer to the patients' lived experience, with the realization that patients themselves are the ones who perform the ethical work of illness.[45]

Rather than starting from the objective features of a clinical situation and asking what a person should do next, narrative ethics focuses on how that person came to be here and where the path forward might lead. What has happened to lead to this situation? What alternative endings to this story can be imagined? The patient's lived experience—including his or her experience of illness—in all its particularity and meaning guides the thinking and judging regarding medical action that ensues.[46] The narrative ethicist is trained to pay close attention to what patients, families, and clinicians say and write about the situation. From literary, linguistic, or social science disciplines, the ethicist learns to recognize the genre, point of view, metaphor, diction, and temporality of a conversation or a written text to understand what the story's content might in fact tell. They comprehend the power and implications of the rhetorical and performative aspects of these accounts.[47] In these ways, the ethicist gradually develops a nuanced sense of what it might be like to be within this story— imagining the forces acting on the patient and other agents in the narrative, using the evidence of conversations with families to construct a mental image of the patient's situation. Gradually, as the careful listener is able to sense the climate of this narrative world and what it might be like to live within it, he or she asks questions that show the patient and family that their world is being taken seriously, respected for what it is, not contested. With this recognition as a basis, the work of narrative ethics can proceed.

What does this practice of narrative ethics look like? To exercise compassion in adjusting treatment to the particularities of *this* patient's life story, to remove the blindfold of a universalist principle of justice and attend to a patient's *specific* needs, indeed to exercise any of the virtues, which are never enacted universally but rather in unique situations with particular persons, requires narrative skill. Stories, Arthur Frank suggests, "give lives legibility; when shaped as narratives, lives come from somewhere and are going somewhere. Narratability provides for legibility and out of both comes a sense of morality—practical if tacit answers to how we should live."[48]

Part of the charge to the narrative ethicist is to identify who the tellers of this story are. The narrative ethicist elicits accounts from those who need to be heard in order to have a full enough view of the patient's situation—family, friends, neighbors, professional caregivers. Using approaches from qualitative research in the social sciences and narrative inquiry from the literary/narratological disciplines, narrative ethicists understand what to do with competing or contradicting versions of situations, and how to seek and find some kind of coherence or at least unity, albeit uneasy, over the full account given.[49] They encourage the participants, including professional caregivers, to each hear one another's accounts and then assess what has been collectively revealed in dialogue with all involved.

Whether the patient is a stranger newly admitted to the hospital or a patient known for decades in a primary care practice, coming to appreciate his or her story from the inside is not an easy or low-stakes act. To enter the unknown world of another insists that one lay down one's own assumptions about the very source of meaning, thereby escaping Powers' straitjacket of the self. It takes the courageous willingness to admit that one's own values and priorities are not supreme. Opposing values and points of view must be honored to be as capable of illuminating the meanings and necessities of life as coherently as one's own. Seeing others fully and faithfully means seeing them in all their particularity, ambiguity, and contradiction while being forced to question one's own convictions. Therefore, to decide to listen, to attend to the other's story, is already to take an ethical stand. To enter the story, the listener must experience its moral complexity in all its ambiguity and challenge to one's own moral sense.

What, now, do narrative ethicists *do* in performing ethics consultations in a hospital or practicing with ethical skill as a clinician?[50] In practice, narrative ethicists have been listening very closely to stories told by patients and their families, searching for the necessary voices that might have been silenced. Some narrative ethicists write these stories down, knowing that the knowledge of complex events is enhanced through acts of representation, like writing, that confer form on what is until then chaotic and formless. Narrative ethicists might suggest that patients and families write or dictate stories so that their stories, too, through representation, can become visible and can aid in envisioning the way forward. By reading these accounts together, patients, ethicists, and clinicians can together discover central but sometimes hidden elements in the situation they face. Narrative ethicists invariably spend time with patients and families to get to know something about the patient's and family's climate, their ways of making sense of things, their habitual means of coming to decisions about important matters. The ethicists sometimes become mediators between the clinicians and the patients, helping them translate to one another what they cannot seem to convey on their own, smoothing the way for frank conversation not dominated by blame and mistrust. Religious scholar and ethicist Larry Churchill writes, "Narrative is a profound mode for understanding ethics consultations, not because it resolves problems, but because it forces us to attend to the human voices, including our own, behind what is being said."[51] Churchill nominates humility as the ethicist's most important virtue, reminding us all of the paucity of answers and the gravity of the questions.

The Narrative Ethics from Literary Studies

We turn now to the second "narrative ethics" to be considered here. Around the same time that narrative ethics surfaced in bioethics, literary studies of the 1980s created its own field of narrative ethics. Rather than the need to solve biomedical quandaries, this narrative ethics became a fundamental inquiry into questions of narrativity and identity. It is crucial for bioethicists to understand literary narrative ethics—crucial for the intellectual, relational, and structural aspects of addressing moral problems in healthcare. In effect, literary narrative ethics supplies the intellectual foundations to the practice of narrative ethics in healthcare settings.

Within literary studies and its branch called *narratology*, a particular focus arose on the relationship between narrative and ethics. This narrative ethics gathered scholars who began to pay fine attention to the ethical relationships between readers and their texts.[52] They came to understand that one cannot read a novel or poem or essay *without* being ethically engaged in both the plight of the characters and the acts of the author in telling about them. Reading, they came to see, is an active process that calls forth ethical discernment from the reader in judging the actions of characters, in assessing the reliability or unreliability of a narrator, in measuring up the moral climate and claims within the story—a world whose moral climate makes claims or poses challenges in one's own life. As the character's consciousness and conscience is exposed in the text, the reader's consciousness and conscience too may be awakened. Literary critics and philosophers propose that the narrative text affords grounds for the serious reader to examine personal choices and realities afresh, for the relationship between a reader and a text forms a context for ethical acts.[53] Although not addressing itself to problems in healthcare, the literary narrative ethics has been a source of knowledge and perspective to which bioethics' narrative ethics owes a tremendous debt.

To read, closely and seriously, embarks the reader on a committed search for the sources of meaning within the text and within the experience of reading it. Literary scholar Adam Zachary Newton writes in his *Narrative Ethics* that narrative ethics "attribut[es] to narrative discourse some kind of ethical status . . . [and] ethical discourse often depends on narrative structures."[54] The reader answers to a moral imperative to open himself or herself to the author's and characters' ways of making moral sense of their worlds. Perilous, such literary work exposes the reader to another's way of making sense of events of life, challenging the reader to accept the proposed "ground rules" within any narrative text and, by extension, within whatever world that narrative text depicts. In the words of literary scholar J. Hillis Miller, "Ethics and narration cannot be kept separate, though their relation is neither symmetrical nor harmonious."[55]

Literary scholar Wayne Booth, author of the seminal *The Rhetoric of Fiction*, stakes out his ethical position in *The Company We Keep* to suggest that books, seriously engaged with, function as friends in the reader's life, and that the reader's gradually developing ethical stance influences what he or she makes of a particular book while each book, in turn, contributes to the further development of that ethical stance.[56] Booth points out that, as is the case with friends, one can accept or reject the company of a book, sometimes as a matter of taste and sometimes as a matter of moral principle. In view of the persuasiveness of violent or sectarian literatures available widely in the media, Booth's caution has been taken seriously as a measure of the power of reading in developing a life-long moral compass.

Literary narrative ethicists remind us that the literary text exerts ethical force not only in its plot but also in its form. Narratologist James Phelan insists that the ethical work of the reader is done not only in weighing moral choices made by characters but also in examining the ethics of representation itself: "I . . . [tie] ethical response to the techniques of narrative itself, as I focus on the links among technique (the signals offered by the text) and the reader's cognitive understanding, emotional response, and ethical positioning."[57] So the dual processes of form and content work on the reader, letting the reader inspect the proposed reality of the world depicted while simultaneously undergoing the personal process of having come to know that world. Reading, in effect, is a laboratory in which the reader comes to know his or her deep-seated modes of judgment—of the beautiful, of the revolting, of the gripping, and of the moral.

From the worlds of psychology and philosophy come complementing means of making sense of the ethics of reading. Originator of the field of cognitive psychology, and more recently of cultural psychology, Jerome Bruner asserts the primacy of a literary form of narrative for meaning-making: "Narrative seems to depend for its effectiveness . . . upon its 'literariness'. . . . It relies upon the power of tropes—upon metaphor, metonymy, synecdoche, implicature, and the rest, to 'expand the horizon of possibilities'."[58] Aristotelian philosopher Martha Nussbaum has been drawn to literary work, especially the late novels of Henry James, as a source of philosophical thought on questions of freedom and responsibility. Her *Love's Knowledge* makes the case that philosophical thought cannot be consummated within philosophical language, and rather requires the putting-into-words peculiar to the novelist to express, and only then to understand, the thoughts embroiled in words: "To show the force and truth of the Aristotelian claim that 'the decision rests with perception', we need . . . texts which display to us the complexity, the indeterminacy, the sheer *difficulty* of moral choice, and which show us, as [Henry James's *The Golden Bowl*] does, the childishness, the refusal of life involved in fixing everything in advance according to some system of inviolable rules."[59] Both form and content of literary works are seen, in these two comments, to be salient to the projects of appreciating moral worlds and being prepared to make some distinctions, if not choices, in their midst.

This excursion into literary study's practice of narrative ethics brings us organically back to the practice of narrative ethics within bioethics. The two types of narrative ethics converge on the realization of the saturation of the moral in everyday life. Whether we listen to the story of a patient in the office or we read the words of a well-wrought novel, we are taking seriously human beings' capacity to formulate, in words, what they are going through. We use the same narrative skills in both the literary and the clinical contexts. Trained to capture the evidence of words, we can try to meet the tellers or writers in their world, at least permitting ourselves to picture what living in that world must be like. Our task as listeners or readers is to experience the full force of the accounts of others, to appreciate the gravity of being exposed to the meaning-making efforts of others, and to become aware of the impact of such accounts on our own moral development.

In teaching narrative ethics within our Master of Science in Narrative Medicine graduate program at Columbia, we teach the literary as well as clinical faces of this practice. In addition to the clinical practice of helping patients, families, and clinicians arrive at fitting decisions about healthcare, teaching narrative ethics entails training in the close reading of literary, legal, and clinical texts. The narrative ethicist has a duty to examine whatever texts or oral communications influence macro-level as well as micro-level discourses about ethical issues, whether in the academic press or in popular and social media. Close reading of clinical ethical cases, of nonfiction accounts of ethical conflicts, and literary representations of the moral issues in healthcare are all important in the development of the narrative ethicist. Understanding the narrative structures of all types of texts and images and following the interplay between the narrative and the ethical enable the learner to identify the intellectual, clinical, and ideological forces at work and to respond thoughtfully to them. Such study exposes learners to the complexities of bioethical discourses in all communicative frames and equips them to help others make sense of the barrage of information on healthcare ethics. Such capacities contribute to both the ethicist's intellectual growth and potential to be of help to individual patients and families within their illnesses.

Perhaps the most consequential aspect of both forms of narrative ethics is to expose the ethical nature of narrative engagement in the world. As the particular illuminates the universal, so the personal ethical dilemma of one patient points to societal and global inequities and widespread threats to safety and equality. Feminist bioethicist Susan Sherwin proposes a "public ethics" that would address urgent global threats ranging from climate change to the escalating wealth/health disparities. Urging bioethics to recognize its responsibilities in facing collective moral threats as well as individual moral dilemmas, Sherwin details the contributions a feminist relational approach can bring to a bioethics of this scale, a contribution irreversibly narrative in nature:

Feminist relational theory looks not only at the behavior of individual patients, providers, and administrators, but also at society and asks how dominant values and institutional options tend to direct individuals in particular directions despite obvious
problems with these options. It encourages us to seek changes at all levels of human
organization, both formal and informal, in pursuit of moral values. As such, it provides an important model for ethicists willing to take on the challenge of developing a
public ethics aimed at guiding humans away from the potential catastrophes ahead.[60]

Such an approach demands far-flung horizons with a capacity for vast conceptual range that can take in not only the predicament of one person or one
institution but also the interconnected genesis of global threats. Sherwin continues to propose that "[w]hat we need is an approach to ethics that encourages
humility regarding our own interpretations without abandoning the value of
searching for reliable guidelines and being willing to promote their discussion
and adoption" (p. 18).

The qualities required of bioethicists—if we are to consider widening their
scope to address the ethics of the collective—resemble the capacities endowed
by both forms of narrative ethics. The discernment of the network of responsibilities and the ability to move from the part to the whole and then back to
the part are, from their genesis, hermeneutic skills built on elemental narrative
powers. To even raise such questions within a society demands the narrative
skills to open conversations, to solicit diverse points of view, and to tolerate the
disagreements without resorting to silencing dissidents. Forms of narrative
competence, these are the interventions that may enable us to raise our ethical
sights above the local toward the contemplation of a justice for more than a few.

Philosophers Jens Brockmeier and Hanna Meretoja propose that "[i]f there
is one point we consider essential for the hermeneutics of narrative, it is the
way in which it brings together engagement with issues of storytelling in linguistic, discursive, and artistic contexts with the wider existential relevance of
narrative practices for our (self-) understanding and being in the world."[61] We
take the growth in both forms of narrative ethics as a signal of the serious study
of engagement, of human contact, of the growth toward the radical humility
to seek the word of one, to see the perspectives of the many, to find means to
accept alien ways of making meaning, and so to live more fully—together with
those with whom we've been thrown—the lives we've been given to live.

The Pedagogy and Practice of Narrative Medicine's Ethics

Narrative medicine is poised to integrate the literary narrative ethics and the
clinical narrative ethics, being a citizen of both worlds, so that the clinical

ethics deliberations can proceed in light of the literary and rhetorical insights now available from narrative study.

Narrative ethics is an ethics practiced with narrative competence, which we define as the fundamental human skill of recognizing, absorbing, interpreting, and being moved to action by the stories of others.[62] This ethics can be practiced both by ethicists/consultants who obtain narrative training and by clinicians whose narrative training enables them to attend carefully to the ethical dimensions of their own practice.

Narrative ethics, in a manner of speaking, *is* narrative medicine practiced in the setting of bioethics. As Frank writes,

> [N]arrative ethics is more interested in preventing breakdowns in mutual understanding from happening in the first place than in adjudicating conflicts over preferred courses of action. The primary focus is to prevent situations from turning into cases. Thus narrative ethics necessarily morphs into narrative medicine, including in its purview how everyday clinical practice proceeds and how well such practice honors people's stories of suffering. . . . Ethics conflict—autonomy being set in opposition to beneficence—can be avoided by a physician who practices narrative medicine . . ."[63]

One way to develop the narrative competence required of narrative ethics is through the study of literature and the development of the skills of close reading. To listen to patients' stories with a view toward understanding how the storytellers find themselves in their present situation requires the same narrative competence used in reading a literary text. We propose that the close reading of great literature develops the narrative competence necessary to understand, through Aristotle's phronesis, moral complexity and ambiguity.[64] Although principlists are fully aware of the importance of attending to the complexities of each unique case, they do not provide guidance on how to facilitate this attention. [65] Casuists focus on the particularities of each case yet do not elucidate the way that narratives are shaped, how they function, what they mean, or how one enters the case at all. Gesturing, in a broad way, to the narrative nature of casuistic reasoning does not get us far.

We teach narrative ethics by teaching narrative medicine—close reading, creative writing, responding to the writing of others, co-constructing narratives. Not only the reading of the text but talking about it and writing in its shadow seem to be required for the reader to achieve dividends of the learning. In the formation of the narrative ethicist, these same powers of sight and meaning, achievable by the close reader and writer, are the necessary equipment for coming to envision and comprehend the meaning-making of patients, families, clinicians, and wider communities. Once they have learned to be close readers, they have the capacity to become close listeners. Once they have strengthened their skills of representation in writing, they can lend this skill to the patients for whom they care and whose accounts they may attempt to configure into a written narrative.

Through these pedagogies, the reader comes to recognize his or her habitual moves in interpretation as well as his or her blind spots, assumptions, and prejudices. The contrasting responses of respected fellow readers need not lead to antagonistic arguments to declare the winner but rather can open mutual examination of the contingent grounds of any one interpretation. Together readers realize the range of possible interpretations, which helps to deliver each one from the peril of certainty. Narrative training is the staple of training in narrative ethics, hand in hand with close and critical attention to the stories that unfold in illness and care, recovery and death.

This pedagogy performs another critical function for those who would practice narrative ethics: it strengthens creativity. We see the importance of the work of imagination in moral life—we cannot choose to live that which we cannot imagine. Clinicians must be skilled at this imagining if they are to provide opportunities for patients to choose among the possible alternatives open to them. To engage in this work is to exercise both ethical discernment and narrative recognition—the *phronesis* of Aristotle to which Ricoeur refers. Narrative recognition or logic does not insist on narrative consistency: often ethical conflicts arise because the way someone has been telling her story no longer fits the changed circumstances of her life. In such a case, the effort is not to make the next story fit the narrative patterns of the old, but to help the patient to imagine new ways to tell and to interpret her story, ways that open possibilities for moving forward rather than living in the past.

We teach that narrative ethics has a responsibility to move toward social justice. The reason to develop the skills of escaping the straightjacket of self is to actively acknowledge and respect otherness. Proposing that reading novels makes possible "the will to believe in the possibility of alterity," literary scholar Dorothy Hale concludes that

> the novel reader's experience of free submission, her response to the 'hailing' performed by the novel, becomes . . . a necessary condition for the social achievement of diversity, a training in the honoring of Otherness, which is the defining ethical property of the novel—and is also what makes literary study, and novel reading in particular, a crucial pre-condition for positive social change.[66]

The understanding of narrative ethics that emerges from the practice of narrative medicine now comes into view. Several qualities surface as part of the practice of a narrative ethics that is itself an aspect of narrative medicine.

Narrative ethics is reflexive ethics: An ethics oriented toward narrative focuses on the ubiquity of moral considerations in healthcare and not only on the moral reasoning that is applied from afar in ethical crises.[67] As a reflexive practice, narrative ethics is lived, in real time, whenever patients and those who care for them work together, enabling the participants to recognize *as ethical* issues that arise and to respond to them throughout their work together. (See Chapter 12 of this volume for a discussion of reflexive clinical practice.) Reflexivity engages a community of witnesses to consider values and to empower moral choices. Here we see narrative ethics' solidarity with feminist ethics and care ethics. As Hilde Lindemann Nelson writes,

> On the theoretical-juridical model, morality is a matter of applying codified rules derived from comprehensive theories as criteria for assessing wrongdoing and making rational choices. The narrative approach . . . sees morality instead as a continuous interpersonal task of becoming and remaining mutually intelligible. It is expressive of who we are and hope to be; it is collaborative in that it posits, not a solitary judge, but a community of inquirers who need to construct ways of living well together. And it is feminist because it offers a means of resisting powerful ideologies, whether these be of gender, medicine, ethnicity, or all three at once.[68]

Although narrative ethicists indeed participate in ethics consultations and contribute to resolving acute quandaries in the lives of patients they have not previously known, those narrative ethicists who are themselves clinicians also practice a tonic form of ethics within the texture of the clinical care itself. Called everyday ethics, slow ethics, or microethics, this form of ethical practice pays attention to the ordinary aspects of patient care instead of the dramatic eruption of quandary situations.[69] In these cases the narrative ethicist is the clinician, not the consultant, and the context of ethical practice is the dutiful professional care of the patient. Mutual, reflexive knowledge between these two develops over episodes of care, be they 30 hours in the Emergency Department, 4 days of an inpatient stay, or decades in the clinic, laying the groundwork for a shared practice of careful listening and recognition.

Emotions and feelings are present and helpful in narrative ethics: Both literary narrative ethics and clinical narrative ethics acknowledge the importance of emotions in an ethical practice. As they examine the processes of reading in neuroscientific and aesthetic terms, narratologists are taking up questions of empathy, affect, agency, and imagination.[70] Questions of the place of emotions and individual patient/clinician relationships in clinical decision making are an important part of narrative ethics as well as of other healthcare practices, including relational ethics and care ethics.[71] Rather than being seen as interfering with clinical judgment, emotions of empathy or compassion are recognized to be a source of care. Issues of self-care for clinicians, moral distress of clinical practice, and what has been called "ethical mindedness" also require complex and conscious handling of and interpretation of emotion in practice, and have reminded narrative ethicists to care for the carers as well as the patients.[72] (See Chapter 2 of this volume for a discussion of the place of emotion in narrative medicine's teaching and practice.)

Narrative practices are not only the therapeutic means, but the therapy itself: The narrative acts of giving accounts of the self, skilled listening to such accounts, and co-creating narratives of illness not only propel toward care but bring about healing. They are not adjunct to the care; they are the care itself. Narrative medicine and narrative ethics are learning from practices arising from gerontology and palliative care that entail storytelling as a germinal part of the care itself. Aging and dying persons come to recognize themselves, frame their life histories in ways that make sense to them and to others, and leave behind something of beauty and singularity.[73] Both narrative medicine and narrative ethics recognize the therapeutic power of the practices of unhampered expression and careful listening. Literary scholar Derek Attridge could have been writing about facing a patient instead of reading a literary work when he wrote that "the impulse to do justice to the work, which means to make it happen anew (and always differently) in one's reading of it, is an ethical impulse: in Levinasian terms, to respond to the other not as a generalizable set of features or a statistic but as a singularity."[74] Achieving the attention and performing the representation constitute the giving of care—care that extends both to the patient and the provider of care.

These reflections on a narrative ethics consonant with the practice of narrative medicine are the beginnings, we hope, of a deepening relationship between the two. In a reciprocity reminiscent of that between narrativity and identity with which we opened this chapter, narrative medicine and narrative ethics can together create concepts and methods to singularize clinical care and ethical care. Both practices have the power to recognize those who participate in care, those who come to be heard, and those who do the work of listening.

Postscript

The effort really to see and really to represent is no idle business
in face of the *constant* force that makes for muddlement.
—Henry James, *What Maisie Knew*

We deliver to patients that which they came to the clinic *for* when we humbly, meticulously, in affiliation listen to what patients say and then do justice to it. Knowing that the presence of *this* clinician and *this* patient will result in a singular outcome, the process of care nourishes both, either with hoped-for relief of suffering or with acknowledgment of having been of use. The technical interventions follow upon this singular, selfless listening. The result will be both the product of and the evidence of a healing relationship between teller and listener.

In an interview describing how she understands her own literary efforts, Toni Morrison says that her "books are about very specific circumstances, and in them are people who do very specific things. . . . The plot, characters are part of my effort to create a language in which I can posit philosophical questions. I want the reader to ponder those questions not because I put them in an essay, but because they are part of a narrative."[75] Reflecting on Morrison's words, the philosopher George Yancy writes that

> Morrison is not depicting abstract and universal truths, but 'accidents of private [and public] history' that philosophically shed light on what it means to be a self. . . . Morrison is able to place the reader into an imaginative *lived* space, a powerful narrative space that is able to articulate modalities of lived existence . . . . Hence, one might say that Morrison posits philosophical questions that are linked inextricably to narrative. After all, our lives are lived narratives, journeys of pain, endurance, contradiction, death, intersubjectivity, suffering, racism, sexism, terror, trauma, joy and transcendence. Avoiding abstract and non-indexical discourse, Morrison reveals the power of literature to embody the flesh and blood reality of what it means to-be-in-the-world.[76]

It is this capacity of literature to embody the reality of being-in-the-world that gives narrative practices in healthcare their powers. A practice of ethics within narrative medicine is creative, shot through with imagination, innovation, and singularity. It is reflexive, where both parties see the self more clearly by virtue of their contact. And it is reciprocal, leaving behind no debt, no lien, no diminishment but instead mutual growth, even at the ends of life. It is a powerful and respectful way for humans to meet—two subjects—to contemplate mystery, to tolerate doubt and fear, to accept help, to recognize love. It is, in the end as in the beginning, the word.

We will give Ricoeur the last word. In his groundbreaking philosophical work *Time and Narrative*, Ricoeur writes: "We tell stories because in the last analysis human lives need and merit being narrated. This remark takes on its full force when we refer to the necessity to save the history of the defeated and the lost. The whole history of suffering . . . calls for narrative."

Notes

1. Brockmeier, *Beyond the Archive*, 181.
2. Ricoeur, "Life in Quest of Narrative," 29.
3. Ricoeur, "Life in Quest of Narrative," 32.
4. Frank, *Wounded Storyteller*, 53.
5. Herman, Jahn, and Ryan, *Routledge Encyclopedia of Narrative Theory*.
6. Robinson, *Narrating the Past*.
7. McAdams, "Role of Narrative"; Bruner, *Acts of Meaning*.
8. Czarniawska, *Narratives in Social Science*; Kreiswirth, "Merely Telling Stories?"; Riessman, *Narrative Methods*.
9. Peters and Besley, "Narrative Turn."
10. Reed et al., "Narrative Theology."
11. Ricoeur, *Time and Narrative*.
12. Hamkins, *Art of Narrative Psychiatry*.
13. Kreiswirth, "Merely Telling Stories?"
14. Ricoeur, "Life in Quest of Narrative," 22–23 (cited hereafter in the text by page numbers).
15. Gadamer, *Truth and Method*.
16. Although this chapter will not treat works other than literary texts, there are parallel critical works in aesthetic and musical theory that contribute to the argument for the ethical dimensions of creative work in other media. See as one example Rabinowitz, "Rhetoric of Reference."
17. See Ricoeur, *Time and Narrative*, vol. 1, especially chapters 1 and 2.
18. Dewey, *Art as Experience*.
19. Cleanth Brooks, *Well Wrought Urn*, 205–6.
20. Gregory, *Shaped by Stories*, 37–38.
21. Powers, "Richard Powers."
22. Murdoch, *Black Prince*, 162.
23. Nussbaum "Introduction," in Murdoch, *Black Prince*, xiii.
24. Beauchamp and Childress, *Principles of Biomedical Ethics*.
25. National Commission for the Protection of Human Subjects of Biomedical and Behavioral Research, *Belmont Report*.
26. Beauchamp, "Principlism and Its Alleged Competitors," 181.
27. Beauchamp, "Principlism and Its Alleged Competitors," 182.
28. Beauchamp, "Principlism and Its Alleged Competitors," 183.
29. Beauchamp, "Principlism and Its Alleged Competitors," 184. Italics in original.
30. For a collection of essays from scholars of various humanities and social science disciplines challenging the dominance of principlism, see DuBose, Hamel, and O'Connell, *Matter of Principles?* See also Charon and Montello, *Stories Matter*; Hedgecoe, "Critical Bioethics"; Irvine, "Ethics of Self-Care"; Jones, "Literature and Medicine"; and O'Toole, "Story of Ethics."
31. Bosk, *All God's Mistakes*, 171.
32. Frank, *Wounded Storyteller*, 147 (cited hereafter in the text by page numbers.)
33. Cole, Goodrich, and Gritz, *Faculty Health in Academic Medicine*.
34. Clouser, "Veatch, May, and Models"; Clouser and Gert, "A Critique of Principlism"; Clouser and Gert, "Morality vs. Principlism"; Gert, *Morality*.
35. Clouser, "Common Morality," 223.
36. Clouser, "Common Morality," 223 (cited hereafter in the text by page numbers).
37. Jonsen, "Casuistry: An Alternative."
38. Jonsen and Toulmin, *Abuse*.
39. Jonsen, Siegler, and Winslade, *Clinical Ethics*.
40. Jonsen, "Casuistry: An Alternative," 243 (cited hereafter in the text by page numbers).
41. Pellegrino, "Toward a Virtue-Based," 254.

42. MacIntyre, *After Virtue*.

43. Pellegrino, "Toward a Virtue-Based," 265 (cited hereafter in the text by page numbers).

44. For discussions of feminist ethics and public ethics, see Sherwin, "Whither Bioethics?" For recent reviews of the development of feminist bioethics, see Scully, Baldwin-Ragavan, and Fitzpatrick, *Feminist Bioethics*. For examinations and critiques of feminist bioethics' contributions to theoretical philosophy, see Nelson, "Feminist Bioethics," and Rawlinson, "Concept of a Feminist Bioethics."

45. Two collections of essays published at the turn of the century helped to state the case for narrative ethics and to state its limits, convening in print authors writing from multiple clinical and theoretical perspectives. See Nelson, *Stories and their Limits*; and Charon and Montello, *Stories Matter*. See also Brody, *Stories of Sickness*; Hunter, *Doctors' Stories*; and Carson, "Interpretive Bioethics."

46. Phenomenologists writing about the ethics of illness have helped patients and clinicians to recognize both the complexity of any one patient's experience of illness and the gulfs that can separate the worldviews and values of patients and professionals. The seminal work of S. Kay Toombs, Richard Zaner, Drew Leder, and, more recently, Havi Carel contribute both theories and methods for clinicians who want to make contact with patients' lived realities and to take them into account as choices are made. See Toombs, *Meaning of Illness*; Zaner, *Conversations*; Leder, *Absent Body*; and Carel, *Illness*.

47. See Tod Chambers's influential study of the literary genre of the ethical case history, *Fiction of Bioethics*. See also literary scholar and patient Kathlyn Conway's probing study *Beyond Words*, which inspects language's capacity or inability to express that which the patient experiences in serious illness.

48. Frank, "Why Study People's Stories?", 111.

49. For background on qualitative research methods of asking questions and arriving at some conclusions, see Hurwitz, Greenhalgh, and Skultans' *Narrative Research*. Kathleen Wells' *Narrative Inquiry* and Elliot Mishler's *Research Interviewing* give strong accounts of narratively based ways to seek underlying unities contained in accounts.

50. See a 2014 Special Issue of *Hastings Center Reports* on narrative ethics, edited by Martha Montello, that collects perspectives from many of the ethicists and clinicians who pioneered these practices from the emergence of the field (Montello, *Narrative Ethics*). Dawson Schultz and Lydia Flasher suggest that the responsibility of the ethicist to get the story straight is an act of clinical phronesis (Schultz and Flasher, "Charles Taylor").

51. Churchill, "Narrative Awareness," S38.

52. For introductions to narratology's narrative ethics, see Newton, *Narrative Ethics*; Booth, *Company*; J. Hillis Miller, *Ethics of Reading* and *Literature as Conduct*; and Phelan, *Living to Tell* and "Rhetoric, Ethics."

53. Attridge, "Innovation"; Montgomery, "Literature, Literary Studies."

54. Newton, *Narrative Ethics*, 8.

55. J. Hillis Miller, *Ethics of Reading*, 2.

56. Booth, *Company*, 38–39.

57. Phelan, *Living to Tell*, 22.

58. Bruner, *Acts of Meaning*, 59–60.

59. Nussbaum, *Love's Knowledge*, 142–43.

60. Sherwin, "Whither Bioethics?", 14.

61. Brockmeier and Meretoja, "Understanding Narrative," 2.

62. Charon, *Narrative Medicine*, 4.

63. Frank, "Narrative Ethics as Dialogical," S16–S17 <<subsequent citations not found>>

64. Neuroscientific studies of the consequences of reading literary fiction support hypotheses that reading serious literature enhances the reader's capacity to recognize or imagine emotional states in others. See Kidd and Castano, "Reading Literary Fiction," and Djikic, Oatley, and Moldoveanu, "Reading Other Minds."

65. See Beauchamp, "Principlism and Its Alleged Competitors."

66. Hale, "Fiction as Restriction," 189.
67. Geisler, "Value of Narrative Ethics."
68. Nelson, "Feminist Bioethics," 505.
69. Truog et al., "Microethics"; Gallagher, "Slow Ethics"; Carrese et al., "Everyday Ethics;" Branch, "Ethics of Patient Care."
70. Leys, "Turn to Affect"; Altieri, "Affect, Intentionality"; Keen, *Empathy*.
71. Initially triggered by the work of Carol Gilligan and Nel Noddings in a feminist theory of moral development, care ethics has developed theoretical and practical guidelines for a radically practice-oriented conception of personal responsibilities of caregivers. See Tronto, *Moral Boundaries*; and van Nistelrooij, Schaafsma, and Tronto, "Ricoeur and the Ethics of Care."
72. See Guillemin and Gillam, "Emotions, Narratives"; Kearney et al., "Self-Care;" and Pauly, Varcoe, and Storch, "Framing the Issue."
73. Kenyon, Bohlmeijer, and Randall, *Storying*; Baldwin, "Narrative Ethics"; Paulsen, "Narrative Ethics of Care."
74. Attridge, "Performing Metaphors," 28.
75. Dreifus, "Chloe Wofford Talks."
76. Yancy, *Black Bodies*, 217–18.

IDENTITIES IN PEDAGOGY

The Politics of the Pedagogy: Cripping, Queering and Un-homing Health Humanities

Sayantani DasGupta

To be at the margin is to be part of the whole but outside the main body.
—bell hooks, *Feminist Theory: From Margin to Center*[1]

Whose house is this? . . . It's not mine. I dreamed another, sweeter, brighter . . . This house is strange. Its shadows lie. Say, tell me, why does its lock fit my key?
—Toni Morrison, *Home*[2]

Introduction

Pedagogical theorists from Paulo Freire to bell hooks to Chandra Talpade Mohanty have argued that teaching and learning are fundamentally political acts.[3] This is no less true in the emerging field of narrative medicine, which is predicated on intersubjective meaning-making between not only listener and teller but also professor and student, such that what happens in the narrative medicine classroom is a parallel process, modeling the sorts of relationships that can happen between professional and patient in the clinic room. However, we must recognize that it is not enough simply to read stories with medical students or have nurses write and share narratives together. This work must be done with careful attention to power and privilege that attends to not simply the texts we read and write together, but the relational texts we live, breathe, and create in our classrooms and workshop spaces. Otherwise, even narrative work within healthcare risks carrying within its practices and pedagogies the potential to replicate the selfsame hierarchical, oppressive power dynamics of traditional medicine that the field is designed to address. Hence, narrative medicine must insist on a hypervigilance against exploitation of the inherent power of professional status. Mohanty writes,

> Education represents both a struggle for meaning and a struggle over power relations ... Education becomes a central terrain where power and politics operate out of the lived culture of individuals and groups situated in asymmetrical social and political spaces ... questions at stake in the academy ... are questions of self- and collective knowledge of marginalized peoples and the recovery of alternative, oppositional histories of domination and struggle.[4]

Is it possible to search for such oppositional knowledge within the health humanities disciplines?[5] What does it mean to, say, crip, queer, or un-home these many fields?

Both cripping and queering have been used in academic and activist circles to imply a movement of certain types of knowledge from margin to center. They imply undermining traditional understandings and opening up alternate perspectives—not just rewriting the perception of disability or queer politics, but reconceptualizing fundamentals of knowledge or action.

I do not identify as crip, queer, or trans*[6] but use these words here in solidarity, as an ally in the struggle and as someone whose work frequently relies upon disability, queer, and trans* activism and theory. As a woman of color, academic, and activist, I recall the 2013 words of Sami Schalk in *Disability Studies Quarterly*:

> Although I do not identify as a person with a disability, I nonetheless have come to identify with the term "crip" as elucidated by feminist and queer crip/disability theorists ... [a] disidentifying process among/across/between minoritarian subjects can allow for coalitional theory and political solidarity. . . . By coalitional theory, I mean theories which are inclusive of multiple minority groups without being limited to only those people who occupy multiply minoritized positions.[7]

I also borrow from David Eng, Judith Halberstam and José Esteban Muñoz's famous question, from the introduction to their co-edited 2005 issue of *Social Text*, "What's Queer about Queer Theory Now?" In this essay they suggest that "the political promise of the term [queerness] resided specifically in its broad critique of multiple social antagonisms, including race, gender, class, nationality and religion, in addition to sexuality."[8] And it is with this broad-reaching understanding of both cripping and queering that I conceptualize this essay, also influenced by postcolonial understandings of "home" and what literary theorist Homi Bhaba calls "unhomeliness."[9] My attempt is to uncover, as Mohanty suggests, radical educational practices that "simultaneously critique knowledge itself" lest any classroom, including those in health humanities, risk becoming a colonizing educational space.[10] I also acknowledge that, even as I write this essay, I may still run the risk of "accommodation and assimilation and consequent depoliticization."[11] Ultimately, I write from what bell hooks calls "the margin as a space of radical openness." In her words, "marginality [is] much more than a site of deprivation . . . it is the site of radical possibility, a space of resistance . . . a central location for the production of counter-hegemonic discourse."[12] Finally, I write with humility from a situated "I" position about my own evolving pedagogical and political practice. This is not to imply that other teachers and scholars do not share my practices.

Crip Politics and the Medicalization of Health Humanities

The first course I ever taught in the health humanities fields was a seminar initially called *Illness Narratives: Understanding the Experience of Illness.* I designed the course as part of the core requirements in the graduate program in Health Advocacy at Sarah Lawrence College.[13] The program had previously offered a course in patient psychology to help future advocates "understand the experience of the ill,"[14] and so I unthinkingly included that phrasing in my course title.

Yet, I designed even that early syllabus with politics in mind. My 2001 course was envisioned to help health advocates understand the experience of illness not through reductive study of "them" by "us," but through listening to the voices of the ill themselves. Additionally, I wanted to break down that artificial binary of healthy professionals and ill patients, allowing future advocates to explore their own personal experiences of illness and caregiving. This act not only reminded my students that there were vulnerable bodies on both sides of the professional relationship but also allowed them to begin identifying their own frames of listening, the personal and professional narratives they were bringing to their future listening encounters. And so that early class incorporated multiple pedagogical modalities, assignments I still use today: the reading of illness memoir, the writing of students' personal illness or caregiving narratives, and the oral history interviewing of individuals with chronic illnesses.[15]

Power and privilege were, from the start, central to my teaching. Influenced by Paulo Freire and bell hooks, I considered myself a co-learner, a facilitator rather than a didactic teacher. I did not believe in what Freire called the banking method of education, the notion that unadulterated knowledge is something that flows straight from professorial lips to be deposited in the vault-like open minds of students. Instead, a desire to acknowledge the expertise my students already brought with them into the classroom deeply impacted my pedagogical choices—from the way I facilitated class discussions to beginning each class with a "business time" during which I could not only field questions but also "take the temperature" of my classroom, feeling out frustrations, curiosities, tensions and interests. These practices stay with me today.

Similarly, the personal narratives of illness and caregiving my students wrote on a weekly basis, assignments which differed weekly in form, genre, or point of view, made room for the personal to impact the academic, for the private to inform the professional in a concrete way.[16] Elsewhere I have written about this exercise as a way to "decenter" the professional as the hero of the medical story, and a way for both healthcare practitioners and patients to embrace corporeal vulnerability.[17] As philosopher Judith Butler has asserted, this kind of decentering of the protagonist-self is an act of profound social justice that leads beyond an egocentric, binary understanding of the world ("us" vs. "them").[18] Although Butler is meditating on US fantasies of national invulnerability and global mastery that were effectively crumbled after 9-11, her words can be equally applied to the fantasies of professional invulnerability that are so common in medical culture: "We cannot, however, will away this vulnerability. We must attend to it, even abide by it, as we begin to think about what politics might be implied by staying with the thought of corporeal vulnerability itself."[19]

Yet, the texts we were reading together in that early class often fell short of the attention to power and hierarchy I sought to infuse in my students. Who has access to language, the time to write, the ability to get published? Whose voices were we not hearing? I was compelled to ask these questions with my students time and again because of the overwhelming class, race, and other privileges of the illness memoirists we were reading—there were few to no people of color, working class people, queer writers, or non–native English speakers in the bunch. I eventually sought out different written and nonwritten narrative genres—from spoken word poetry about cerebral palsy and sickle cell anemia to film about disability and post-polio syndrome to graphic memoirs about everything from childhood cancer to caring for an ill elderly parent. But I ultimately had to confront the realization that no matter how radical I thought I was being by "listening to the voices of the ill" rather than the voice of the medical establishment, the very parameters and limits of the terms "illness," "disease" or "patienthood" confined me to a very narrow field of study.

It was disability studies and disability activism that gave me the language to critique my own teaching. As someone trained in traditional medicine, I felt bound to a medicalized view of illness, disability, and health, whereby all the texts I assigned were filtered through a medicalized lens. I use "medicalization" here to imply the ways that individuals with disabilities, diseases, or embodied differences have been categorized as "sick" and placed under the jurisdiction of the medical establishment and medical professionals. This model views difference solely through the lens of impairment and is undoubtedly related to what sociologist Arthur Frank has critiqued as medicine's investment in the restitution narrative: the belief at all conditions are treatable through medical intervention, which then returns the "sufferer" to the condition of health and "normalcy."[20]

It was disability theory that helped me understand the risk for medicalization of our field. If mainstream medicine is predicated on the relationship of someone called a "patient" to the health provider and healthcare industry, then the nature of the patient's illness, disability, or other embodied difference is necessarily defined by the clinician and the parameters of diagnostic categories. The power of definition lies outside the self, then, and with the provider and the medical establishment. Although we speak often in narrative medicine and other health humanities fields about listening to and honoring the voices of patients, the challenge made to the binary of "clinician" and "patient" itself must continuously be emphasized.

In health humanities classrooms, learners and facilitators speak often of mutuality in the medical relationship, the necessity for clinicians to consider that, as oral historian Alessandro Portelli has suggested,

> An inter/view is an exchange between *two* subjects: literally a mutual sighting. One party cannot really *see* the other unless the other can see him or her in turn. The two interacting subjects cannot act together unless some kind of mutuality can be established. The field researcher, therefore, has an objective stake in equality, as a condition for a less distorted communication and a less biased collection of data.[21]

This formulation regarding oral history can be extended to clinicians and teachers working at the intersection of humanities and healthcare. Healing and teaching are fundamentally intersubjective inter/views and, as such, experiments in equality. Equality here does not imply that physicians, nurses, or scholars give up their knowledge and authority; rather, it implies putting ourselves in a place of mutuality and transparency in order to promote a better care of our students, clients, and patients, and a more satisfactory professional relationship for ourselves.

But what about an equality not predicated on patienthood or diagnostic categories at all? What about the life of the ill or disabled individual outside of any relation to medical professionals or institutions? Or the person who cannot, or will not, be diagnosed? Disability studies provides health humanities a "citizenship model" of embodied difference as opposed to only the "patient model."[22] As disability scholars including G. Thomas Couser have noted, the social model of disability is one that suggests all human beings have differing abilities; what is disabling is lack of equal physical, economic, and sociocultural access.[23] This is a model that understands embodied and psychological differences outside of its relationship to the medical establishment or the normative constrictions of health. It is a model that places the power of identification and definition with individuals themselves rather than necessarily with clinicians or diagnostic categories. The social model of disability also potentially makes room for that which may be considered illness or disability by others but is not necessarily considered either by the individuals in question. One case in point is the experience of (big D) Deafness, a cultural category of (non-ill, non-disabled) linguistic difference that differentiates itself from (little d) deafness, which is alternately considered an impairment or disability.[24] The Deaf community identifies itself as a linguistic minority, a culture which, like ethnic or sexual minority groups, has a history of oppression and threatened erasure—from Alexander Graham Bell and other oralists who opposed the teaching of sign language, and even the intermarrying of deaf individuals lest they create a "deaf variety of the human race," to the present day use of cochlear implants as well as movements away from teaching sign language and toward lip reading.[25] The resistance of the Deaf community to being considered ill or disabled is a political choice that highlights our challenge: how do we make room in our fields to honor the experiences of those who do not consider themselves "ill" (or disabled) at all?

Cripping my syllabus meant changing its title (I called it *Illness and Disability Narratives* and dropped the notion of "understanding the experience," which seemed particularly totalizing) as well as its content. Rather than a series of memoirs written by individuals possessing different medical diagnoses, I began to conceptualize my syllabus as an ever-expanding series of circles—with the self in the middle, surrounded by circles of family, community, culture, and sociopolitics. Over the course of the semester, then, there weren't weeks dedicated to diseases or particular variations of disability, but rather to works in a variety of genres and forms addressing issues of body, voice, and self, caregiving practices, or embodiment and cultural identity.

Rather than seeking the assuredness of fixed answers, I was—and continue to be—transparent with my students about my own discomforts. What does it mean to teach a course called "Illness and Disability Narratives?" Is such a formulation necessarily making equivalent two states of being that, at least from the disability theory side, are diametrically opposed? And what about experiences such as Deafness, in which community members identify as neither ill nor disabled? What does it mean to teach such a course, which critiques medical power and privilege, in a field called "narrative medicine"? Are our classes, as Chandra Talpade Mohanty has written about women of color in the academy, a superficial nod to diversity without fundamentally challenging the frame within which we are teaching?[26] It continues to be a concern that keeps me critical of my own positionality within this field and this work. In the words of Audre Lorde,

> For the master's tools will never dismantle the master's house. They may allow us to temporarily beat him at his own game, but they will never enable us to bring about genuine change. Racism and homophobia are real conditions of all our lives in this place and time. I urge each one of us here to reach down into that deep place of knowledge inside herself and touch that terror and loathing of any difference that lives here. See whose face it wears. Then the personal as the political can begin to illuminate all our choices.[27]

Is it possible to truly incorporate a disability studies perspective and a medical perspective? This is a question I continue to explore in this work.

Queer Politics and the Problems of Intelligibility

In early 2014, transgender actress Laverne Cox appeared on the cover of *Time Magazine* next to the headline "The Transgender Tipping Point."[28] As trans* activism has gained more attention in the mainstream press in recent years, I too have reached a "tipping point" in understanding the politics of health humanities and my own responsibilities as a teacher in the interdisciplinary field.

In 2013, I took the *Narrative, Health and Social Justice* graduate seminar I had taught for some time in Columbia's master's program in narrative medicine and offered it also as a senior undergraduate seminar through the Center for Comparative Literature and Society's Medicine, Literature and Society track at Columbia. (Eventually, I would also offer this course to undergraduates through the Center for the Study for Ethnicity and Race.) During one session when we discuss bodies and embodiment, we ask ourselves questions like "whose bodies 'count'?" and "whose bodies are discounted?" For this session, I had my class watch, as I usually do, Kate Davis' 2001 documentary *Southern Comfort*, which chronicles the dying of rural Georgia native Robert Eads from uterine and cervical cancer—due partially to physicians who refused to see a transgender man (with "female" reproductive organs still intact) in their offices. The film is powerful and allows the class to discuss medical neglect, transgender communities, and physician prejudices, as well as the ethics of Davis' filmmaking—which avoids a voyeuristic, sensationalizing view of Eads and focuses on Eads' relationship with girlfriend Lola (a transgender woman) as well as their network of transgender friends, Eads' "chosen family."

Alongside Davis' documentary I had the students—as always—read the work of Judith Butler on both medical gender assignment surgeries for infants with "ambiguous genitalia" and her classic work on gender as "a performative act." In Butler's words, "We act and walk and speak and talk in ways that con-solidate an impression of being a man or being a woman . . . We act as if that being of a man or that being of a woman is actually an internal reality or some-thing that is simply true about us, a fact about us, but actually it's a phenom-enon that is being produced all the time and reproduced all the time."[29]

In my graduate seminar I would usually begin our class discussions the week we watched *Southern Comfort* by showing a clip from a very different film, Duncan Tucker's 2005 *Transamerica*,[30] a cross-country road trip buddy film in which a transgender woman named Bree (played by non-trans* actress Felicity Huffman) takes a cross-country road trip with a teenage son she conceived in the past but did not know about. The clip begins with Huffman practicing a "feminine" voice, then getting dressed in a stereotypical pink skirt suit and stockings, painting her nails, brushing her hair, practicing a stereotypically "feminine" walk, and the like. Huffman's character then ends up in a psychia-trist's office, where she has to jump through the hoops of proving her diagnosis with GID (gender identity disorder) in order to earn a physician signature on the paperwork that will allow her to undergo transitional surgery.

My goal in showing this clip is usually to get students thinking about gender as performativity as well as medicine's role in policing the gender binary. Included in the clip is the following exchange between Bree and her doctor:

"The American psychiatric foundation categorizes gender dysphoria as a very serious mental disorder."

—Doctor

"After my operation not even a gynecologist would be able to detect anything out of the ordinary about my body. I will be a woman. Don't you find it odd that plastic sur-gery can cure a 'mental disorder'?"

—Bree

Despite the clip's potentially critical portrayal of how (gender) queer bodies are medicalized and how trans* people are forced to submit to reductive diag-nostic categorizations, my sophisticated undergraduate students were beyond frustrated with *Transamerica*. I will never forget the words of one student, who was not himself trans* but identified himself as an ally of the commu-nity. Forget the issue of whether Felicity Huffman should have been given the role over a trans* identified actress, this student argued that the film's focus on binary gender signifiers (pink clothes, nails, etc.) was typical of a *cis*-dominant society's voyeuristic fascination with trans* bodies—particularly trans* genitalia. "The film only reinforces the idea that trans* folks are obligated to make themselves intelligible in that way to everyone else," argued my student. Unlike *Southern Comfort,* he suggested, mainstream films like *Transamerica* did very little to move the conversation away from physical transitioning, and in fact only reinforced the rigidity of the gender binary. A trans* individual, this student argued, was only intelligible to the mainstream when either one of two binary genders is firmly on the way from one to another. There was no room in such narratives for challenging the gender binary itself, no space for gender fluidity and those who would seek to obscure rather than illuminate any sense of "understanding" of their gender and body by others.

Much moved by my undergraduate student's comments regarding the demands of intelligibility and recognition, I began guiding the class discussion on *Southern Comfort* and trans* health issues with a 2014 clip of transgender actress and activist Laverne Cox being interviewed by Katie Couric. To Couric's rather pointed questions about her transition, genitalia, and surgeries (or lack thereof), Cox refused to answer, instead saying,

> The preoccupation with transition and with surgery objectifies trans people. And then we don't get to really deal with the real lived experiences—the reality of trans people's lives is that so often we are the targets of violence. We experience discrimination disproportionately to the rest of the community. Our unemployment rate is double the national average; if you're a trans person of color it's four times the national average. Rates of homicide in the LGBT community are highest among trans women. And if we focus on transition, we don't get to talk about those things.[31]

The demand to "know" the Other's "true self"/"true body" is of course a characteristic of the surveillance state. As opposed to the disciplinary control of Foucauldian biopower, modern day surveillance is predicated on a surveillance assemblage where obtaining knowledge about the other is of paramount importance.[32] Also useful here are Judith Butler's comments about recognition-as-power:

> If the schemes of recognition that are available to us are those that "undo" the person by conferring recognition, or "undo" the person by withholding recognition, then recognition becomes a site of power by which the human is differentially produced.... The question of who and what is considered real and true is apparently a question of knowledge. But it is also, as Michel Foucault makes plain, a question of power.[33]

Butler's comments about recognition deepen our understanding of the tension between Katie Couric's desire to know about transgender bodies and Laverne

Cox's demand that she leave that question obscured and instead attend to transgender lives.

Un-homing Narrative Medicine: Pedagogical Frames

To write the Couric/Cox conversation onto postcolonial relations, let me take a moment to discuss a text that examines both gender and sexual identity as well as racial and imperialistic relations. Consider David Henry Hwang's 1998 play *M. Butterfly*, a play I read with narrative medicine graduate students in a course called "Embodied Borderlands: Diasporic Fictions and Narrative Medicine." In the play, recognition of the colonized by the colonizer is an imaginative enterprise whereby the "Other" is conceptualized by the imperialistic "Self" using maps of Orientalism and racial binarism.[34] Hwang's play uses the real-life story of Rene Gallimard, a French diplomat imprisoned for treason after it was discovered he was for years passing governmental secrets to his Chinese lover. Central to Hwang's play and Gallimard's actual trial was the Frenchman's claim that he was never, over the course of a 20+-year relationship, aware that his lover Song Liling was a man presenting himself as a woman. In Hwang's play this is due, for the most part, to Gallimard being in love with not a real man or woman but his imagined conception of the perfect "Oriental" woman: the self-sacrificing, exotic, and loyal Madame Butterfly. When, at the end of the play, Song insists on revealing his unclothed (male) body to Gallimard, the following exchange takes place:

GALLIMARD: . . . what exactly are you?

. . . . . .

SONG: I'm your butterfly. Under the robes, beneath everything, it was always me. Now, open your eyes and admit it—you adore me.

. . . .

GALLIMARD: You showed me your true self. When all I loved was the lie. A perfect lie, which you let fall to the ground – and now, it's old and soiled.

SONG: So—you never loved me? Only when I was playing a part?

GALLIMARD: I'm a man who loved a woman created by a man. Everything else—simply falls short. . . . I am pure imagination. And in imagination I will remain. Now get out![35]

Here, then, is a complication of the colonizer's demand to know the subaltern body. In Gallimard's case, what he wants is the "Eastern woman" of his fantasy and for Song to be the canvas, the mirror upon which to cast this imagined figure. When Song wants to show his lover his "true" body, Gallimard is repulsed. Gallimard, perhaps like Couric, wants to know the Other but only on his own terms and through his own frames. Anything beyond that narrow set of parameters is rendered unrecognizable ("get out!").

What is the implication of these understandings about the gender binary, as well as the demands of intelligibility upon "other" bodies, and the work of narrative medicine and health humanities? On the subject of intersubjectivity, narrative medicine at Columbia has been deeply influenced by the work of philosopher Emmanuel Levinas. Among other things, Levinas reminds health humanities practitioners not to totalize but to approach the Other with "that sense of humility toward that which we do not know—the face of the Other. The face we cannot know but to which we are responsible."[36] With Levinas' cautions in mind, how can we understand another who does not occupy fixed spaces on either side of socially constructed binaries, those whose identities obscure these very categories—the gender queer individual, the culturally Deaf family, the ill clinician, the listener who also must tell, the Other who is simultaneously the Self? Our goal must be to challenge such binaries of difference.

Indeed, as I have discovered in my grappling with health humanities pedagogy through the lens of crip and queer understandings, there is a potential violence in making ourselves at home in these seemingly immutable categories. Consider: in health humanities classrooms and workshops all around this country, students/participants are often asked to read, write, and share together. Yet, when conducted without attention to the power of the pedagogy, such workshops risk becoming environments of surveillance. Despite allowing a sense of humility and mystery toward the Other who is understood to be the patient, health humanities workshops potentially demand an emotional vulnerability and candor from preclinical and clinical students that is akin to the demands of intelligibility made upon trans* bodies. If workshop/classroom rules are not clearly articulated—including the possibility to opt out of sharing aloud one's in-class writing—facilitators risk creating unsafe environments and stifling narrative medicine's possibilities of revelation and self-discovery.

Novelist Iris Murdoch once wrote that that "a novel must be a house fit for free characters to live in."[37] Writer Alice Munro suggests that "a story is not like a road to follow . . . it's more like a house. You go inside and stay there for a while . . . discovering . . . how the world outside is altered by being viewed from these windows."[38] To enter a narrative and have one's perspective of the world altered is at the heart of narrative medicine. Yet, are all homes equally welcoming? How, in the process of entering such narratives, does difference—in identity, in power, in body, in history—*among* narrative medicine practitioners and students get understood? Without attention to the power of the pedagogy, narrative-based teaching in health humanities risks being the exact opposite of "homely," particularly for those clinicians, students, and scholars whose identities, bodies, or ways of being in the world place them at the sociopolitical margins.

In response to Murdoch's claims about fiction's "homeliness," literary theorist Homi Bhabha asks, "[W]hat kind of narrative can house unfree people? Is the novel also a house where the unhomely can live?"[39] Bhabha's concept of the "unhomely" in postcolonial experience can be extended, and we can ask ourselves: "What kind of narrative can house marginalized peoples? Is narrative medicine a house where the unhomely can live?"

The bioethical implications of clinicians writing about patients is a topic of much discussion in the health humanities fields, particularly in the age of social media.[40] Equally pressing, however, are the bioethical implications of asking our health humanities students to write and share about themselves in our classrooms. Of particular concern to me in this essay is how such self-revelatory exercises, conducted without attention to difference, structural power, and the privacy of students, is potentially an act of violence and surveillance.

So, what are pedagogical frameworks to help teachers and facilitators better enable an ethical practice of health humanities work? I would venture that the three pedagogical pillars supporting socially just narrative practices are narrative humility, structural competency, and engaged pedagogy.

NARRATIVE HUMILITY: THE ROLE OF THE FACILITATOR

I first wrote about the term *narrative humility* in 2008, adapting the idea from Melanie Tervalon and Jann Murray-Garcia's term *cultural humility,* which they suggested as an alternative to traditional approaches to cultural competency in medicine.[41] Tervalon and Murray-Garcia argued that medicine tends to reify culture into fixed facts, which encourages practitioners to approach cultural background as something they can completely understand. Instead, they suggested that practitioners acknowledge how their own backgrounds affect the ways in which they interpret the views and values of others. Narrative humility in medicine extends this notion to all narratives a clinician encounters, not just those of people identified as cultural "others." Indeed, even those patients who seemingly share a clinician's social positions and identities must be approached with humility—a sense of wonder and the understanding that some aspect of their stories will necessarily be unfamiliar or unknowable. Narrative humility in medicine suggests that rather than looking out and learning all there is to know about racially marginalized or other communities, clinicians begin by looking inward and becoming aware of our own prejudices, expectations, and frames of listening.

Narrative humility in health humanities practice requires that we teachers and facilitators reflect on our own power when we teach and elicit narratives from our students. If I am teaching students who depend on me for their grades, how can I ensure that they feel both safe sharing their reflective writing and comfortable opting *not* to share? Do I see myself as a didactic instructor or, as educator Paulo Freire would suggest, a co-learner? How do I understand my own prejudices and expectations, ensuring that all participants' voices are heard? Do I approach with defensiveness or openness those students who disrupt my plans or disagree with my teachings? Faculty facilitators determine and define the parameters of their classrooms with every small decision, including how we open the class, how much we speak, and whom we call upon. Establishing classroom safety, delineating classroom rules regarding confidentiality and community responsibility, and paying attention to how social power plays out in the group are critical roles that a narrative medicine facilitator must play, and a stance of humility is one way for a teacher or clinician to attend to these issues of personal and sociocultural power.

STRUCTURAL COMPETENCY: NARRATIVE CONTEXTS

Structural competency is the notion that structural forces (for example, poverty, food availability, or gender-based violence) are just as important for physicians to consider as physiological determinants of disease.[42] In the work of health humanities, structural competency involves understanding not only patients' but students' individual stories against wider narratives of sociopolitical and cultural power. Which stories are usually told and heard in hospitals and medical schools? Which are silenced or marginalized? How is, for example, a trans* student's narrative heard by *cis*-gendered faculty colleagues, if at all? Might a faculty member's decision to use only binary gendered pronouns (he/she) without asking for students' preference make such a student feel vulnerable and unsafe in the classroom? What are the broader structural forces that may impact that person's ability to speak honestly in a workshop setting— will they be subject to harassment or differential treatment in the hospital or educational institution?

ENGAGED PEDAGOGY: THE ARCHITECTURE
OF HEALTH HUMANITIES

Engaged pedagogy is a teaching philosophy written about extensively by bell hooks. In her words, "To teach in a manner that respects and cares for the souls of our students is essential if we are to provide the necessary conditions where learning can most deeply and intimately begin."[43] Caring for the souls of our students seems a tall order, but it has practical manifestations. What sorts of ways do we as teachers and facilitators welcome our students and their role in the collaborative learning enterprise? Even in a short workshop setting, I find it impossible not to do some kind of introductions, both to understand to whom I am speaking and as a first step in acknowledging students'/participants' roles as co-creators of the educational enterprise. In a longer-term classroom setting I often spend the first few weeks privileging interpersonal dynamics and the community-building aspects of the classroom.

Engaged pedagogy also demands that classroom safety comes again to the fore. Collaboratively decided classroom rules, an attention to group dynamics, and a reiterative process of checking in with students is critical to an engaged pedagogy. So too is attention to what we teachers ask of our students. For instance, a writing exercise that asks students to describe an incident of personal suffering might feel appropriate at the end of a semester-long class, but it could be overwhelming during a one-hour single-session workshop with no closure or communal "safe space" established with the group members. If we are training for a more attentive, engaged, and affiliated clinical practice, then we must model this intersubjectivity in our classrooms and workshops.[44]

Yet, even as I invoke the health humanities classroom as a parallel process, a blueprint for dynamics in the clinic room (whereby teaching in nonhierarchical, empowering ways models for clinical students nonhierarchical, empowering relationships with their future patients), I would also suggest that an engaged pedagogy means, perhaps, moving away from the rigid walls of a narrative (medicine) "home" altogether and realizing that each of us—patients, clinicians, facilitators, teachers, participants, students—understands the work of narrative medicine slightly differently. And that boundarylessness is, in fact, narrative medicine's strength. The way that I, with my particular identity and perspective, teach narrative medicine in New York is necessarily different from the way my colleagues may teach in my own institution and certainly from the way it might be taught by someone else in, say, Mumbai or Sydney or London. Un-homing narrative medicine is also acknowledging its flexibility and malleability, and the fact that this work depends deeply on process, on a collective experience of striving together rather than on any reified and fixed frames.

Conclusion

Cripping, queering and un-homing narrative medicine are acts which remind us that the true potential of health humanities fields lies in their ability to evolve through self-critical analysis. The work of narrative medicine is perhaps not about finding a "home" at all, but about embracing the state of being "unhomed," both at and ultimately beyond boundaries. The work of narrative medicine pedagogy, then, is in the interstitial spaces between multiple states of being—healer and ill, citizen and patient, teacher and student—while simultaneously finding spaces away from such reductive binaries. The coauthored space of narrative work can no longer be considered a singular "home" of any sort, but rather a multiply layered space and time—a heterotopia that not only affirms difference but, as Foucault suggests, provides an alternative to authoritarian power and oppression.[45] Or perhaps the narrative medicine classroom is ideally akin to what postmodern thinker Edward Soja calls a "thirdspace"; that is, a space

> . . . in which everything comes together . . . subjectivity and objectivity, the abstract and the concrete, the real and the imagined, the knowable and the unimaginable, the repetitive and the differential, structure and agency, mind and body, consciousness and the unconscious, the disciplined and the transdisciplinary, everyday life and unending history.[46]

For me, this work of narrative medicine is both deeply personal and deeply political. It is a way to teach and continue to learn truths about power, meaning, witnessing, collectivizing, and growing. In the words, again, of hooks, "We come to this space through suffering and pain, through struggle. We know struggle to be that which pleasures, delights, and fulfills desire. We are transformed, individually, collectively, as we make radical creative space which affirms and sustains our subjectivity, which gives us a new location from which to articulate our sense of the world."[47]

I would like to thank and acknowledge all my colleagues and students in narrative medicine, but particularly my former students/now cherished colleagues Rebecca K. Tsevat, Anoushka A. Sinha, and Kevin J. Gutierrez, who have been instrumental in furthering my understanding the politics of narrative medicine pedagogy. An earlier version of some of these thoughts was coauthored with these three fine scholars in Academic Medicine *(2015).*

Tsevat, R. K., Sinha, A. A., Gutierrez, K. J., & DasGupta, S. "Bringing Home the Health Humanities: Narrative Humility, Structural Competency, and Engaged Pedagogy." *Academic Medicine* 90(11) (2015): 1462–1465. Permission to reprint portions of this essay in this chapter is granted by Walters Kluwer Health, Inc., of Lippincott Williams & Wilkins for *Academic Medicine*.

Notes

1. hooks, *Feminist Theory*, preface to the first edition, xvi.
2. Morrison, *Home*, 1.

3. See Freire, *Pedagogy of the Oppressed*; hooks, *Teaching to Transgress*; Mohanty, *Feminism without Borders*.

4. Mohanty, *Feminism*, 194–95.

5. I use the more encompassing term *health humanities* to include narrative medicine, medical humanities, literature and medicine, and other similar fields. For more, see Jones, Wear, and Friedman, *The Health Humanities Reader*.

6. Trans* with an asterisk is used here to imply a broad range of non-*cis*-gendered identities, including but not limited to those who identify as transgender, transsexual, gender queer, agender, third gender, genderfluid, two spirit, etc. I also use the terms *crip* and *queer* here in solidarity with communities who have reclaimed those otherwise derogatory terms as spaces of political identification.

7. Schalk, "Coming to Claim Crip."

8. Eng, Halberstam, and Muñoz, "What's Queer," 1.

9. Bhaba, "World and the Home."

10. Mohanty, 195.

11. Mohanty, 195.

12. hooks, *Yearning*, 206.

13. The first such graduate program in the country. www.slc.edu.

14. I use illness as opposed to disease in this essay, following the lead of Arthur Kleinman, who has discussed disease as implying physiological impairment and illness as encompassing far more—the entirety of the individual's life context.

15. See DasGupta, "Teaching Medical Listening."

16. See DasGupta and Charon, "Personal Illness Narratives."

17. See DasGupta, "Decentering."

18. See Butler, *Precarious Life*.

19. Butler, *Precarious Life*, 29.

20. See Frank, *Wounded Storyteller*. See also DasGupta, "Medicalization."

21. Portelli, "Research as an Experiment," 31.

22. See the work of G. Thomas Couser and others for a discussion of the models of disability—the moral or spiritual (disability caused by moral failing), the medical (disability as impairment in need of medical intervention), and the social (we all have differing abilities; what is disabling is the discrimination or the lack of access).

23. See Couser, *Recovering Bodies*.

24. See Lane, "Constructions of Deafness."

25. Although the Deaf community's position against cochlear implants was initially quite adamant, there is some increasing acceptance of cochlear implants.

26. See Mohanty, *Feminism without Borders*.

27. Lorde, "The Master's Tools," 112.

28. See Steinmetz, "Transgender."

29. Butler, "Your Behavior Creates."

30. *Transamerica* 2006

31. Couric, "*Orange is the New Black*'s Laverne Cox."

32. See Haggerty and Ericson, "Surveillant."

33. Butler, *Undoing Gender*, 2, 27.

34. See Said, *Orientalism*. See also Frantz Fanon's *Black Skin, White Masks*, where he discusses how metaphoric understandings of race (black = bad, white = good) helped justify the French colonial project.

35. Hwang, 89–91.

36. Irvine, "The Other Side," 10.

37. Murdoch, "Sublime and Beautiful," 271.

38. Munro, *Selected Stories*, 8.

39. Bhaba, "World and the Home," 142.

40. See Ofri, "Passion and the Peril."

41. See DasGupta, "Narrative Humility"; Tervalon and Murray-Garcia, "Cultural Humility."
42. See Metzl, "Structural Competency."
43. hooks, *Teaching to Transgress*, 13.
44. See Charon, *Narrative Medicine*.
45. See Foucault, "Of Other Spaces."
46. Soja, *Thirdspace*, 5.
47. Hooks, *Yearning*, 209.

PART

CLOSE READING

CHAPTER 7

Close Reading: The Signature Method of Narrative Medicine

Rita Charon

Narrative medicine is committed to developing deep and accurate attention to the accounts of self that are told and heard in the contexts of healthcare. Whether in settings of individual clinical care, health promotion, or global health activism, our deepest mission is to improve healthcare by recognizing the persons who seek help with their health. Along with the accuracy of recognition come the powerful consequences for the person—of having been heard, of having achieved an unimpeded and free voicing of the matter at hand.

From such diverse fields outside of healthcare as literary criticism, anthropology, oral history, phenomenology, consciousness studies, and aesthetic theory, narrative medicine has developed methods that strengthen the capacity of the clinician to recognize the patient by attending closely to what he or she conveys. Toward the goal of a full, nonjudgmental, generative reception that is informed by all aspects of what a teller tells—in words, silences, gestures, position, mood, prior utterances—the attentive listener absorbs what is given and can then *return* to the teller a representation of what was heard. As if to say, "This is what I think you told me," the listener reflects back in affirmation his or her witnessed version of a conversation, giving the teller a view, as a starting point, of what might have been told.

The consequences of attentive and accurate listening in a clinical practice can include deep companionship between teller and listener, mutual investment, reciprocal clarity, and affiliation—ideally hallmarks of healthcare itself. That such listening was perhaps better achieved in the time of Hippocrates and Galen and Chekhov than in contemporary practice alerts us to deep-seated tensions within a contemporary bioscientific ethos that challenges the particular with the universal, the personal with the corporate, and the intimate with the mechanized.[1] Earnest efforts have been made by health educators over the past several decades to impart listening skills and psychological/affective insight to trainees in many of the health professions.[2] Many disciplines and practices have been recruited to improve the listening performance of clinicians: communication studies, literature and medicine, improvisational theater, health psychology, discourse analysis, and linguistics. Despite the range of sources and skills bent toward the effort to improve clinical listening, patients continue to complain that their doctors, at least, don't listen to them, and so patients find their way to alternative healers, even if they need to pay directly for their services, *because* these practitioners are better able to attend to what they say. Narrative medicine evolved from and has learned from these many teaching projects to strengthen the capacity for accurate, clinically useful listening, bringing to the effort its particular commitment to the acts of reading, the discovery potential of writing, and the intersubjective contact made possible by stories.

The Origin and Fate of Close Reading

> It is difficult
> to get the news from poems
> yet men die miserably every day
> for lack
> of what is found there.

—William Carlos Williams
Asphodel, *that Greeny Flower*

Narrative medicine's recognition of attention as a requirement for empathic and effective care of one person by another—whether or not this occurs in a healthcare setting—accounts for our deepening examination of the acts of reading. Both a model for and an avenue toward attention, close reading fortified with attention to its subjective dimensions has become narrative medicine's laboratory and training ground.

Literary scholar Rita Felski writes in *Uses of Literature* that "[t]he practice of close reading is tacitly viewed by many literary scholars as the mark of their tribe—as what sets them apart, in the last instance, from their like-minded colleagues in sociology or history. . . . A sharply honed attentiveness to nuances of language and form . . . simply is, in Rorty's phrase, what we do around here."[3] A term with a history of contention, *close reading* is both a brand-name term for a movement within literary criticism that arose in the 1920s and flowered among the New Critics of the 1940s and 1950s and a generic term for attentive, critical, careful reading. In the following section I will briefly rehearse the history of the appearance of the term and summarize some of the controversies that continue to surround it and will then describe in detail why narrative medicine recognizes close reading as an inspiration and method for respectful and effective healthcare.

Like other transformative ideas, close reading has had many beginnings.[4] In the period between the world wars, this new form of criticism arose when literary scholars sought a fresh examination of the processes of literary acts. The earliest writings about close reading, and the first use of the phrase, were published in the United Kingdom by literary scholar I. A. Richards, starting in the 1920s with the publication of *Practical Criticism* and *Principles of Literary Criticism*.

Richards sought to consider the nature of the thought and experience undergone by the reader. Protean, his work spanned the study of Peircean semiotics, the psychology of interpretation, the philosophy of rhetoric, and the individual consequences of aesthetic experiences.[5] A poet himself, Richards probed not only the meaning of the words of a poem but also the means by which language gives birth to thought and feeling through signs, symbolism, perception, and aesthetic beauty. He proposed radical views on the function of literary criticism, emphasizing attention to individual readers' interpretive process in addition to the attention to the text itself, and asserting therapeutic dividends to the reader who integrates conflicting perceptions into an aesthetic whole. Richards took his conceptual start by contesting Kant's notion that the aesthetic realm exists separate from ordinary life. "Ever since 'the first rational word concerning beauty' was spoken by Kant, the attempt to define the 'judgment of taste' as concerning pleasure which is disinterested, universal, unintellectual, and not to be confused with the pleasures of sense or of ordinary emotions, in short to make it a thing *sui generis,* has continued."[6] Instead, Richards passionately proposed, starting in *The Meaning of Meanings* co-written by C. K. Ogden in 1923 and then in *Principles of Literary Criticism*, that the sense of beauty is available to all humans, that they depend on it to live their ordinary days, and that there are no powers of seeing restricted to the "professional" seers. Richards sought to bring the experience of beauty back to ordinary life:

> When we look at a picture, or read a poem, or listen to music, we are not doing something quite unlike what we were doing on our way to the Gallery or when we dressed in the morning. The fashion in which the experience is caused in us is different and as a rule the experience is more complex and, if we are successful, more unified. But our activity is not of a fundamentally different kind.[7]

Richards saw that human consciousness is capable of aesthetic acts even without formal training or artistic gift, and that one uses ordinary experiences as works of art. Accordingly, his interest in literary criticism, his "practical criticism," was founded on the desire to return to readers the dividends of authentically undergone aesthetic experience. He taught his poetry classes at Harvard by distributing four poems per week. "Extremely good and extremely bad poems were put *unsigned* before a large and able audience."[8] The matter of the course was furnished by the responses to these poems anonymously submitted, in writing, by the undergraduate students. Their own aesthetic responses to the texts—where they were driven in mind and mood and sense of form—were treated as more authoritative than anything written by experts about the work or the artist. If "What is art *for*?" was close reading's foundational and eternal and brave question, the answer focused on the interior experiences of the readers themselves.

A student and then colleague of Richards in the development of close reading, William Empson, delineated the aspects of literary texts that make them literary. First published in 1930, his *Seven Types of Ambiguity* spearheaded the practices of seeking the paradox, tone, irony, and antinomies in poetry, turning the critical tide away from the time's conventional philological and archival approaches to texts toward a fine and focused examination of the complexities of the text itself.[9]

From the beginning, the continents clashed on the nature of this new form of literary activity. In the United States, starting in the 1940s, notably in the South, close reading was championed by John Crowe Ransom, Cleanth Brooks, T. S. Eliot, Robert Penn Warren, and their associates—an effort tinged for some of them with a nostalgia for the by-then bygone Southern agrarianism.[10] This literary movement of the early 1950s valorized extremely focused readings, mostly of poems, with no attention to the contexts of the poems or to objective correlatives in the life experience of the poet. In an effort to systematize the reading of poetry toward a scientific analysis, the New Critics proposed that seeking the author's intention in writing or the reader's emotional response to a text—what they called the *intentional fallacy* and the *affective fallacy*—could misdirect the critic's effort to understand the poem.[11]

Brooks' *The Well-Wrought Urn* offered extensive literary commentaries on ten poems, all of them English, from the seventeenth century to the 1940s. The ten included works of Donne, Shakespeare, Milton, Herrick, Pope, Gray, Wordsworth, Keats, Tennyson, and Yeats. Unlike Richards and Empson, the American New Critics were not interested in the reader's situation. They modeled an ivory-cool cognitive approach to the poem, minimizing the presence of either the poet or the reader in the development of meaning. For example, in discussing Robert Herrick's poem "Corrina's going a-Maying," Brooks writes:

To say that Herrick "communicates" certain matters to the reader tends to falsify the real situation. The old description of the poet was better and less dangerous: the poet is a maker, not a communicator. He explores, consolidates, and "forms" the total experience that is the poem.[12]

Over time, the positions of the American and British close readers influenced one another, not tempering their conflicting positions but enlarging and complicating their own scopes of vision. The 1960 edition of Brook's and Warren's *Understanding Poetry*, initially published in 1938, states in the Preface: "Poetry gives us knowledge. It is a knowledge of ourselves in relation to the world of experience, and to that world considered, not statistically, but in terms of human purposes and values. . . . The knowledge that poetry yields is available to us only if we submit ourselves to the massive, and subtle, impact of the poem as a whole."[13] They highlight for this edition considerations of the contexts of the poem's creation, its historical moment, and the actions of the individual readers in recognizing the implications of the form. Hence, the history of close reading not only maps profound disagreements on what it means to read a poem but also the literary process of interrelation and influence.

The 1970's and 1980's cataclysmic theoretical revolutions in literary studies—the influence of the anthropology and linguistics of Claude Levi-Strauss and Roman Jakobson;[14] the structuralism of Roland Barthes and Jonathan Culler;[15] the deconstructive turn ushered by Jacques Derrida, Jean-François Lyotard, and Julia Kristeva;[16] the influence of Marxist theories of history of Fredric Jameson;[17] the impact of the post-Freudian psychoanalysis of Jacques Lacan;[18] and the vision of Michel Foucault's macroanalyses of power and system[19]—transformed readers' understanding of what they do when they read. The response of those schooled in New Criticism was marked at the start more by resistance than excitement, for, as summarized by Andrew DuBois,

[T]he move into theory proper is marked by a move into linguistics and a break from aesthetics. This may be why so many critics considered theory detrimental to the reading of literature, since "reading" and "literature" are intertwined not only with aesthetics but with aesthetic *appreciation*. To remove this as a grounding critical consideration was by some accounts tantamount to the annihilation of reading as we had known it.[20]

Despite such reservations, with the benefit of contemporary theory, literary scholars of the time found new means to closely examine the words on the page, now in view of all that might be hidden in the subtexts or historical/political/psychological shadows of the work. The massive and generative turns that culminated in the postmodern era made possible a raft of probing reading approaches that took account of social power, individual identity, and political dominance and powerlessness. Such schools of theory as New Historicism, feminist criticism, queer studies, Marxist criticism, autobiographical theory, reader-response and reception studies, and psychoanalytic methods of criticism widened the ground on which the writer and reader were visualized to stand and expanded the range of questions one could ask of a text and its actions.

Close reading has received sustained critique, both at the time of its rise in the 1950s and more recently by cultural studies scholars, autobiographical theorists, and world literature proponents. Some charged that New Criticism, through its careful attention to a small selection of texts, endorsed a narrow and elite canon of works, restricted in general to white males writing in English, as suitable to study. If only the words on the page matter, others alleged, the reader need not contextualize the work by time or space or person. Such matters as race, language, class, or gender are seen to not come in for the attention they require of the reader.

Despite these critiques, close reading has never been abandoned in the classroom and the academy but has sequentially been informed, fortified, challenged, and sharpened by intellectual and creative cultural movements.[21] Seasoned by a postmodern awareness of the indeterminacy of language and the contingency of meaning and reference, close readers continue to examine what they do when they read. In the preface to their 2003 study called *Close Reading*, Frank Lentricchia and Andrew DuBois write that they intend to

> represent and undercut what we take to be the major clash in the practice of literary criticism in the past century: that between the so-called formalist and so-called non-formalist [especially "political"] modes of reading . . . The common ground, then, is a commitment to close attention to literary texture and what is embodied there. We emphasize the continuity, not the clash of critical schools . . . We like to imagine an ideal literary critic as one who commands and seamlessly integrates both styles of reading.[22]

Not only has the classroom teaching of close reading survived into the present, but the critical conversation about it has proliferated as well. Lentricchia's and DuBois' hope may be, to some extent, fulfilled as current studies of close reading combine formalist concerns and methods with cultural/political ones. Stephen Best and Sharon Marcus introduce a 2009 special issue of *Representations* entitled "The Way We Read Now" with a discussion of the reversal of Paul Ricoeur's hermeneutics of suspicion, in reign during the rise of theory, that instructed the critic to dig below the surface of the text in a chronic state of seeming paranoia that any meaningful aspect of a text would have been suppressed.[23] Such symptomatic reading—seeking signs of disease or malice within the text—is being replaced, they suggest, with forms of "surface reading" that might disavow the need to master the text and all its secrets and, rather, to discern its manifest intricacy and pluripotency—in effect, another turn of the spiral toward attention to the words on the page. D.A. Miller notices "too-close reading" as an obsessive distraction for the reader who cannot ignore anything in the text, and yet finds himself in a state of being hailed, almost in friendship, by a work of art so closely known, as if the work of art knows him.[24] Such formulations of contemporary reading, articulating new conceptions of the nature of both "close" and "reading," join to form a lineage of studies moving away from reading as suspicion toward a recognition of reading as reparation, recognition, and pleasure.[25]

Accompanying these movements within criticism is an explosive attention to the role of emotion and empathy in reading, two central and contested dimensions in the original emergence of close reading.[26] Consciousness studies, theory of mind investigations, neuroscientific investigations of brain activity, and psychological probings into literary actions have attracted interest and funding toward explicating the biological consequences of reading and writing.[27] Banner headlines are made of studies proving that reading fiction, but not nonfiction, triggers empathic activity in the brain of the reader.[28] Neuroscientists try to pinpoint the areas of the brain responsible for these findings, even though the currently available imaging methods are still quite primitive. The existence of such bodies as "The International Society for Empirical Research in Literature" and such fields as "Scientific Study of Literature" alert literary scholars and neuroscientists of a new effort, to some troubling and to others promising, to master the machinery of reading as if its performance was indeed housed only in the brain.

Despite the excesses of the reductionist tendencies to map profound human experiences with brain imaging tests, this upsurge in interest in the emotional and moral consequences of reading heralds promise.[29] It seems to me to be a latter-day recuperation of reader-response studies, a school of critical interest that arose in the 1970s, peaked in the late 1980s, and has been rarely discussed since the turn of this century.[30] Reader-response, during its brief tenure, sought to understand the interior activities of the reader. Formulations of the transactions between reader and text as both aesthetic and moral (Louise Rosenblatt), Proustian descriptions of the trance-like experience of being possessed by a book (Georges Poulet), psychological studies of characterological moves made by the reader (Norman Holland), interest in the workings of interpretive communities of readers (Stanley Fish), phenomenological investigations of readers' experiences (Wolfgang Iser), gendered studies of reading (Elizabeth Flynn and Patricio Schweickart), probing of the subjective experiences of reading (David Bleich), and locating readers' personal responses within the process of rhetoric (Booth) composed a vital and productive realm of criticism. Reader-response was a departure from New Criticism's objective and analytic goals toward an interest in the subjectivity of reading and a commitment to explore and understand it.[31]

Our adoption of close reading as a central method for narrative medicine training and practice blends multiple currents in these decades of study of the ways we read. The fine, disciplined examination of formal features of poetry or prose cannot be overlooked in any serious reading or hearing of texts. In addition, the attention to emotion that arose in reader-response study and now continues in some of the subjective and philosophical studies of literary acts is pivotal to a singular understanding of the transaction between *this* text and *this* reader. The intersubjective contact among members of an interpretive community, whether in a graduate course or on the hospital wards or within a dyad in clinical care, is made possible through this contemporary version of close reading that is fortified with attention to the reader himself or herself. By adopting a critical stance that combines the timeless practice of close reading with attention to the roles of emotion and intersubjectivity in how the reader reads, we hope to be able to maintain deep disciplinary roots in the major movements of literary criticism and reading theory while contributing to clinical work's examination of its complex sites of written and oral textuality. We hope to move toward Lentricchia's and DuBois' state of "command[ing] and seamlessly integrat[ing] both styles of reading," bringing Richards's commitment to the ordinary reader's experience, Brooks's laser concentration on the formal characteristics of a text, a reader-response awareness of the complexity of the reader/text transaction, and the postmodern fluidity among schools of political and cultural criticisms to learn how we experience texts, what happens to us as a result of our reading, and how acts of reading change the world.

Why Narrative Medicine Is Committed to Close Reading

In an essay in the 2007 Modern Languages Association's *Profession*, feminist scholar Jane Gallop writes that "Close reading ... learned through practice with literary texts, learned in literature classes, is a widely applicable skill, of value not just to scholars in other disciplines but to a wide range of students with many different futures. Students trained in close reading have been known to apply it to diverse sorts of texts—newspaper articles, textbooks in other disciplines, political speeches—and thus to discover things they would not otherwise have noticed."[32]

If close reading helps persons "to discover things they would not otherwise have noticed," perhaps it might help clinicians to notice what their patients try to tell them. The close reader, as Tompkins suggests, becomes gradually more receptive to appreciating texts outside of the literature class. She continues: "This enhanced, intensified reading can prove invaluable for many kinds of jobs as well as in their lives." Transcending the conventional boundaries of close reading, narrative medicine reading practices reach beyond literary texts to examine and try to understand visual and musical arts, personal conversations, the mood in a room, or the silent communication of performance and gesture.[33]

The dividends for narrative medicine in close reading are found in those features that distinguish it from casual, technical, or information-seeking reading. The close reader absorbs a text, squandering nothing. Whether reading a novel, a lyric poem, or a paper in *JAMA*, he or she notes the genre, the diction, the temporal structure, the spaces depicted, and the metaphorical and musical work being done with the words. The close reader registers who is telling the text's story—whether first-person or third-person narrator, whether or not this narrator is involved in the action of the plot, whether remote, familiar, reliable, inviting, or combative. The close reader appreciates the text's meter and rhythm; he or she recognizes when the text alludes to some other text outside of itself. As if in conversation with the author, the reader is aware of his or her own place in the text, asking questions about the contract with the author that emerges from the text. What duty, the reader asks in the key of narrative ethics, do I incur by reading this book?[34]

Close reading thickens and complicates the effects of the words on the page. The text is treated as a thing of beauty, an occasion of bliss, a created object of both rare delicacy and raw power. Alternatively, it might be experienced as noxious, revolting, denigrating of values held closely by the reader. Or it may be received with indifference, the reader impervious, despite effort, to the forces of the text. Sometimes a reader encounters a book he or she does *not* want to be inhabited by. Literary critic Wayne Booth, who championed the field of ethical criticism, emphatically reserves the right of any reader to refuse to become the kind of reader being demanded by a particular book. You simply close the book.[35] All of these aspects of the text contribute to its ultimate meaning—for this one reader—and help to expose what this reader undergoes by virtue of reading it.

We have shown at Columbia that rigorous close reading can be taught and learned in clinical settings, where its dividends have been found to enhance patient care.[36] But teaching healthcare professionals how to be close readers does far more than improve their interviewing skills. Here is where we find the transformative potential of our practice of narrative medicine. The close reader gradually discovers that the world within the text—be it novel, news-paper story, one's own diary, or an account of illness given by a patient in the emergency room—is real. The creative acts of representation—in writing or telling or painting or composing—do not merely reflect something real but create something real. A work of art results in a product, not a copy. Radical, disturbing, a challenge to reductive objectivity, the realization of the created-ness of the real by and in language can shock the unprepared newcomer to the acts of reading. Rigorous training in close reading—at least narrative medi-cine's version of close reading—improves readers' capacity for attention but also revolutionizes the reader's position in life from being an onlooker check-ing the log of past events to becoming a daring participant in the emergence of reality. The trainee comes to realize that, until told or written or in some way represented, events remain unheard, unconfigured, and therefore imper-ceptible. Such unformed chaotic experiences will not allow themselves to be known. But once configured by language or image or composition, once form has been conferred onto the unformed, the chaos is discernible both by those who witness it and those who hear accounts of it. Once represented, the chaos is at least potentially comprehensible. It will then have been recognized.

Close reading became one of the narrative medicine's foundational meth-ods for its teaching and practice because it serves all the various uses of the reader's skill. For sure, close reading prepares a student to read complex liter-ary texts with attention and skill and even to read or hear accounts of illness with nuance and sophisticated comprehension. At the same time, it fulfills a far more weighty duty. It not only suggests but demonstrates that one's acts as a person who cares for the sick arise from the same "self" as that person who is transported by a Rothko painting, a Bach partita, a novel by Virginia Woolf, or a graphic novel by Alison Bechdel. The close reader becomes, in the end, more deeply and powerfully attuned to all that may lie in awareness and outside of awareness, in consciousness and out of consciousness, in body, in mind, and whatever is left once those two are accounted for; in relation to the voice and the presence of the other. Close reading may be a threshold to a life fully lived.

Close Reading and Its Progeny, Attentive Listening

Close reading develops the capacity for attentive listening. Henry James's dictum to novelists, "Try to be one of those people on whom nothing is lost," can be said to readers; it can also be said to listeners.[37] Time and again, in the office getting to know a new patient, I have the remarkable and identifiable experience of "tuning in," of letting what is being said—usually some form of account of illness—wash over me and wash into me. I submit to it, I relax my vigilance regarding the clinical duties that bristle around any new recitation of illness (the frantic search in the mind for the things to look for in a particular disease, the humiliating ignorance of a medication the patient might name, the anxiety to hear about a thorny symptom) to simply absorb all that is being made manifest. As the shift occurs from "listening like a doctor" to "listening like a reader," my self shifts within my body and consciousness. I roll my chair away from the computer. I let my hands sit in my lap. Instead of being on an edge of ignorance and challenge, I feel summoned by the patient—is it her account? Is it her words? Is it her presence? Is it her action in having come to me because she thinks maybe something good will come of it?—to what feels like a different self, my readerly self. I think it is the difference between being a judging outsider who is being put to the test to know what to do about a problem and being a welcoming receiver of its mystery, willing to sit within all its doubts.

This sequence in the office is not unlike a sequence of close reading. The same alert, creative presence is needed by the reader or the listener; the same attention to all features of the narrating are awakened; the same intimacy between creator and receiver of the narrative is achieved. But close reading is far easier to talk about than is close listening, and maybe this is why we start there. When the words are on a page, when all heads in the seminar can bend over those words and read them simultaneously, each reader undergoes a parallel experience, or at least a personal experience that begins with a parallel ignition and can be inspected. When one person has a conversation with another person and others listen to or hear about the conversation, the passive listeners are simply not having the same experience as the conversant. A conversation cannot be shared in the way that a text can. Perhaps this is why we start with the reading, even if our ultimate destination is the listening.

Reading is teachable. The reading can be watched as one makes one's way down an inch of text, once and then again and then again, noticing the verb tenses, putting rectangles around particular words or phrases, drawing lines to connect images that travel together, gleefully getting the pun or the internal rhyme or, mouthing the words, hearing the words spoken aloud, undergoing the meter, relishing the rhythm. When students or colleagues do this in groups, each participant comes to know something about his or her own reader-response while reaping the valuable dividend of witnessing how the minds of his or her colleagues work as well. Reciprocal, these recognitions lead to individual clarity and intersubjective transparency.

As one reads a story—or watches a film, or attends a theatre or dance performance—one takes in countless aspects of knowledge, perception, and emotion. The beholder opens the self to the creator, offering the full use of the self's equipment as a receiver and decoder of that which is offered. Not that the readers or audience members are radar screens or satellite dishes in space, but rather that there is nothing squandered in the evidence available in the telling or performing being given.

The habits of close reading furnish means of crossing the gap of unknow-ingness between one individual and another. Literary scholar and writing teacher Peter Parsisi notes that "[t]he real object of literary study is not to bring readers a message, but to bring them into a mode of attention."[38] The writer writes, and then the reader reads, with the always mysterious inhabita-tion in the reader of the thoughts and views and sensations and impressions of the writer. That is to say, the thoughts and views and sensations and impressions of the writer are, in the oddest way, absorbed by the reader in order that they be experienced from within. It is as if intense and repeated reading can lead the reader to feel that he or she has somehow ingested the writing—eaten it up, engulfed it with amoeba arms, made it become part of self. Virginia Woolf writes almost mystically about this process in many of her essays, describing the site of reading as a powerful synchrony of personal and historical time, making possible travel beyond the bounds of mortality.[39] Roland Barthes describes the "pleasure of the text" and the bliss of reading in ways that illuminate this pro-cess of ingestion, asserting the corporeal components of these literary acts.[40]

These intersubjective processes explain the always startling discovery of students new to close reading who find themselves writing endless sentences replete with parentheses and em-dashes as they encounter Henry James for the first time. Or they are surprised by the slippery stream of naturalistic imagery that unintentionally spools into their term papers after a semester with *To the Lighthouse*. This is not as mysterious as it sounds. Elements of language like temporal structure, diction, imagery, narrative situation, plot, and voice carry messages back and forth from writer to reader. They are either the message's bottles or the messages themselves. Not a little interpretive work has to be done, but in our teaching we have observed that readers new to close reading can become quite adept at careful, slow reading in a relatively short period of training. If the reader is introduced to those elements of text to look for, he or she rather quickly becomes attuned to the temporal, imagistic, generic, spatial, perspectival aspects of a text or image or spectacle.

These skills of the attentive reader are then transferrable to the skills of the attentive listener. I learned this from a patient who had been under my care for around ten years, a woman with hypertension, back pain, and a history of breast cancer.[41] She had faced her breast cancer squarely, almost matter-of-factly, underwent a lumpectomy in her left breast, and completed a course of hormonal therapy. We celebrated her achievement of her five-year cancer-free period. Some years passed, and she developed a second cancer in her left breast.

Although she soldiered through a mastectomy and additional chemotherapy and recovered physically from the surgery, she developed anguishing fear that the cancer would again recur. She visited her breast surgeon or me almost weekly, anxious about small changes in her breast tissue and certain that a third cancer was underway.

I remember so clearly the day she described powerfully her sense that something was waiting in the wings, as if about to pounce. I remember leaning against the sink in the examining room, listening to her words, taking in her panic at this invisible pursuant. Knowing her quite well by then, I took the chance to wonder aloud if it was dying that she feared. We talked about dying, about the certainty of it, about the fear that surrounds it. I remember realizing how much I myself was deriving from this frank and unafraid opening-up of the subject of death. We found a way to be together in the forecast of death, even though hers felt much closer to her than, at that moment, mine felt to me. She realized that the recurrence of her breast cancer had tormented her with the unspoken—until now—certainty that she will at some point die. This conversation, oddly, brought peace to her, for she felt she understood more clearly what it was that had brought her such anguish. I wrote a description of this situation, trying to better understand it myself. When I showed her what I had written, when she read the story and when she helped me to make it even more accurate, she learned even more herself about what she had undergone. Her repeated visits to her doctors for reassurance became no longer necessary, and to the day on which I write this she is healthy and remains at peace.

I see, in retrospect, that my listening to her that day included the close reader's attention to metaphor and figural language, to tone, to mood. I am grateful that I did not surrender to the instrumental means of reassurance, "But look, your cancer markers are not elevated. Your repeat mammogram is fine." Instead, her words and her mood and her actions revealed to me the presence of another truth, a lurking fear that had yet to be perceived. Like the kind of listening I might do in a narrative inquiry interview on a qualitative research project, I was trying to treat her utterance as a unit, with an underlying unity despite the ruptures of paradox. Our conversation that day added to the good we have done to one another since then, for it strengthened the ground of relation between us that a more conventional medical approach would not have been able to achieve.

The Interior Processes of Close Reading

If close reading crosses the gap of unknowingness between two people, it also is a means of crossing the gap between what one consciously knows and the "unthought known," that which is known outside of awareness.[42] There are many avenues toward knowing one's unthought known—interpreting one's dreams, psychoanalysis, and aesthetic creation are perhaps the most powerful ones. Close reading too can reveal aspects of knowledge and self otherwise out of awareness. Like the writer or artist who embarks on a creative process without knowing where it will lead, the close and creative reader embarks, with every book, on an uncharted process toward discovery.

The opportunities afforded by close reading bring the reader to look attentively at his or her own ways of making meaning. How does my mind work? What are its practiced or chosen or fated moves? Readers come to know, if they *watch themselves read*, how their own cognitive and affective and characterological methods converge to create meaning. Whether reading or listening or acting, the person is using his or her singular means of recognizing stimuli, experiencing them, ordering them in some characteristic way, and feeling his or her way toward coming to conceive what, perhaps, this phenomenon is about. When the analysand talks while the analyst listens and silently participates, he or she has recourse to the second person's frame of mind. When the reader reads, he or she has recourse to other readers who have read the text, to other texts the author wrote, to other times the reader himself or herself has read the text. And so the close reader is accompanied on the readerly journey, not necessarily by another person who will actually say things back, but by a similarly attentive presence—the self increasingly known.

Many mysterious processes occur through close reading. How does it happen that a reader, reading a novel or poem written centuries ago in a foreign language, can recognize herself in a character or a situation in this fiction?[43] Why is it the case that a reader might feel a powerful bond of intimacy with an author long dead? It may seem unusual to propose that absorbing the words of another— perhaps dead for centuries, perhaps writing in a language unknown to the reader, perhaps living in one's exact time and place—can expose something powerful about the reader to the reader himself or herself. How can it be that when I read Henry James, I see with such otherwise unavailable clarity aspects of my own peril? It is not exactly recognition. There is little similarity between this master of nineteenth- and twentieth-century American fiction and me. Yet, his sentences open up some view of myself to myself. In their cadences, their never-endingness, their ever-receding conclusions, their always-qualifying second and third and fourth thoughts, I find some familiarity, some belonging, some kinship not in belief or way of life but, instead, in turn of mind. My close reading of James entitles me to appreciate some of the ways in which my own mind works. Roland Barthes describes this phenomenon in *The Pleasure of the Text*, a description that reassured me about that which I underwent at the hands of my author: "The text chooses me, by a whole disposition of invisible screens, selective baffles: vocabulary, references, readability, etc.; and lost in the midst of a text (not *behind* it, like a *deus ex machina*) there is always the other, the author."[44]

I am visited now, in my mind, by one of my Master of Science in Narrative Medicine students. He is a successful corporate man-of-the-world, manager of a large unit in the public relations office of a prominent healthcare company. He was smitten by Félicité in Flaubert's "A Simple Heart." This businessman was exquisitely drawn to the frail yet hardy self-contained peasant woman who loved, in the end, her stuffed parrot. The enigmatic resonance between reader and character can be a spring of deep meaning and self-recognition for the attentive reader. Another student is a physical therapist who created and directs an integrative healthcare practice providing physical therapy, acupuncture, massage, and other modalities of care. He had never read modernist British fiction and felt, early in his narrative medicine training, that he didn't know how and couldn't really learn how to read Virginia Woolf. But he found himself transported into *To the Lighthouse*, quite against his expectations. He could not get enough of the novel, of other writings by Woolf, and when he wrote about her works in his papers for me, he discovered, in Woolf's characters and forms, critical aspects of himself:

> Woolf places her novel in the interior lives of her characters, the place that is unheard, unspoken. She allows us to be inside the mind and soul, inside the anxieties and emotions, the place in each of us that is invisible to the world, the place in an individual that is separate from the other. This is the only space in which this novel could exist. Time and space are connected as one, a chronotope, as Bakhtin says in *The Dialogic Imagination*, "The intrinsic connectedness of temporal and spatial relationships are artistically expressed in literature . . . It expresses the inseparability of space and time (time as the fourth dimension of space)" (84). In *To the Lighthouse*, the space and time exist in the interior lives of the characters.

Such sightings of the self occur when readers allow themselves to be taken into a text, not as acts of will but as aesthetic surrender. Not without effort and skill, this committed and close reading gradually opens the reader to self-expression and self-examination. In Wayne Booth's terms, we come to know ourselves through "the company we keep."

Close Reading Enacts the Principles of Narrative Medicine

Several overarching principles that govern narrative medicine as a whole have been pivotal in our development of a commitment to close reading as a signature method for the field: (1) action toward social justice; (2) disciplinary rigor; (3) inclusivity; (4) tolerance of ambiguity; (5) participatory and nonhierarchical methods; and (6) relational and intersubjective processes. In a reflexive arc, these principles warrant our adherence to close reading as a practice, while our close reading deepens our commitment to the principles. Our fidelity to these principles appears in the design and execution of our graduate program, the design and execution of our curriculum in the College of Physicians and Surgeons of Columbia University, the performance of our externally sponsored research projects, and in our many collaborations with national and international partners. By articulating the contribution that each one of these governing principles makes to our work in close reading, I hope to exemplify the contributions close reading makes to the field as a whole.

Action Toward Social Justice: I start with the most overarching goals of our work: narrative medicine is committed first to just and effective healthcare. I need not rehearse here the evidence that ill health is tied to inequality, racism, sexism, and other injustices. I need not detail the forms of trauma, violence toward persons, state violence, corporate or personal greed, and deprivation that are the root causes of much of the world's suffering and disease. Our creation of narrative medicine was from its start an effort to bring equality to healthcare—across class, gender, ethnicity, sexual preference, and health status lines. We see close reading as a critical tool in seeking healthcare justice. The capacity to imagine the situations of others is prelude to acting on their behalf and to developing the receptive stance of the respectful and humble witness. At its best, this is what close reading does.

Disciplinary Rigor: In conceptualizing narrative medicine's commitment to close reading, Maura Spiegel and I relied on some of the foundational critical approaches that inspect, analyze, or theorize the acts of reading. The more rigorously our work is located within the disciplines of literary criticism and narratology—and their ever-expanding neighboring disciplines like relational psychoanalysis and cognitive neurosciences—and the more fluent we and our students become in both contemporary critical discourses and the lineage of ideas from which they arise, the more engaged our work becomes in the currents of the day and the more likely it is that our own efforts in narrative medicine will be responsive, responsible, heard, and consequential. Accordingly, one goal in teaching and practicing close reading in narrative medicine is to welcome students and colleagues into the critical community of ideas, controversies, and discourses regarding textuality and narrative acts and to learn how such ideas influence the world of healthcare. Without limiting ourselves to one narrow school or approach to literary criticism and narrative theory, we try to open doors to complex formulations of what happens when a reader reads a text or a listener hears a tale.

A rigorous foundation in theory and its articulation obviates a tendency to only "read for the plot," to overlook issues of power, or to develop anemic or puny readings for lack of robust conceptual models. Not theory for theory's sake, our practice calls upon tested and emerging perspectives on the texts or aspects of literary action we study so as to attain full benefit of the interpretive community of which we are part.

Inclusivity: Our principles include inclusivity of theoretical approaches, genres, artists, and perspectives, exposing students and colleagues to the geography of critical approaches, texts, and textual practices. As individual scholars, each of the faculty has developed loyalties and preferences—mine for a Jamesian narratology and a psychoanalytically inflected practice of reading, for example—but our teaching attempts an inclusivity that will extend beyond the particular chosen specialties of the individual faculty members. We and our students try for an intellectual and personal flexibility, not restrictive and not judgmental. The inclusivity extends beyond intellectual frameworks to include aesthetic tastes, areas of interest, forms of intellectual and creative activity, and specific goals sought.

Tolerating Ambiguity: Ambiguity is a constant in our work and a required aspect of our teaching and practice of close reading. A position of non-totalizing elemental contingency undergirds our reading of literary texts, our responding to one another's creative writing, and our witnessing of events in healthcare. Colleague Sayantani DasGupta has written extensively about narrative humility, the awareness of the impossibility of knowing accurately what another's account fully encompasses. "We cannot ever claim to comprehend the totality of another's story, which is only ever an approximation for the totality of another's self. . . . Narrative humility acknowledges that our patients' stories are not objects that we can comprehend or master, but rather dynamic entities that we can approach and engage with, while simultaneously remaining open to their ambiguity and contradiction, and engaging in constant self-evaluation and self-critique."[45] Whether a story is heard in a clinic office or a novel by James, the receiver of the account of the other can only approximate, near, guess, wonder about what the source of the story might have had in mind. That receiver is also attuned to the impact of that story on himself or herself—challenging beliefs, supporting assumptions, raising worries about the self, awakening memories, giving pleasure, giving pain. In *The Ethics of Ambiguity*, Simone de Beauvoir observes that "to attain his truth, man must not attempt to dispel the ambiguity of his being but, on the contrary, accept the task of realizing it. . . . To say that [existence] is ambiguous is to assert that its meaning is never fixed, that it must be constantly won. . . . It is because man's condition is ambiguous that he seeks, through failure and outrageousness, to save his existence."[46] Attuning oneself to ambiguity, then, is a movement within the development of the human self that narrative medicine in all its facets tries to support.

Central to the clinical as well as the critical enterprise, tolerating ambiguity encourages a generosity toward discord in which opposing readings or interpretations can coexist and be contained by a community of practice, whether a graduate seminar or an ambulatory clinic staff. Such collective "containing" confers on the group itself the power to tolerate difference, to open each individual to obscure dimensions of the matter at hand, and to see one's position more clearly. The following two principles—participatory methods and relational processes—follow from the recognition of ambiguity and doubt at the heart of the enterprise.

Participatory and Nonhierarchical Methods: Narrative medicine undertakings do their best to embrace participatory egalitarianism. In teaching and learning close reading, the doors must be open at all times for singular interpretations, opposing readings, vigorous shifts in one's own understanding of a stretch of text. It has seemed to me that close reading *in particular* brings out the absolute requirement that all take part, that no voice stays unheard, and that all in the group have equal time. These standards lead to some rather heated sessions that can be lived through without rupture because the group has created the collective means to tolerate the disagreement.

When we teach close reading—whether in the required "Methods of Narrative Medicine" graduate seminar or in medical center seminars or workshops at Columbia and elsewhere—the premium is on each participant's undergoing and registering his or her own reading experience. I find myself often asking of participants, "What did you undergo by virtue of reading this text?" We typically read texts aloud a great deal, examining the words in fine detail for whatever narrative features might seem to be key. We then write in the shadow of the text we are reading as a powerful means to discover what we are learning or feeling through our close contact with it. When one person reads aloud what he or she has written, the others in the group respond to the writing, taking the opportunity to share individual reactions and to add to what the writer might learn in the process of the work. By these means, the focus of our teaching of close reading remains participatory, developing the agenda to include the tendencies of us all.

The ultimate goal of a participatory and nonhierarchical principle is power symmetry. There are limits on the symmetry—teachers grade students' papers, attending physicians evaluate medical trainees. And yet, those granted the conventional power position in such dyads can choose to alter routines toward egality. Since clinical or university routines favor conventional power asymmetry, if only implicitly, those who seek nonhierarchical participation have to break step and challenge convention. We hope that our practices and those of like-minded colleagues can effectively challenge the inbuilt hierarchical systems within the academy and healthcare systems, or at least channel a growing awareness of the high costs of fragmented groups in silos with little to bridge their divides.

Relational and Intersubjective Processes: Learners learn together. Selves become selves in relation to others. The isolated, deracinated, up-by-the-bootstraps individual is a fantasy concocted by those fearful of human contact. Narrative acts of telling and listening or writing and reading affirm that there is no work of art without a spectator; as James writes in an essay on the novels of George Eliot, "the reader does quite half the labor."[47] We even more boldly claim the presence of narrative co-construction in professional, pedagogic, personal, and societal transactions: the listener or reader or spectator is an active shaper to that which is told or written.

Close reading is a specific illustration of relationality and intersubjectivity. The mysterious processes described above whereby a reader is chosen by an author, whereby a reader "ingests" the thinking and feeling of an author and makes it part of self, or whereby a reader recognizes himself or herself in the fictional characters imagined by a stranger are instances of the inevitable and irreversible human contact occasioned by close reading. Medical students at Columbia University are, at the beginning of their medical studies, often unused to narrative medicine methods. When they participate in the required curriculum in narrative medicine, joining in small, rigorous, participatory seminars on literary arts, visual art, or philosophical topics, they are surprised by the intimacy and transparency developed with their classmates. A qualitative research study of medical students' responses to their narrative medicine seminars documented the importance of the intersubjective processes by which these seminars were taught:

> I . . . feel like the most important thing is getting us to realize how to work with our classmates and talk with them and work outside of the normal classroom mentality, and realize that there are these people we can go to when . . . we do struggle with death and dying, it's not us doing it alone.[48]

The clinical routines of narrative medicine as both practiced and taught are influenced by practices of narrative therapy and relational psychotherapies. In facing the complexities of Virginia Woolf's *To the Lighthouse*, our close reading graduate seminar relies on concepts and practices of narrative psychologists and relational analysts including Michael White and Stephen Mitchell.[49] The boundaries are permeable between a narrative approach to close reading and a narrative approach to close listening in a therapeutic setting. This is not to suggest that readers diagnose their characters or their authors or texts. Rather, it suggests that the processes that obtain between reader and writer are as singular, as formative, and as transformative as are those between a person and his or her therapist. Training in close reading is indeed a powerful prelude or preparation for the clinical work of coming to know, care about, and develop affiliation with a patient, a student, or a psychotherapeutic client.

These six overarching principles illuminate both the processes of reflection on and growth of our field. As narrative medicine matures, the field encompasses more and more explicitly questions of trauma, state violence, global health inequities, and health disparities. Our partnerships with the Columbia University Oral History Research Office and with the storytelling project *Narativ* have led to participation in international work to hear silenced voices and to amplify evidence necessary for a just world. One example is an educational and advocacy project addressing healthcare for marginalized populations, including Europe's Roma population. Our growing engagement with the Veterans' Administration in the United States emerges from the commitment to respond to trauma, especially trauma suffered in our name as Americans. The focus on intersubjectivity and bearing witness to others' suffering poise narrative medicine to respond skillfully to accounts of trauma and injustice, equipping the listener with the resource of nonjudgmental attention.

We realize that the polarization of the world politically, culturally, economically, religiously, and nationalistically increasingly fractures any kind of underlying human unity—it is Sunni versus Shia, Ukraine versus Russia, 99% versus 1%. (Oxfam reports, in 178 Oxfam Briefing Paper, that "those richest 85 people across the globe share £1 trillion, as much as the poorest 3.5 billion of the world's population.")[50] We have gradually come to recognize that the *having* of a human body gives us a rare ground of unity—we share the same body, we have the same organs, we are prey to the same diseases, and we all will die. In a world where grounds for diplomacy seem to be disappearing, matters of physical and mental health may be now the most promising portfolios within which to develop commonalities of values, meanings, and goals. Our bodies may be the only thing left that we truly, globally share. It is no accident that much of global justice work today is related to physical or mental suffering, whether inflicted by the state or by natural disasters. Our bodies are becoming both the instance of care and the tools of care, and eventually perhaps an egalitarian healthcare will be seen as an avenue not just toward healthy bodies and minds but toward healthy worlds.

The idea that one person can understand what another person says or means is the deepest part of science and the deepest part of art. This idea is the groundspring of language, of beauty, of knowledge, of government, of culture, and of love. In the shadow of that meta-perspective of human experience, we place our work in narrative medicine at a series of boundaries, realizing that the effort is always to bridge the divides, to seek the permeability, to unlock the channels that might provide unexpected benefit to both sides. Whether the two sides of the divide are psychopharmacology and psychoanalysis, a doctor and a patient, a war veteran and a nurse, or two readers reading one poem, the effort is to transcend the partisan or defensive, toward contact with one's partner not in argument or agreement but in paradox, a contact that will not nail answers but will craft vessels for thought. In the process of the craft comes relation.

What we do when we do clinical work as nurses, physical therapists, or doctors includes what we do when we read. Hand in hand with the gait training and diabetes management comes Felski's "sharply honed attentiveness to nuances of language and form," comes the aesthetic sensations of beholding an original creation, comes the affective and emotional processes that, if nothing else can, can open the pores between the subject and the object, the seer and the seen, the person seeking care and the person offering it.

Coda

Fiction-writer Aleksander Hemon visited Columbia to present our Narrative Medicine Rounds in the spring of 2014. He read almost in its entirety his personal essay "The Aquarium" that details the events of the illness and death of his infant daughter Isabel from brain cancer.[51] The aquarium of the title is the green-glass tank in which he and his wife and daughter felt trapped:

> One early morning, driving to the hospital, I saw a number of able-bodied, energetic runners progressing along Fullerton Avenue toward the sunny lakefront, and I had an intensely physical sensation of being inside an aquarium: I could see outside, the people outside could see me inside (if they somehow chose to pay attention), but we lived and breathed in entirely different environments. Isabel's illness and our experience had little connection to, and even less impact on, the world outside. (pp. 201–202)

In the discussion after his reading, a novelist asked him a daunting question: "What is writing *for*?" Hemon answered, "To make contact, to bring about engagement." I couldn't help but ask, a few questions later, "What is healthcare *for*?" Without a beat, Hemon replied, "To make contact, to bring about engagement."

Close reading brings us to a brink—of identity, of knowledge of self, of knowledge of other. It transports us, it summons us, it liberates us from narrow precincts. Once equipped with the not insubstantial skill it takes to do well, close reading provides a chance for permeable contact with other persons, other times, other viewpoints, other selves. There is no wonder in our minds that it is a signature method for the work we want to be able to accomplish in the care of the sick and in the effort, more widely conceived, of making contact, of bringing about engagement.

Notes

1. See Hurwitz, "Form and Representation," for a summary of case history genres through the ages, which reflect the styles of listening deemed critical to the clinical enterprise along the way. See also Starr, *Social Transformation of Medicine*; Relman, *When More Is Less*; Gawande, *Being Mortal*.
2. Such textbooks as Newell, *Interviewing Skills for Nurses*; Lipkin, Putnam, and Lazare, *The Medical Interview*; Cassell, *Talking with Patients*; Fortin et al., *Smith's Patient-Centered Interviewing*; and Coulehan and Block, *The Medical Interview*, are among many such guides to eliciting clinical histories and achieving interpersonal rapport needed to understand the patient.
3. Felski, *Uses of Literature*, 52.
4. North, "What's New?"
5. Ogden and Richards, *Meaning of Meaning*; Richards, *Richards on Rhetoric*.
6. Richards, *Principles of Literary Criticism*, 11. The internal quotations in this excerpt from Richards are quotations from Hegel's *History of Philosophy*.
7. Richards, *Principles*, 16–17.
8. Richards, *Principles*, 4.
9. Empson, *Seven Types of Ambiguity*.
10. Ransom, *New Criticism*; Eliot, "Tradition and the Individual Talent"; Cleanth Brooks, *Well Wrought Urn*; Cleanth Brooks and Warren, *Understanding Poetry*.
11. The two influential essays by Wimsatt and Beardsley, "The Affective Fallacy" and "The Intentional Fallacy," are collected in *The Verbal Icon*.
12. Cleanth Brooks, *Well Wrought Urn*, 74–75.
13. Cleanth Brooks and Warren, *Understanding Poetry*, xiii.
14. Jakobson and Halle, *Fundamentals*; Levi-Strauss, *Structural Anthropology, Vol. 2*.
15. Barthes, *S/Z*; Culler, *Structuralist Poetics*.
16. Derrida, *Of Grammatology*; Lyotard, *Postmodern Condition*; Kristeva, *Desire in Language*.
17. Jameson, *Political Unconscious*.
18. Lacan, *Écrits*.
19. Foucault, *Order of Things*.
20. Lentricchia and DuBois, *Close Reading*, 34.
21. See Parisi, "Close Reading, Creative Writing"; Bialostosky, "Should College English."
22. Lentricchia and DuBois, *Close Reading*, ix.
23. Ricoeur, "Freud and Philosophy"; Best and Marcus, "Surface Reading."
24. D. A. Miller, "Hitchcock's Understyle." See Ferguson, "Now It's Personal," for a study of too-close reading as a means of being hailed by a work, in a simulacrum of friendship.
25. Sedgwick, *Touching, Feeling*; Jurecic, *Illness as Narrative*; Philip Davis, *Reading and the Reader*.
26. See Reddy, *Navigation of Feeling*, for a history of the emotions, and Leys, "Turn to Affect," a critique of the adoption of neuroscientific means of characterizing emotion or locating its production in the brain. See also Keen, *Empathy and the Novel*, and the growing body of work on theory of mind in Zunshine, *Why We Read Fiction*.
27. See Kandel, *Age of Anxiety*; Chalmers, *Conscious Mind*; Dehaene, *Reading in the Brain*; Oatley, *Such Stuff as Dreams*.

28. Kidd and Castano, "Reading Literary Fiction."
29. Felski, *Uses of Literature*; Rudnytsky and Charon, *Psychoanalysis and Narrative Medicine*; Brockmeier and Carbaugh, *Narrative and Identity*; J. Hillis Miller, *Reading for Our Time*; Royle, *Veering*.
30. Harkin, "Reception of Reader-Response."
31. For milestones of the work in this complex field, see Rosenblatt, *Literature as Exploration*; Poulet, "Criticism and Experience"; Holland, *5 Readers Reading* and *Dynamic of Literary Response*; Fish, *Is There a Text?*; Iser, *Act of Reading*; Flynn and Schweickart, *Gender and Reading*; Bleich, *Subjective Criticism*; Booth, *Rhetoric of Fiction*. Tompkins's *Reader-Response Criticism* is an authoritative anthology and introduction to the field.
32. Gallop, "Historicization of Literary Studies," 183.
33. Tompkins, *Reader-Response Criticism*.
34. J. Hillis Miller, *Ethics of Reading*; Booth, *Company We Keep*.
35. Booth, *Rhetoric of Fiction*, 138.
36. See Charon, Hermann, and Devlin, "Close Reading and Creative Writing"; Devlin et al., "Where Does the Circle End?"; Sarah Chambers et al., "Making a Case."
37. James, "Art of Fiction," 390.
38. Parisi, "Close Reading, Creative Writing," 65.
39. See Woolf's "Reading," "How Should One Read a Book?" and "On Re-Reading Novels."
40. See his *Pleasures of the Text*, and the essay "Reading" in *The Rustle of Language*.
41. I have written elsewhere, with the patient's supervision and her permission to publish, about what she and I learned together. She has given me permission to share her story for the benefit of other patients. Charon, "Membranes of Care."
42. Bollas, *Shadow of the Subject*.
43. Felski, *Uses of Literature*. See also the scholarship on enchantment and disenchantment in literature including Bennett, *Enchantment of Modern Life*.
44. Barthes, *Pleasure of the Text*, 27.
45. DasGupta, "Narrative Humility," *Lancet*, 980, 981.
46. de Beauvoir, *Ethics of Ambiguity*, 13, 129.
47. Stein, *Appreciation*; James, "Novels of George Eliot," 485.
48. Eliza Miller et al., "Sounding Narrative Medicine," 339.
49. Michael White and Epston, *Narrative Means*; Mitchell, *Relationality*.
50. Wearden, "178 Oxfam Briefing Paper."
51. Hemon, "Aquarium."

CHAPTER 8

A Framework for Teaching Close Reading

Rita Charon

I had the chance to read David Foster Wallace's magisterial novel *Infinite Jest* with a group of first-year medical students. In between dissecting their anatomy cadavers and learning of brutal diseases that take lives, they'd read Wallace's edgy leave-nothing-left-unseen PET scan of ordinary life exposing the surreality, the madness, the faceted fractaled epiphanic that can sometimes be fleetingly seen amid the cynical, the fantastic, and the habitual.[1] One student softly said on our third session, "Reading this is making me see more of what goes on every day, but I can't tell yet what that will cost me." We all appreciated his wondering, sharing in his uncertainty of the value and cost of sight.

His question hinged on both the text we were reading and the way in which we read it—closely, every word counts, keeping track of temporal, spatial, metaphorical, allusive, affective, structural aspects of the 1079-page novel at once. We were doing with this literary text something not unlike what they were doing with the dead human body that had been entrusted to them, respecting the architecture while taking it apart, comprehending that there is a life in its unity that cannot be seen in its parts, yet one must see the parts in order to see the whole. Hermeneutic, their efforts with this novel became a model for a form of dynamic and creative *thought* that registers detail while constructing pattern, that tolerates chaos, that is moved by proportion and balance and contrast, that is led to remember things, that colors itself with emotion, and that appreciates the presence of the thinker in the thought.

I wished I had had the evidence to tell my student that seeing more of what goes on every day expands the life you lead, gains you access to more truth and beauty than otherwise will come to you, wounds you, arouses you, introduces you to your self-always-in-the-making, lengthens your life not by days but by the depth to which each instant is lived. I told him that we have some evidence that the kind of seeing that comes from close reading adds to our capacity to see life as it happens, and that the seeing of it is but the prelude to the living of it.[2]

One Way to Teach Close Reading

There are probably as many methods of teaching close reading as there are methods of teaching human anatomy. I do not propose here to survey the methods, but will propose some of the ingredients necessary to impart this skill. Being a close reader requires abstract thought, textual judgment, psychological insight, and a surrender to being carried away by a book. Doing close reading entails the commitment to believe, initially with not much evidence, that the time and effort devoted to reading a particular book will be repaid in pleasure, wisdom, questing, or finding. It entails a particular kind of freedom—the freedom to abandon oneself to an unknown, to place oneself in the hands of an agent not even present at the transaction. It entails the confidence that one can summon forth the width and depth of knowledge needed to make sense of the work. The close reader squanders none of the evidence of meaning from any linguistic, structural, metaphorical, allusive, poetic, or rhetorical aspect of either a sentence or an utterance. Literary scholar Edward Said writes that in the music of Bach, "every note counts. . . . The formal concept is articulated assertively and consciously, from the large structure to the merest ornament."[3] This is true of written compositions, and it is arguably true of spoken or performed language as well.

As a reader starts to read, he or she gets oriented to a set of features encountered in almost any text: time, space, genre, metaphor, voice, mood, and a relationship with the text itself. These features can be artificially separated from one another for the sake of seeing each clearly. Not unlike what a pianist must do in practicing a piece separately for the right hand and the left hand, a close reader can read a section of text attending in particular to one or another of these cardinal features so as to perceive at the level of detail what the text is doing. One can inspect a text for its temporal scaffolding, then its sensory detail, then its diction, metaphors, narrative strategy, voice, or mood. The reader fortifies the inspection of these textual features with a knowledge of salient elements of literary criticism, narratology, and philosophy. When all these aspects of the text are then combined, the reader has achieved a deep and unforgettable grasp of what that text has done. By paying detailed and disciplined attention to each of several narrative features of texts, readers find doors into them—whether read, heard, or written by themselves.

To practice narrative medicine requires the skills of close reading. As ongoing study demonstrates the mechanisms and intermediates by which close reading leads to close listening, and as we learn how close listening improves the effectiveness of ordinary healthcare, we will eventually have robust evidence of the salience of readerly skills to healthcare. Through our research program in narrative medicine at Columbia, we are learning more and more about the consequences of our teaching methods. Our learners find, through training in narrative medicine, greater affiliation with colleagues and patients, greater awareness of their own personal predicaments or predilections, deeper curiosity about what they witness, braver curiosity about what they themselves undergo, and a lovely sense of beauty caught in the work they do.[4]

The following sections are devoted each to teaching a specific narrative feature of text, worth inspecting in detail, whose inspection is enhanced through rigorous training and study of some works of literary theory and narratology. Over a course of study—a semester-long graduate seminar, a weekly faculty development project, or a clinical preceptorship for medical or nursing students—learners can become familiar with some of the compass points in considering temporal structures, spatial elements, figural language, or narrative strategies. Although the specific list of features is not static and will be tailored to the individual teaching goals, settings, and texts, the practice of rigorous training in these multiple avenues toward meaning continues to repay narrative medicine teaching and to deepen the consequences for teacher and for student.

In the examples that follow, I describe teaching sequences that examine several of the cardinal narrative features—time, space, metaphor, and voice. In brief summaries I suggest some of the urgent issues related to each of these features, trying only to identify the foundations within a disciplined intellectual framework of literary and narrative theory for further study. For each feature I have chosen a particular text and describe an actual situation teaching the text to a group of learners—graduate students, social workers, physicians, and so forth. It goes without saying that the teaching setting dictates which narrative features are chosen, how deeply to delve into the theoretical backgrounds, and how much time would be devoted to each of these features. I hope that the following portraits of actual teaching give readers an understanding of how the conceptual foundations of narrative medicine are borne out in pedagogical practice.

Choosing Texts and Writing Prompts

We are often asked on what criteria we choose the texts we teach in narrative medicine. First, there is absolutely no need to restrict the teaching to texts that treat illness or medicine or health. It is arguably easier to teach non–medically inflected texts, since the clinical or illness-related dimensions of a text can sometimes deflect attention from considerations of form. Choosing texts that have nothing to do with illness can emphasize that we are not focusing on content or plot in our seminars, but rather we are examining how the words do what they do and how to cultivate habits of noticing all that is held in a poem, a story, or an utterance in a conversation.

In order to effectively engage a group of learners in consequential work on a text, the text must repay attention. It has to be a "great text," however one can adequately define that. The fiction, poem, play, visual image, or musical composition has to support repeated visits, surprising the reader not only with aspects that were hidden upon former readings but also exposing to the reader how he or she has changed since that last reading. The work we might teach has depth, dimensions, internal resonances, and ambiguities. The figural language is alive, provocative, subtle, building throughout the work. There is a temporal complexity, with flash-forwards or flashbacks, with time travel or overlapping periods of time. One can productively examine the verb tenses and moods in searching out the meaning or impact of the work.

With intention, we include voices typically silenced by the culture at large. This includes wide ranges in culture/ethnicity of the writer, language, class, and time period. Postcolonial theorist Gayatri Spivak's subaltern speaks in narrative medicine teaching.[5] Bringing voices of the dispossessed or disenfranchised into the learning challenges the power asymmetries of conventional healthcare. Works that confront issues of injustice, that open up violences to inspection, that address situations of bias can marry practice to principle in our teaching. While conveying literary and clinical skills, narrative medicine simultaneously poses questions of power: Who is at home in this text or in this classroom? Whose voice is recognized? Who might be absent? The selection of texts is informed by the needs of the pedagogy, the social and cultural examinations underway in the classroom, and the effort to cultivate equitable power relationships within the learning setting and, ultimately, the clinical setting.[6]

If the text is a visual or aural one, parallel considerations arise. The second movement of Robert Schumann's Violin Concerto in D opens with a strain that weaves in and out of the minor key. As if effortlessly, the music moves from sunlight to darkness, the shift sometimes within a measure, with an absence of jar between major and minor. The effect on the careful listener is to apprehend the simultaneity of these moods, to accept the non-exclusivity of what are often perceived as opposing moods. I will sometimes teach to a series of Mark Rothko "bars of color" paintings. The abstract expressionism of these paintings precludes questions of content altogether, enabling a group of viewers to be summoned into the buoyancy and balance and aliveness of the deeply saturated pigments. It is beyond contemplation. It is transport.

Certainly, the teacher chooses texts that accord with the goals of teaching—first-person accounts in a seminar on relationality or texts that open up to inspection the reader/writer contract in a course on narrative ethics. The preferences of the class, both teacher and learner, certainly come into play. One teaches well the texts one loves, and the pedagogical habit of including texts that have been proposed by the learners is always repaid by deepening the collaboration and egality within the class.

Our narrative medicine practice has evolved to include creative writing in almost all our teaching.[7] As I demonstrate in the examples offered below, inviting students to engage in spontaneous creative writing in the shadow of—or in the light of—a closely read text widens the dimensions of power of the text. After a class discussion of a text, the facilitator offers a writing prompt and invites all students to take 4 or 5 minutes to write spontaneously, then and there, to the prompt. Unlike prompts that might be offered in a composition class or a professional writing seminar, these prompts are short, expansive invitations that aim to open the mind. The more evocative and ambiguous the prompt the better, for the student is not being told what to write about, how to write about it, or what points need to be covered in the writing. Instead, each student is free to surrender to the text's capacity to transport its reader.[8] By writing to these prompts, the students begin to appreciate what the reading is doing to them—what interpretations are aroused, what moods summoned, what allusions heard, what memories unlocked, what beauty discovered, what ideas stirred. In listening to students read aloud what they have just written and in responding to one another, the students realize how they themselves use form to express content—one writes a list while another writes a prayer; one starts at the end and writes backward while another writes entirely in the subjunctive mood; one writes with an intimate access to the consciousness of a protagonist while another writes from a detached, impersonal narrative position. They thereby come to recognize that their own creative process is not altogether intentional but emerges—form and content—in the chaos of the process of writing itself.[9] We have found this uniting of reading and creative writing to be the most direct way for students to develop the skills of close reading and, as a dividend, to come to comprehend what they themselves do with words. They realize that they as writers need committed readers to show them what they have done, and they experience the reciprocity of the creative processes of reading and writing.

Time

From the beginnings of curiosity about how stories work, narrative studies have been obsessed with time. From Saint Augustine's *Confessions* (Book XI), written in 398 C.E., we learned of the slim knife-edge of the present between memory and anticipation. "There be three times; a present of things past, a present of things present, and a present of things future. . . . present of things past, memory; present of things present, sight; present of things future, expectation. . . . But time present how do we measure, seeing it hath no space? It is measured while passing, but when it shall have passed, it is not measured; for there will be nothing to be measured. But whence, by what way, and whither passes it while it is a measuring? whence, but from the future?"[10] Such dreadful uncertainty in the face of the lived experience of time perhaps signals the start of what has become existential or phenomenological considerations of the human condition. Over the centuries, Augustine's questions attracted the best minds of their times in theology and philosophy: Giambattista Vico's *The New Science* in 1744 reconceptualized time, history, and ideas as creative processes; Henri Bergson's *Time and Free Will* in 1889 considered duration and succession as factors of human consciousness that are dependent on the conscious human living witness; Bertrand Russell sought concepts from early twentieth-century physics and psychology to conceptualize "those immediate experiences upon which our knowledge of time is based."[11] Hand in hand with philosophical considerations about the nature of time have arisen questions about the human's capacity to represent it. From literary scholar Georg Lukács, we learned that the novel was invented in order to solve the problem of time: "In the novel, meaning is separated from life, and hence the essential from the temporal; we might almost say that the entire inner action of the novel is nothing but a struggle against the power of time."[12]

Such investigations emerging from religious studies, philosophy, and literary studies intertwined with investigations of the natural world's phenomena, of the interrelation between time and space in gravity, velocity, and duration. Einstein's 1915 theory of relativity altered every subsequent experience of our understanding of the "flow" of time, influencing radically and irreversibly our narrative and experiential conceptions of what it means to live in time and space. As articulated more recently by philosopher Paul Ricoeur, "[T]ime is both what passes and flows away and, on the other hand, what endures and remains."[13]

Narratological examinations of temporality following Augustine, Vico, Bergson, and Russell have become among the mainstays of narrative theory: Mikhail Bakhtin's *Dialogic Imagination*, Gérard Genette's *Narrative Discourse*, Frank Kermode's *The Sense of an Ending*, Percy Lubbock's *The Craft of Fiction*, and Paul Ricoeur's *Time and Narrative*.[14] Ricoeur's proposal that "*time becomes human to the extent that it is articulated through a narrative mode, and narrative attains its full meaning when it becomes a condition of temporal existence*" (italics in the original) rings as a manifesto that narrativity's mission is tied irrevocably to time.[15] Perhaps more influential in investigating the workings of time than the theorists have been the literary artists themselves. The modernist inventions of Virginia Woolf and James Joyce, the heroic exploits of memory of Proust, the surreality of Beckett and Borges, the poetics of Shakespeare, John Donne, and T.S. Eliot have been the laboratories for a linguistic depiction of time's paradoxes.[16] In teaching close reading in the Master of Science in Narrative Medicine program at Columbia, we usually read Woolf's *To the Lighthouse*— slowly, over an entire semester—as our textual grounding in examining not just time but space, voice, metaphor, mood, and intersubjectivity as well.

Finally, in the evolution of narrative medicine we find ourselves moving beyond the textual to examine the narrative nature of time in visual arts and music. Narrative medicine students and scholars have written about the parallels between *To the Lighthouse* and the Cubism of Picasso and Braque that emerged at around the same time. We are attuned to the means of temporal distention achievable through Baroque counterpoint and jazz improvisation. The contemporary medium of the graphic novel alters both time and space by allowing for unuttered passages of both time and space gaping in the gutters. And, in a turn back to the human body, we heed the efforts to extend life span through technological interventions, to seek stem cell immortality's help in producing one's own replacement organs ad infinitum, to alter biological clocks to enable middle-aged women to conceive, or to extend the adolescent's growth period indefinitely. Such scientific exploits are, in the end, cultural contributions to the lived experience of time that must be integrated into one's concept of being if one is, indeed, to continue to live in one's present.

I want to depict a recent narrative medicine teaching session that dramatizes some of these considerations of the search for time within texts. This seminar took place in New York Presbyterian Hospital's Social Work Services department. Around 12 to 15 social workers from various parts of the large hospital meet monthly for a session of close reading and creative writing. On this day, our text was "the death of fred clifton" by Lucille Clifton:

> the death of fred clifton
> 11/10/84
> age 49
> i seemed to be drawn
> to the center of myself
> leaving the edges of me
> in the hands of my wife
> and i saw with the most amazing
> clarity

> so that i had not eyes but
> sight,
> and, rising and turning,
> through my skin,
> there was all around not the
> shapes of things
> but oh, at last, the things
> themselves.[17]

What do we readers experience in reading this poem? The economy of the words, of the line lengths, even of the number of lines seems out of proportion to the event depicted. It seems, my readers found, that the "i" of the poem, whoever that might be, was in the very duration of the poem dying. Perhaps our status as healthcare professionals led us to interpret the poem in corporeal ways, but most of us present that day envisioned a bed in an intensive care unit, or perhaps a hospice, where a man is dying and his wife is holding on to his earthly presence. The "rising and turning,/ through my skin" seemed, mystically, to invoke a kind of rising of the soul at that moment of death. I recalled to the group that I once taught this poem to a group of intensive care doctors. One very promptly identified the "rising and turning,/through my skin" as what nurses do when they reposition patients in their beds to avoid skin breakdown. This physician later in the session wrote a deeply metaphorical and existentially ringing testament to the meaningfulness of life, demonstrating the combination of the literal-mindedness that comes inevitably with clinical work and a simultaneous making of personal and contextual meaning in its midst.

We wondered about the voice of the poem. Is the poet, who shares the last name of the man who dies, ventriloquizing her dying husband's voice? Is she trying to imagine what he is going through? If so, we wondered if the event of death was being unduly sanitized or sanctified by depicting it as a kind of secular resurrection. Was it just wishful thinking? We wondered what the "edges of me" might be—could it be material possessions, or progeny, or perhaps the unpaid mortgage or, perhaps, even the body itself? Could it be the future? Despite the grave setting, most of the readers experienced a mood of intimacy and peace in reading the poem. "I can almost see love," said one social worker.

Our discussion kept circling around questions of the "now." The speaker "seemed" to be drawn to the center of self, and then "saw" with clarity and "had" not eyes but sight. These past tense verbs attest to this account being given as a retrospect. But the final lines "oh, at last, the things themselves" felt as if they were uttered in the very act of witnessing. It was as if the past caught up to the present, as one of the readers said. If this poem was published by

Lucille Clifton in 1987 and fred clifton died in 1984, we wondered whether this was an elegiac effort to bring the dead man backwards from death back to life. The pivot of this poem, oddly, seemed to occur in the penultimate line, with the evocative, "oh, at last."

We then set out to write for 4 minutes, understanding that everyone would be invited to read aloud what he or she had written. The prompt I gave was, "Oh, at last."

One social worker writes:

> At the end of my life
> I find myself no longer in fear
> Did I ever suspect, when imagining
> this for so many years
> that I could be
> released
> at the end
> ready
> free of anxiety and mournfulness
> at how I couldn't bear to leave you.
> Alas, no fear.
> If only I had known.

Both plot and form of Clifton's poem have inspired this writer. The economies of words, lines, and line lengths, including two one-word lines, are adopted here. However, the situation of the poem's speaker is reversed, with the "I" seeming to be the writer addressing a beloved "you." The mood of serenity is replaced by tension or regret. Unlike Clifton, this writer writes most of the poem in the present tense—"I find myself no longer in fear." I was stunned by the word "Alas." It seemed a paradoxical regret, in some peculiar way signaling that the writer craved fear. Was it supposed to be "at last"? I asked. The writer and I continued our conversation by e-mail after the session:

Yes, "alas" suggests regret. I have so many thoughts about it—having feared death because I am surrounded by young dying people every day for years and years. As I get older, I am not the fierce, solo protector of my son. Always fighting for him. Really he is a man and so confident and independent—maybe I am saying I won't be so needed ever again. . . . Those stages of my life will be over and "alas" there will be so much less to lose at the end of life.[18]

We left this work more deeply than ever shrouded in the mystery of Clifton's poem, now with the help of the creativity of one of our members to so complicate the presence or absence of fear at the time of death. The poem, and the writing in its shadow, enabled at least this writer to experience, acutely, her own position in Augustine's triumvirate and to predict, with such courage, the ambiguities of loss and need and fear.

Another writes:

> Oh at last—he has found his peace. Oh at last—*we* have found our peace. Going on for days like that was torture. Torture to see and hear. He seemed uncomfortable in his body, in his own wrinkled skin. Sitting up, laying down, grabbing for things, calling to people. He seemed ready to go, but there also seemed to be just one more thing. Did he want to hear her voice one last time? She hesitated . . . and then . . . at last—she made her way to his bedside, whispered the words he was longing to hear .. and as she left . . . so did he.

Again, this writer borrows the concepts and even some of the words and details from Clifton's deathbed poem to construct a dark version for herself. The sensory detail of the paragraph—"sitting up, laying down, grabbing for things, calling to people"—brings the reader immediately into this tortured scene. It is indeed a familiar one for these hospital social workers. That our writer can depict a deathbed scene without divulging its nature—work or life—makes the writing all the more clearly a creative act and not a confession or case report.

Here is why that matters. In the setting of healthcare, writing is usually used instrumentally to convey to colleagues the clinical facts of a case. Writing about or talking about patients seems by nature either a professional duty to inform teammates about a patient's clinical status or a sign of personal distress, as when clinicians join support groups to help them deal with burnout or medical error. In narrative medicine sessions, in contrast, the focus is on the creative process. A participant is not necessarily writing something to unburden himself or herself of it or to communicate to another what is known. Rather, the writing act becomes a form of self-discovery as well as reciprocal recognition. In the case of this response to Clifton's poem, both the writer and the listeners have interpretive leeway to contemplate this final act: Was it forgiveness? Was it a final letting-go of hostilities? Was it a long-awaited apology? The hidden stays hidden, the whispered will not be transcribed, as the onlookers, including us listeners, are given a chance themselves to puzzle through the puzzles of being.

Space

To move from time to space introduces the force of gravity, the awareness of mass, a bow to dimension. Although time is indeed experienced by the body and perhaps created by the condition of mortality (Do angels or ghosts experience time? Could Einstein have conceived of relativity were he not mortal?), it cannot be touched or felt or located. Space, on the other hand, is irrefutably material. What space adds to time was expressed unforgettably by Russian literary theorist Mikhail Bakhtin in his 1937–38 "Forms of Time and of the Chronotope in the Novel." In a dazzling epiphany, Bakhtin merged time and space into the concept of the *chronotope*: "In the literary artistic chronotope, spatial and temporal indicators are fused into one carefully thought-out, concrete whole."[19] Giving examples of such chronotopes as the road, the threshold, the castle, the parlor, and the encounter, Bakhtin encourages his reader to experience time passing within specific spaces: "Time, as it were, thickens, takes on flesh, becomes artistically visible; likewise, space becomes changed and responsive to the movements of time, plot, and history" (p. 84). Putting to literary use Bergson's suggestion in 1889 that "time, conceived under the form of an unbounded and homogeneous medium, is nothing but the ghost of space haunting the reflective consciousness," Bakhtin alerted readers and writers to means to expand the consciousness both in the perception and the representation of whatever might be called reality.[20] Within narrative medicine, the notion of the chronotope is immensely helpful. It solidifies the abstract categories of time and space into palpability. The chronotope provides a means of finding meaning, as the merging of time and space is required for events or situations of any kind to be perceivable and then representable: "It is precisely the chronotope that provides the ground essential for the showing-forth, the representability of events. And this is so thanks precisely to the special increase in density and concreteness of time markers—the time of human life, of historical time—that occurs within well-delineated spatial areas" (p. 250).

Sometimes trumping even time, place and space in a novel draw a reader into its narrative world, awakening the senses to experience the "real" of the text. E.M. Forster captures in a few sentences in *Aspects of the Novel* the power of space to convey meaning to a reader. He writes that *War and Peace* "has extended over space as well as over time, and the sense of space until it terrifies us is exhilarating, and leaves behind it an effect like music. After one has read *War and Peace* for a bit, great chords begin to sound. . . . They come from the immense area of Russia."[21] Human beings, as embodied creatures, themselves occupy space and so are partial to other things that do. Forster suggests that Tolstoy's "bridges and frozen rivers, forests, roads, gardens, fields, which accumulate grandeur and sonority after we have passed them" recognize the human being who reads, in effect "making space" for that reader to walk into the frame of an imagined realm (p. 39).

Inspecting the space described in a literary text or depicted in a work of visual art can provide a key to the meanings hidden within. Virginia Woolf's novel *The Waves* is in its fiber "about" time—the plot is time, the drive is time, the very structure of the novel alternates descriptions of hours of one day—from dawn to night—with decades of the characters' lives—from childhood to death. And yet, the intimacy and surprise of the spaces carefully wrought by Woolf carry the imaginative cargo—children hiding under the currant bushes, snails in their cathedral shells, a forlorn mother trapped into her domestic life like a fenced-in tree are the pictures that stay with one after reading the novel.[22] French phenomenologist Gaston Bachelard awakened literary scholars to the poetics of space in his book by that name. Close and loving study of such spaces as huts, nests, and shells enabled Bachelard to consider the deepest drives of the creature to be held in space, to create a room of one's own, to both be sheltered and to hail others to enter and be sheltered. "Space that has been seized upon by the imagination cannot remain indifferent space subject to the measures and estimates of the surveyor. It has been lived in, not in its positivity, but with all the partiality of the imagination."[23] Our spaces, Bachelard proposes, declare something otherwise unsayable about our forms, our gravity, our vulnerability, and our spread.

Studies of the human use of space reveal deep-seated meanings in how we occupy our domains, how we describe them, how we experience them, and even how we endure them. Narrative medicine is itself a nondualistic effort to appreciate the spatial nature of a body, both within its individual biological frame and within its social and political and professional frame. Healthcare, we know, has to be directed toward the body-who-is-the person/the person-who-is-the-body. There is no other way. A non-narrative reductionist medicine risks overlooking the spatiality of the body when it theorizes biological disorders or offers treatment for those disorders at the level of the organ or the tissue or the cell. (Subspecialists caring for a seriously ill patient are wont to try to absolve their organ from guilt in a clinical downturn—cardiologist says, "it's not the heart;" nephrologist says, "it's not the kidneys.") The messy body with its unique appetites and passions and disorders and senescence can interfere with the drive toward clean logical reduction. The distinction between *place* and *space* proposed by sociologist Michel de Certeau is helpful here. A place (*lieu*) is geometrically defined by its coordinates. Two things cannot be in one place at one time. A *space* (*espace*) "exists when one takes into consideration vectors of direction, velocities, and time variables. Thus space is composed of intersections of mobile elements. It is in a sense actuated by the ensemble of movements deployed within it. . . .

In relation to place, space is like the word when it is spoken. . . . In short, *space is a practiced place.*"[24] Reductive medicine treats the human body like a place. Narrative medicine treats the human body like a space.

Borrowing ways of thinking from the literary scholars, the modernists, the phenomenologists, and the sociologists, let us enter the narrative medicine classroom to see how space enters our teaching. This teaching took place in the Master of Science in Narrative Medicine graduate program, in the required core course in close reading called "Methods of Narrative Medicine." This was one of several seminar sessions on the narrative features of space, for which the class had read works, among others, of Bachelard, Bakhtin, de Certeau, Ricoeur, and Woolf cited in this chapter.

Our text is an excerpt from Henry James's *Portrait of a Lady*. Isabel, a penniless young girl from Albany, NY, is brought by her wealthy aunt to meet her British relatives. On the evening of her arrival at Gardencourt, her ancestors' manor on the Thames, Isabel's cousin Ralph brings her to see the paintings in the gallery:

> She asked Ralph to show her the pictures; there were a great many in the house, most
> of them of his own choosing. The best were arranged in an oaken gallery, of charming
> proportions, which had a sitting-room at either end of it and which in the evening
> was usually lighted. The light was insufficient to show the pictures to advantage, and
> the visit might have stood over to the morrow. This suggestion Ralph had ventured
> to make; but Isabel looked disappointed—smiling still, however—and said, "If you
> please I should like to see them just a little." She was eager, she knew she was eager
> and now seemed so; she couldn't help it. "She doesn't take suggestions," Ralph said
> to himself; but he said it without irritation; her pressure amused and even pleased
> him. The lamps were on brackets, at intervals, and if the light was imperfect it was
> genial. It fell upon the vague squares of rich colour and on the faded gilding of heavy
> frames; it made a sheen on the polished floor of the gallery. Ralph took a candlestick
> and moved about, pointing out things he liked; Isabel, inclining to one picture after
> another, indulged in little exclamations and murmurs. She was evidently a judge; she
> had a natural taste; he was struck with that. She took a candlestick herself and held it
> slowly here and there; she lifted it high, and as she did so he found himself pausing
> in the middle of the place and bending his eyes much less upon the pictures than on
> her presence. He lost nothing, in truth, by these wandering glances, for she was better
> worth looking at than most works of art.[25]

What a rich paragraph, inviting the reader to enter this space, a place that is duly described geometrically but "actuated" by the encounter of Ralph and Isabel. The close reader notices the presence of the disembodied narrator with its own set of judgments and assessments, hovering not far from the protagonists, eavesdropping and transcribing both their spoken words and their thoughts. More specifically, the reader notices the shifting access to consciousness that moves from what Isabel "knew" to what Ralph "said to himself." Simultaneously, the reader pays attention to the socioeconomic details offered by the setting, learning that Ralph lives the life of the moneyed class. This short excerpt gives a reader a glimpse into the erotic potential of this encounter, that Ralph is taken with his cousin's physical presence as well as with her aesthetic taste. And Isabel declares herself to be a woman of will, not easily put off from doing what she wants to do.

But all these characterological and narratological and erotic features take a back seat to the striking element in the excerpt: the light. The reader *sees* this scene by virtue of the play of candlelight and lamp-light on the paintings— described so memorably as "vague squares of rich color"—and on their heavy frames, on the polished floor of the gallery, and on the person of Isabel. This detailed description of one aspect of the setting's space imprints the scene in the reader's mind and grants entry into its precincts. The lighting director gets credit here for the impact of the excerpt.

In an effort to allow my students to experience further the consequence of this writerly decision by James, I invited them to join me for the next three minutes in writing to a prompt:

> "Write about an event or a situation solely in terms of its light."

Knowing that we would be invited to read aloud what we wrote in the three minutes, the students and I set to work. One student wrote about a car accident on a rainy highway at night. Another wrote about how the lights in a new operating room made it possible for the surgeon to see inside the abdomen and how, in retrospect, the old operating room had been perilously dark. One wrote about a New York City sunset shrouded in clouds and made all the more dramatic by virtue of the cast. One, a practicing nurse, wrote the following:

> I awake suddenly surprised by the alien glow in the room which is piercing the otherwise charcoal air—charcoal owing partly to the street lamp light sneaking through the slats in the window blinds. It was a planetary glow. As I make my way to the hall and beyond the darkness shrouds me until I come to her room. The space is black, pitch black. A small frosty orb sheds just enough light for me to see the soft rise and fall of the quilt on the far side of the room. All is well.[26]

As we listen to the writer read this paragraph aloud, we triangulate with her into the scene, each reader drawn by this alien, planetary glow to follow the figure's movement toward another orb's illumination of the tides of sleeping health. We meet one another in the scene, joining as co-readers with the writer of our text. The writer was surprised by the result of the writing, not "aware" of the illuminatory aspects of this remembered scene until prompted to do so. We see the Jamesian traces in the writing in the long, ever-qualified sentences and the density and prolongation of imagery—shrouds, orbs, far side of the moon. After this text was read aloud, we readers sat in its appreciation. The comments in the seminar, as I recall, had nothing to do with the sleeping child or the parent's vigilance. The comments had to do with the writing itself—its layers of detail, its ability to enforce stillness, simply its beauty.

By writing about space in the shadow of a great text that does so, my students and I experienced the power of an evocation of space to create mood, meaning, context, and even plot. We will be all the more attuned to spatial details in literary texts for the impressions and meanings that they may carry. Were we to continue reading *Portrait* together, we would be prepared to attend to how these two people become "vague squares of rich color" for one another, and how the characters will proceed to behold one another with exactly the kind of mystery and unknowingness that Isabel demonstrates toward the paintings and that Ralph demonstrates toward Isabel.

Voice

Who tells a narrative? To whom is the narrative told? To pay attention to *voice* in a narrative is to ask simultaneously many complex questions about the creator (writer, teller, performer) of a narrative, the narrator chosen by the creator to present the narrative, the role of the receiver (reader, listener, beholder) and the creator in the narrating act, and the contact made between the creator and the receiver. The concept of voice emphasizes that narratives are given from one to another, that the gift of a narrative is absorbed through a language of some sort, be it the words themselves or their mood or tone or music. Voice is originally a physical category, having been usurped for conceptual work within literary studies but carrying still its reference to the sound produced by the flow of air over this particular set of vocal cords and through this particular oral cavity; as such, voice is registered not only by the thinking brain but also by the listening and discerning aesthetic ear. Voice need not come from one individual but can be emitted by a Greek chorus, collective social minds, plural minds, or from non-human animals or machines or other entities that can be imagined to speak.[27]

Voice is a sociocultural and ethical concern as well as a literary one. When psychologist Carol Gilligan studied the ways women talk about moral decision making and found them to be different from the ways men talk about these matters, she called her pioneering study *In a Different Voice*.[28] Claudia Rankine's *Citizen: An American Lyric,* subtitled after a genre of speech, exposes racism not only in chasms of justice and privilege but in unequal "addressability," describing ways in which social violence is inflicted through invisibility and silence.

> When the stranger asks, Why do you care? you just stand there staring at him. He has just referred to the boisterous teenagers in Starbucks as niggers. Hey, I am standing right here, you responded, not necessarily expecting him to turn to you.
>
> He is holding the lidded paper cup in one hand and a small paper bag in the other. They are just being kids. Come on, no need to get all KKK on them, you say.
>
> Now there you go, he responds.[29]

In their seminal book *Narrative Identity,* Jens Brockmeier and Rom Harré describe the authorial voice in terms of moral and social contexts and commitments:

> Stories are told from "positions," that is, they "happen" in local moral orders in which the rights and duties of persons as speakers influence the location of the prime authorial voice. They must be heard as articulations of particular narratives from particular points of view and in particular voices. The significance of this perspectivalism is yet to be fully appreciated.[30]

Gilligan, Rankine, and Brockmeier each recognize the power of voice in narrative life. The voices of the women who spoke to Gilligan conveyed not just the words they said, but far more global properties of values, position, and stance. Rankine provides the raw data of racism in the words that are said that themselves inflict the violence. She quotes Ralph Ellison to say, "Perhaps the most insidious and least understood form of segregation is that of the word."[31]

Brockmeier and Harré's exhortation to heed the positions from which a voice emits and to consider the rights and duties of the speakers is particularly salient to the voices heard, elicited, and often silenced in the healthcare setting. Power asymmetries of class, race, gender identity, preferred language, and health status all complicate the hearing-out of persons marginalized on any of these bases. One is enough to silence a person. Healthcare professionals can overlook the challenges faced by patients in being heard at all—speaking a language other than the dominant one, not being fluent in the diction of bureaucracy, holding nontraditional beliefs about health and life style. Patients and family members can be too easily silenced if they ask too many questions, want too much evidence, or challenge medical opinion. The steep power hierarchies of healthcare, dominated by physicians and, increasingly, corporate interests, can cause profound imbalances of privilege and influence, allowing for a medical imperialism that prevents both patients and other healthcare professionals from being heard.

Since Aristotle considered the concept of mimesis and catharsis in *Poetics*, the literary study of voice and its larger parent concept *point of view* or *perspective* have been among the foundational questions posed by narratology and, by extension, by narrative medicine.[32] The near history of the contemporary study of voice began when the Russian formalists, including Vladimir Propp, studied the narrative structure of Russian folk tales in the 1920s. They distinguished between *fabula*, the events described in an account, and *syuzhet*, the text produced to represent those events. A similar distinction was made later by the French structuralists using the terms *histoire* and *récit*. Such literary distinctions illuminate the ordinary work of healthcare, as Kathryn Montgomery Hunter suggests in her depiction of the case presentation in medicine: "Rather than a transparent account of "reality," its highly organized, conventional structure imposes meaning upon the events it sets in order."[33]

In his 1972 *Narrative Discourse: An Essay in Method*, Gérard Genette proposed that there are three elements to consider in studying a narrative: story, narrative, and narrating.[34] His concept of *story* paralleled the *fabula* and *histoire* to describe the events themselves, while his *narrative* paralleled the *syuzhet* or *récit* as the textual representation of those events. However, the third term, *narrating*, complicated the binary distinction between the "real" of *fabula* and the representation in *syuzhet*. Paying attention to the human acts of emitting and receiving a narrative account exposed the unpredictable, pluripotent, ambiguous, perspectival nature of not only human perception and representation but also human relation.

Reader-response criticism arose to provide a conceptually complex account of the events in Genette's *narrating*, combining linguistic with psychoanalytic and aesthetic attention to the acts of the "speaking" author and of the "listening" reader.[35] The works of critics as varied as Roland Barthes and Walter Benjamin added to our understanding of what the reader does with the words of the writer.[36] We now realize, in the wake of poststructuralism and deconstruction, that events do not stand still to be recorded, that the "real" is created by virtue of its being perceived and represented, that the perspective of the perceiver alters what is perceived, and that *in the narrative act of representing an event does the event itself occur.*[37] When novelist and critic John Berger looks at the blue sky while he floats in the municipal swimming pool, he notices the drift of the cirrus clouds. "The movement of the curls apparently comes from inside the body of each cloud, not from an applied pressure: you think of the movements of a sleeping body."[38] These thoughts may or may not have come to the swimmer as he gazed at the clouds but perhaps only when he represented his having gazed. He goes on: "The longer I gaze at the curls, the more they make me think of wordless stories. Wordless stories like the stories fingers may tell, but in fact here stories told by minuscule ice crystals in the silence of the blue." The *fabula* here is a meteorological or atmospheric science event. The *syuzhet* is a remarkable meditation not only on the cirrus clouds but on the nature of subjectivity and narrativity itself. I remember that, upon reading these lines, I myself underwent something. I felt a movement in my insides, like a settling, a stilling, a curling up of some creature within me, peaceful and activating at the same time. My acts as a reader contributed to the meaning of this narrative, and my reception of Berger's text will never be replicated by another reader's reading. This is the power of the narrating.

The typology of Genette's story/narrative/narrating has been supplanted by more robust conceptual frameworks for describing and theorizing perspective, focalization, position, slant, and other aspects of narrating acts.[39] Nonetheless, Genette's realization that the act of narrating has a pride of place in understanding stories enables those who live through stories (which excludes none of us) to problematize, critique, and recognize stories' tellings and receivings. We are then in a position to fulfill Brockmeier's imperative: to examine the contexts within which narratives arise in social situations, power relationships, historical times, political realities, emotional charges, and intersubjective space.

I doubt there is any narrative medicine teaching session that does not examine the voice of the narrator or narratee. I have chosen a session held in the hospital for a multidisciplinary group of healthcare professionals representing medicine, social work, and health education. The text I chose was the poem "Wait" by American poet Galway Kinnell.

>
> Wait
> Galway Kinnell
>
> Wait, for now.
> Distrust everything, if you have to.
> But trust the hours. Haven't they
> carried you everywhere, up to now?
> Personal events will become interesting again.
> Hair will become interesting.
> Pain will become interesting.
> Buds that open out of season will become lovely again.
> Second-hand gloves will become lovely again,
> their memories are what give them
> the need for other hands. And the desolation
> of lovers is the same: that enormous emptiness

carved out of such tiny beings as we are
asks to be filled; the need
for the new love is faithfulness to the old.

Wait.
Don't go too early.
You're tired. But everyone's tired.
But no one is tired enough.
Only wait a while and listen.
Music of hair,
Music of pain,
music of looms weaving all our loves again.
Be there to hear it, it will be the only time,
most of all to hear,
the flute of your whole existence,
rehearsed by the sorrows, play itself into total exhaustion.[40]

"Wait, for now," the poem's first line, commands, in the imperative mood, a response from the reader. Throughout the poem, the speaker issues orders to a listener addressed in the second person. As we read and discussed this poem in the seminar, we wondered about this listener: who is the "you?" Is it the person reading or hearing the poem him or herself? Might the speaker have the audacity to be ordering *us* to wait, to distrust, to trust, to wait, to not go too early, to wait, to listen, to be there? Is there another character in the poem, unseen, but listening to these commands? Intercalated among the commands are forecasts, almost fortune-telling in quality—Personal events will become interesting again. Hair will become interesting. These lines make the listener wonder about that "you"—why might personal events not have been interesting until now? Or might the poem be an interior monologue addressed to the speaker himself or herself?

We readers noticed the spaces between the imperatives, where the speaker's emotional life becomes audible. That second-hand gloves are lovely by virtue of their remembering other hands they've held suggests some experience with love or friendship, connections that were valued. Who but a lover who has lost would know of the enormous emptiness of that desolation? When the speaking pronoun moves from the implied "I" of the command-giver to the "we" of tiny beings asking to be filled, the chasm between speaker and listener is crossed, both for the "you" in the poem's story space and the listener reading or hearing the poem from outside it. The pluralizing "we" connects these two listeners while it connects them with the speaker.

The second stanza continues to address the listener in the second-person, but the plural address in "music of looms weaving all our loves again" signals an intimacy between the poem's speaker and the poem's "you," whether these are two different entities or a self-speaking monologue.

The group of participants at this hospital seminar spent a long time talking about wind instruments. Flutes are played by blowing across the orifice of the mouth-hole to animate the column of air within the instrument, rather like creating a sound by blowing across the mouth of a bottle. Unlike a recorder or clarinet, where the musician's breath enters the instrument, the flute's sound is already "within" the instrument and the musician brings that sound to audible life. This seemed to matter to us for that last crowning image, "the flute of your whole existence." Sorrow picks up its instrument—you—and rehearses you until you or the sorrow is exhausted. We were awed as we examined this image closely, aware of the implications about the power of sorrow, about personal agency, about how one comes to know or "hear" one's own life, about the "you" that must be rehearsed within each one of us.

My participants all work in the hospital, many of them in oncology. The references to hair and pain signaled to them the very concrete side effects of cancer treatments. Although by no means limiting their reading to the context of illness, reading "Wait" together gave this group the dividend of looking squarely at the kind of waiting their patients do all the time. To see within this poem the allusions to life outside the illness—the lovely gloves, the buds out of season, the emptiness of the loss of love—reminded them of life's ongoingness despite or even because of serious illness.

Our discussion had centered on questions of voice as I've been discussing it—speaker position, the identity of the "you" in the poem, imperative moods, and reader response. My prompt, therefore, was: "Write about the person this poem is written to."

In four minutes, we read to one another what we had written. The group was unevenly split between those who wrote about specific patients near death whose wait would probably be their last one and others who imagined waits of different kinds, far away from the hospital. A physician wrote about a suicide by a young airplane pilot who chose to down a plane filled with passengers in the Swiss Alps. Most participants wrote about real persons, either themselves or others, in their personal lives or their hospital life.

The following paragraph was written by an educational specialist and graduate of our Master of Science program. The writer imagined the poem's "you" as a "she," gave her a history, a present, and almost a future:

> She sits there in the white hospital bed, feeling the thin mattress, rough sheets—
> smelling hospital, hearing hospital. Last year at this time, she was finishing school,

looking forward to the future. Last summer, she was drinking with her friends in the woods, laughing at the stars. Last winter, she was in college, reading and writing, addicted to the feeling of her brain racing from the intensity and exhaustion. Last month, she was rewriting her reality—someone stole her notebook of life, so she had to start over. Last week, she was feeling her scalp, shiny, sterile, like the hospital room. Last night, she ripped her new notebook to shreds—page by page. The last hour. . . .[41]

The accomplishment here was to have, in four minutes, invented a world. The writer has done exactly what might help to lift the veil on the mysterious "you": she imagined her. This short piece of fiction demonstrated to the other participants how an uncertainty about voice can spur creativity. Borrowing some words from the poem, notably exhaustion, the writer provided exquisite sensory detail in all segments of the protagonist's narrative. We smell the hospital; we hear the laughter; we see the stars, we recognize the thrill of thinking. When the crime occurs, the illness the felon, the book disappears, the hair disappears, and we readers / listeners are left on the precipice of this person's mortality, she whom we have seen laughing at stars entering her last hour on earth.

What did my participants learn from this hour and a-half? We learned to delve into a text, learning how to *find* the narrating act itself. We experienced the different meanings each one of us attributed to the poem based on our impressions of the voices in the poem. We argued about the likelihood that the speaker was speaking to itself, or that the "you" was meant to be us readers. Through the multiple perspectives represented around the table, we all increased our awareness of interpretive range. In particular, this poem helped the session's participants to formulate questions and ideas about "who speaks?" and "who listens?"—perhaps coming away at the end of the class better prepared, on hearing or reading a story, to wonder about the teller, to wonder about the consequences of this teller meeting this listener, and maybe to wonder about the listener too.

Metaphor

"Metaphor [is] the creation of resemblance by the imagination. . . . Resemblance in metaphor is an activity of the imagination; and in metaphor the imagination is life," writes poet Wallace Stevens in his artistic manifesto, *The Necessary Angel*.[42] Uncannily combining the intellect with the imagination, metaphor requires a fresh sighting of reality by the originator and stimulates it in the interpreter, releasing all around its potential for meaning. Stevens continues: "[Resemblance] touches the sense of reality, it enhances the sense of reality, heightens it, intensifies it. . . . In this ambiguity, the intensification of reality by resemblance increases realization and this increased realization is pleasurable. . . ." (pp. 77, 79).

Finding the resemblance among things is the origin of figural language. Metaphor, metonymy, tropes, rhetorical devices, and analogies are some of the many figural ways in which language conveys thought or perception from a creator to a receiver in excess of its content. Understanding the opening to the Gospel of St. John, "In the beginning was the Word," requires the reader to search for what the word "Word" might point to beyond its ordinary meaning. Literature and art, from cave-dwellers' paintings on, have relied on their languages' capacities to allude, to refer, to compare, seeing similarities where others may not see them and hence exposing the previously unknown.

Novelist Walker Percy wrote that we humans "must know one thing through the mirror of another."[43] Metaphor defamiliarizes the actual, making of it a mirror by virtue of placing things side by side that do not seem to belong side by side. Literary scholar Derek Attridge describes the activity of reading a metaphor as "the registering of an anomaly, the searching for a sense that would fit with the literary context, the experience of strangeness that is produced, the richness of the meanings made possible by the indeterminacy of the metaphor."[44] As readers encounter an unusual or unexpected comparison of a thing with something unlike it, they undergo an event; they perform a creative act of their own.

Because indeterminacy is at the source of metaphor—is the thing described as being something else not itself, or can it be both itself and something not-itself?—the understanding of metaphor is filled with ambiguity. Perhaps the originating impulse is not to seek similarity but to seek opposition, in search of the unresolvable tension that itself may represent the reality Stevens yearns for.[45] Perhaps metaphor is misunderstood if it is considered only to be a form of figural language; maybe, as early New Critic William Empson asserted, "[M]etaphor, more or less far-fetched, more or less complicated, more or less taken for granted (so as to be unconscious), is the normal mode of development of a language."[46] The vitality of the contemporary critical conversation about metaphor attests to the indeterminacy not only of metaphor itself but also to the tension that surrounds efforts to analytically tame it. Not open to manipulation or domination, the metaphor resists reduction and defies capture.[47]

What, though, is metaphor *for*? Stevens would say that metaphor is for thinking and feeling at the same time. Empson quotes poet, anarchist, and art critic Herbert Read that the metaphor is "the expression of a complex idea, not by analysis, not by direct statement, but by a sudden perception of an objective relation."[46] A surprising answer to my question comes from novelist, essayist, and Jamesian Cynthia Ozick who asserts that "[M]etaphor belongs less to inspiration than to memory and pity. I want to argue that metaphor is one of the chief agents of our moral nature, and that the more serious we are in life, the less we can do without it."[48] These viewpoints enlarge the mandate of this form of expression. It may be our way of achieving a unity of sorts, not just in the poems we write or read but in the acts of perceiving, interpreting, narrating, recognizing, and being in the world.

One of the many consequences of the revolutionary intellectual upheavals of the twentieth century—rise of critical theory, the deconstructionist turn, the linguistic turn, the narrativist turn, now the cognitive turn—has been the opening up of interest in metaphor to a vastly enlarged community of scholars and practitioners. Of late, the cognitive turn has opened the study of metaphor to the linguistic and psychological analysis of "basic conceptual metaphors," which are conventional metaphors ("life is a journey") found in the spoken or written discourse of any culture in which it is sought.[49] Literary studies in general, and narrative medicine in particular, have much to learn from these novel means to study what humans do with words, for our clinical work does not unfold in the domain of belles lettres or written work alone, but rather in the hurried yet consequential spoken conversations that take place in settings of healthcare.

Metaphor and other forms of figural language are necessary angels in achieving the goals of narrative medicine. Whether listening to a patient, reading an operative report, studying illness narratives, or reading *Wings of the Dove*, the receiver who relishes metaphor, who gets its combination of memory and sensation, of analytic thought and free association, will do justice to the text. Those readers or listeners not yet attuned to listening for the brilliance of metaphor will hear but half of what is produced.

I turn now to a teaching session in the "Methods of Narrative Medicine" seminar in the masters program at Columbia, which combines the study of close reading with practical training in how to teach narrative medicine. My 11 students and I have been reading two novels slowly through the spring semester, sometimes as little as 30 pages per week. Along with Virginia Woolf's *To the Lighthouse*, the seminar reads Manuel Puig's *Kiss of the Spider Woman*. Maura Spiegel and I chose these two novels for slow reading to give our students a rich contrasting combination of genres, narrative situations, period, interests, social contexts, and ways of doing things with words.

This session took part during a discussion of *Kiss of the Spider Woman*. Puig sets his dramatized novel in an Argentinian prison. Using almost entirely dialogue, Puig gives voice to Molina, a gender-fluid prisoner convicted of corrupting a minor, and Valentin, a revolutionary Marxist activist and now a political prisoner, as they get used to being cellmates. To pass the time, Molina describes movies he has seen to Valentin. Puig writes from a leftist stance, having himself been imprisoned in Argentina on sexual charges during the repressive regime.

Several pages into the novel the reader realizes that these two characters, who seem to be just talking about a movie, are in some kind of detention:

> —Wait a minute. . . . Is there any water in the bottle?
>
> —Mmm-hmm, I refilled it when they let me out of the john.
>
> —Oh, that's all right then.
>
> —You want a little? It's nice and fresh.
>
> —No, just so there's no problem with tea in the morning. Go on.
>
> —Don't worry so much, we have enough for the whole day.
>
> —But I'm getting into bad habits. I forgot to bring it along when they opened the door for showers, if it wasn't for you remembering, we'd be stuck without water later on.[50]

The reader pieces together a scene in a cell of some kind. Because there is no expository narration, it is up to the reader to learn the state of affairs from these two voices. Gradually, the reasons they have been jailed become known. The addition to the dialogue of footnotes about homophobia and repressive governments adds complexity and contradiction to the plot. The novel slowly reveals itself as a revolutionary statement. This stretch of dialogue opens Chapter 2:

> —You're a good cook.
>
> —Thank you, Valentin.
>
> —But you're getting me into bad habits. That could hurt me.
>
> —You're crazy, live for the moment! Enjoy life a little! Are you going to spoil our dinner thinking about what's going to happen tomorrow?
>
> —I don't believe in that business of living for the moment, Molina, nobody lives for the moment. That's Garden of Eden stuff.
>
> —You believe in Heaven and Hell?
>
> .
>
> .
>
> — There's no way I can live for the moment, because my life is dedicated to political struggle, or, you know, political action, let's call it. Follow me? I can put up with everything in here, which is quite a lot . . . but it's nothing if you think about torture . . . because you have *no* idea what that's like . . .
>
> —But I can imagine. (p. 27, horizontal ellipses in the original)

Themes of state violence, elitist privilege, official corruption and greed, and isolation and interiority flood the novel. Marginalized persons are punished

for cultural habits and life styles and imprisoned by societal prejudices. Those
in open revolt against the prevailing political power structure are silenced. In
effect, the prison where the novel is set is itself a metaphor for corrupt societal,
political, and economic forces that control the lives of all.

Each week I post a writing prompt about the week's reading on an electronic classroom Website. The students are asked to not only post a response
to the prompt but also to read one another's postings before seminar meets.
My writing prompt midway into the novel was: "Describe Molina's and
Valentin's cell."

Here is one of the postings to that prompt:

> The novel unfolds with little direct description of Valentin and Molina's cell, and yet
> in the distance between and around these characters, in the narrative space, a sense of
> place is created. The first allusion to a cell is the "black panther . . . stretched out in its
> cage" (3), an image from the movie Molina is recounting to Valentin. Puig does not tell
> us outright that the two men inhabit a similar cage, but he lays the base coat, or puts
> down the bass line so that as he fills in present-moment detail, adds snips of melody
> here and there, the physical setting of the novel comes into clearer and clearer focus.
> Little by little there are clues that—like the panther—Valentin and Molina are them-
> selves in a cage, a prison cell. . . . . Although Puig reveals gradually and in sparse detail
> where these characters are and why they came to serve time in this Argentine prison,
> he creates immediately and with great impact the emotional and imaginative reality
> of this world. Puig paints in the reader's mind in the first page of the text (3) that we
> are in a mysterious space "Something a little strange," a dangerous space "the panther
> . . . pacing back and forth . . . watching to tear her to pieces," a vexed space "having
> trouble with shading in the drawing," a sordid space "driven by some other, still uglier
> instinct." By the time we get to page 49, landing securely in the 1969 politically dan-
> gerous "Right here in Buenos Aires," we have been suffused in the mysterious, danger-
> ous, troubled, sordid Buenos Aires of the mind.[51]

This student adopts stylistic forms of Puig in the posting—the litany of
spaces mysterious and dangerous and vexed, without conventional punc-
tuation separating the individual items, mimic formal aspects of parts of the
novel. Both by content and form, the student represents a reception of the
many ambiguous resemblances—between cages, between the movie and reality, between Buenos Aires the city and the Buenos Aires of the mind. Other
students described the cell itself in precise sensory detail—the placement of
the cots, the quality of the light, the foul smell of the wax candle. Together,
the group assembled a powerful representation of both the concrete and the
figural cell, bringing one another evidence and interpretations that exploded
the rich metaphorical content of the novel. Because they were alive to the

resemblances, they received the multiple contradictory messages of the text itself and, therefore, were prepared to be left by this work in a state of ambiguity, unresolvable except through the imagination—left forever wondering, forever choosing among alternative endings, accepting that that very state of doubt was, no doubt, the hoped-for destination of the creator of the work.

Conclusions and Room for Further Thought

I have brought you on a tour of some of the narrative medicine teaching practices in presenting close reading. We are encouraged by the ability of our graduate students and clinical colleagues to present literary or visual texts to their own students once they have gained some facility themselves.[52] In such settings as high school classes, family support groups, and seminars for clinical trainees and pre–health professions students, they are able to engage groups of learners, choose texts, select prompts, and respond to the writing that is produced in the process.

Our goals are to increase the capacity of our learners to notice things, to be curious about words, to enter alien narrative worlds without fear or indifference, to gain insight into their own characterological moves in interpreting stories, and to be open to the beauty of what they receive. We are not trying to raise future novelists or poets in our classes; we know that not all our students will with glee read the conceptual essays and books we assign. Yet, the effort to teach close reading is repaid over and over by the attention given to patients, the respect offered to a healthcare team colleague, the self-knowledge gained by the deep relationships that form among group members, and the sense that they are not alone—in their work, in their studies, in their lives.

My medical students and I came to the end of *Infinite Jest* just as the school year came to a close. What we gained in the 1079 pages together was awe at this brilliant and suffering author, tenacity to remain in a narrative world no matter how bleak or ugly it becomes, and unspoken gratitude that we had accompanied one another through the stunning ordeal. Such are the dividends of narrative medicine teaching. The only unanswered question for my students and me is what enormous novel to read together next.

Notes

1. Wallace, *Infinite Jest*.
2. Keen, *Empathy and the Novel*; Kandel, *Age of Insight*; Kidd and Castano, "Reading Literary Fiction."

3. Said, "The Music Itself," 7.
4. See outcomes studies of narrative medicine teaching at Columbia: Arntfield et al., "Narrative Medicine as a Means"; Eliza Miller et al., "Sounding Narrative Medicine"; Devlin et al., "Where Does the Circle End?"; Charon et al., "Close Reading and Creative Writing."
5. Spivak, "Can the Subaltern Speak?"
6. See Tsevat et al., "Bringing Home."
7. Charon et al., "Close Reading and Creative Writing."
8. Gerrig, *Experiencing Narrative Worlds.*
9. Berthoff, "Learning the Uses."
10. Augustine, *Confessions*, 258–59.
11. Vico, *The New Science*; Bergson, *Time and Free Will*; Russell, "On the Experience of Time," 212.
12. Lukács, *Theory of the Novel*, 122
13. Ricoeur, "Life in Quest," 22.
14. Bakhtin, *Dialogic Imagination*; Genette, *Narrative Discourse*; Kermode, *Sense of an Ending*; Lubbock, *Craft of Fiction*; Ricoeur, *Time and Narrative.*
15. Ricoeur, *Time and Narrative*, vol. 1, 52.
16. The countless studies of time in modernist fiction cover the vast territory of philosophy and aesthetics. For studies of time in *To the Lighthouse*, see Banfield, "Time Passes." See also Woolf, "Reading." See Borges, "A New Refutation of Time."
17. Clifton, "the death of fred clifton," from *Collected Poems of Lucille Clifton*. Copyright © 1987 by Lucille Clifton. Reprinted with the permission of The Permission Company, Inc, on behalf of BOA Editions, Ltd., www.boaeditions.org.
18. The writer read this paragraph and gave me permission to reproduce the poem and the contents of the e-mail in this chapter.
19. Bakhtin, "Forms of Time," 84.
20. Bergson, *Time and Free Will*, 99.
21. Forster, *Aspects*, 39.
22. Goyal and Charon, "In Waves of Time."
23. Bachelard, *Poetics of Space*, xxxvi.
24. Certeau, *Practice of Everyday Life*, 117.
25. James, *Portrait of a Lady*, 60–61.
26. The student/writer granted me permission to reprint this text.
27. See Palmer, *Social Minds in the Novel*; Richardson, *Unnatural Voices*; Ryan, *Possible Worlds.*
28. Gilligan, *In a Different Voice.*
29. Rankine, *Citizen*, 16
30. Brockmeier and Harré, "Narrative: Problems and Promises," 46.
31. Rankine, *Citizen*, 122.
32. For detailed overviews of the concept of voice and its related concept perspective, see David Herman, *Story Logic*; and Chapter 7, "Point of View in Narrative," in Scholes, Phelan, and Kellogg, *The Nature of Narrative*. Wallace Martin's elegant *Recent Theories of Narrative* reviews the developments of the rise of narrative theory, including point of view.
33. Kathryn Montgomery Hunter, *Doctors' Stories*, 63.
34. Genette, *Narrative Discourse.*
35. Tompkins, *Reader-Response Criticism.*
36. Barthes, *The Rustle of Language*; Benjamin, "The Storyteller."
37. Hayden White, *Metahistory*; Barthes, *Rustle of Language*; Lyotard, *Postmodern Condition*; Derrida, *Of Grammatology*; Cixous, "Laugh of the Medusa."
38. Berger, "One or Two Pages," 127.
39. See Phelan, "Dual Focalization," for an overview of contemporary theories of focalization.

40. Kinnell, "Wait," from *Mortal Acts, Mortal Words*, by Galway Kinnell. Copyright © 1980, renewed 2008 by Galway Kinnell. Reprinted by permission of Houghton Mifflin Harcourt Publishing Company. All rights reserved.

41. The author of this text gave me permission to reprint the work in this volume.

42. Stevens, *The Necessary Angel*, 72.

43. Percy, "Metaphor as Mistake," 99.

44. Attridge, "Performing Metaphors," 25–26.

45. See Harries, "Metaphor and Transcendence," for a discussion of "collision vs. collusion" in the creation of poetic metaphor.

46. Empson, *Seven Types of Ambiguity*, 2.

47. See the several journals committed to the study of metaphor, including *Metaphor and Symbol* and *Metaphor and the Social World*. See Special Issues on metaphor in *Critical Inquiry* (Autumn 1978) and *Poetics Today* (Fall 1999).

48. Ozick, "Moral Necessity of Metaphor," 63.

49. George Lakoff and Mark Johnson's seminal *Metaphors We Live By* is arguably the starting point of social science's interest in metaphor. See Fludernik, "Metaphor and Beyond," for her introduction to *Poetics Today*'s special issue including essays by such leaders in the field as Raymond Gibbs, Mark Turner, and Gilles Fauconnier, who describe the evolving investigations of psychologists and cognitive scientists in metaphors of ordinary life. The field already has arrived at efforts to bridge the cognitive approach to the literary approach in such movements as "conceptual blending" and "cognitive poetics." See Stockwell, *Cognitive Poetics*; Turner, "The Cognitive Study of Art"; Jackson, "Issues and Problems."

50. Puig, *Kiss of the Spider Woman*, 8.

51. The student/writer of this paragraph gave me permission to reproduce it here.

52. Moran, "Families, Law, and Literature"; Spencer, "All Creatures"; Hellerstein, "'The City of the Hospital'."

PART

V

CREATIVITY

CHAPTER 9

Creativity: What, Why, and Where?

Nellie Hermann

Creativity in Our Everyday Lives

What is the most creative thing you've done so far today?

I ask this of a group of Narrative Medicine graduate students and then of a group of healthcare professionals at an intensive weekend workshop held in New York City. They write for three minutes, and then a handful of people share what they have written with the group. The responses range wildly, from a description of the decision of which tie to wear to what makeup to put on, a shared moment with a stranger on the subway, the choice to enjoy the view from a New York City bridge, or an impromptu stop at a bodega to get orange juice. After we hear the writing, I ask them to use these responses as a springboard to brainstorm what we think creativity **is**—it's a word we all know when we hear it, but what does it really mean? Again the range is wide: thinking outside the box, being flexible, being open, breaking down boundaries, coming up with new ideas. One participant says: "The nature of life." So, okay, I ask them then, if creativity is all of these things, and if we can see it in our lives in all of these ways, then why do people so often, especially in the world of healthcare, say that they are not creative? Why is creativity so often thought to be foreign, other, not-me, not this? Why has the word *creativity* become so scary to so many people?

The question is a complicated one, with very deep roots, not to be answered in a brief exploration with a large group of people nor, for that matter, in this chapter; for our purposes here it is enough to simply state that healthcare in particular has a vexed relationship to the notion of creativity. This vexed-ness exists for many reasons, many of them valid, many of them concerned with the serious nature of the work of health and illness and the perceived need in that work for the maximum amount of control. People in the healthcare world are far more willing to embrace the phrase "reflective writing" than they are "creative writing," for example, even though these two categories are closely related (more on this in a bit). People get nervous around the notion of a creative doctor—I have heard trained professionals and lay people alike say things like "no one wants a doctor who makes things up" or "I don't want my doctor getting creative with my care," as if the ability to think creatively means that you act unethically at your job. This kind of thinking reveals a misunderstanding of what creativity is and how it works in all of us.

It should be acknowledged that the word *creativity* is quite in and of itself flawed, as it has come to mean so many things to different people. It is one of those words that seem too big and broad, and in fact should probably be broken into a number of different words. Whole books, whole sections of libraries are devoted to what this word means. Many artists, those involved in the making of art, believe that a "creative act" specifically refers to the moment when something is made that previously did not exist—those that believe this might be right to argue about whether buying an unexpected orange juice at a bodega constitutes creativity. But these recounted moments are ones where participants' minds were engaged in acts of thinking differently than usual, in acts that quicken the spirit—and it is this that I mean in this chapter when I use the word creativity. Psychologist Rollo May, author of *The Courage to Create*, writes: "When we engage [in looking at] a painting . . . we are experiencing some new moment of sensibility. Some new vision is triggered in us by our contact with the painting; something unique is born in us. This is why appreciation of the music or painting or other works of the creative person is also a creative act on our part."[1] I use the word creativity here in a similar fashion; new moments of sensibility and vision can be born in us in a myriad of different ways. Acknowledging that the word is flawed, our purpose here is to interrogate this word so that it might be seen to be as expansive as it is, and so that more people can and will see the ways they are already using it in their lives.

Let's think about the average patient/doctor encounter: the patient tells the doctor (or other healthcare provider) a narrative of what has been happening in his life, what symptoms and troubles have brought her to seek help. The provider listens and then examines the patient, gathering more evidence to feed the diagnosis and the treatment plan that will follow. In performing this process the doctor must necessarily listen for certain details that mean more than others, thinking through what may not be being said and asking follow-up questions to fill in those gaps. This work—performing a differential diagnosis based on the evidence at hand, determining what further evidence is needed, weighing the things that can't be known, and understanding the possibility that certain things are wrong or misleading—this work *is in itself creative*. It necessitates a form of thinking that is complicated and is, as is explored elsewhere in this book, narrative in nature. Kathryn Montgomery Hunter, in her book *Doctor Stories*, writes that "medicine is fundamentally narrative":

> "Physicians take [a patient's] story, interrogate and expand it, all the while transmuting it into medical information. Sooner or later they will return it to the patient as a diagnosis, an interpretive retelling that points toward the story's ending. In this way, much of the central business of caring for patients is transacted by means of narrative."[2]

And, I would add to this, in the creation and interpretation of narrative the central business is transacted by means of creativity. It is akin to reading a mystery novel (Montgomery Hunter herself uses Sherlock Holmes as an ongoing example in her book), gathering the clues to guess at how the plot turns out, forming a hypothesis that may or may not match reality. This kind of information gathering, synthesizing, and hypothesizing is creative work.

Dr. Stuart Firestein, a professor of neuroscience at Columbia University, has written a book called *Ignorance: How it Drives Science* (Oxford: 2012), in which he argues that scientists are in fact driven by ignorance rather than by facts—ignorance here meaning "a particular condition of knowledge: the absence of fact, understanding, insight or clarity about something."[3] He writes that conducting science is in fact something like searching for a black cat in a dark room—very difficult, especially when it often turns out the cat isn't even there—and argues that "a tolerance for uncertainty, the pleasures of scientific mystery and the cultivation of doubt"[4] should be embraced by more people and understood to be part of all scientific projects. The argument for uncertainty and ignorance that Firestein puts forth is again an opening into a much bigger discussion, one that is necessarily occurring with greater frequency and urgency as healthcare training in our country becomes more and more "evidence-based" and numbers-driven. Ambiguity, doubt, uncertainty, and, as Firestein argues, ignorance: like it or not, these are facts in the healthcare world, creeping around every corner and chasing every decision. In part this is where the creativity enters in, as we need the human mind to place the puzzle pieces together.

Of course all of us wish we were always dealing in absolutes when it comes to our own health. But knowing this is not the case, my guess is we would all choose a provider with a depth of understanding, a tolerance for ambiguity, and a capacity for seeing more than one possibility in a patient's presentation.

Isn't it better to acknowledge the uncertainties than to pretend they don't exist? Of course I don't mean that a doctor should bring every uncertainty into a room with the patient, or even always acknowledge all of them to him/herself—but acceptance, on some level, of the preponderance of doubt in the work is, I would argue, a necessity for strength in the face of it.

Over the years in narrative medicine we have come to see more and more that our work is about reawakening the creativity that lives in all of us. When we go into a room and lead others in an exercise of reading and writing, we are encouraging everyone in that room to be creative: to put down their rigidly held convictions and engage in an exercise where there is no "right" answer, to allow themselves to be swept into something different, something they may not be able to see the end result of. Ultimately we hope that in doing so, and in then examining what they have done, participants in such exercises might realize and reconnect to the creativity they use and express every day in their work and their lives and thereby bring this creativity to other endeavors and to other encounters.

Toward what end, you ask, is this creativity being awakened and being spread? This is what I will explore throughout this chapter. I will focus most specifically on the reasons why we write as we do in the clinical context, but it should be said that the underpinnings behind the writing we do can (and should) be applied to any other sort of applied creative work as well.

In *The Courage to Create*, Rollo May writes: "Whereas moral courage is the righting of wrongs, creative courage, in contrast, is the discovering of new forms, new symbols, new patterns on which a new society can be built. Every profession can and does require some creative courage. . . . The need for creative courage is in direct proportion to the degree of change the profession is undergoing."[5] This quote seems to me to summarize everything else I might have to say about the use of creative work in healthcare, a field made up of many professions undergoing enormous change.

What is Creative Writing For, Particularly in the Clinical Context?

Among the many formats available for narrative medicine work, one of the most common is for a group of people to read a short piece of writing together—a poem or very short story or prose excerpt—and then, after closely examining that piece of writing together, to write for a few minutes to a prompt that arises from the piece that has just been examined. After writing, participants are invited to share what they have written with one another and to respond to what they hear in one another's work.

There are of course many variations on this format—the work can be done using visual art, film clips, music, really any form of expression—but one thing that does not change is the need for writing to be done. And often it is the writing that people are most perplexed about—reading together, talking about a work of art together, this people can more easily grasp, but the writing part is less immediately understood. So this has become the question that I find myself most often trying to answer: Why writing? Why should doctors, or medical students, or anyone in the healthcare community know anything about how to write?

Writing is, at root, an externalizing act. When we write, we bring what is inside to the outside; we put words, however indirectly or metaphorically or imperfectly, to what's inside of us, feelings or experiences that previously were not concrete. Language *is* the realization of thought—it is how thought comes to be in the world, and it is the way that one recognizes it (this idea is taken up in more detail in Chapter 4). As Miguel de Cervantes once said, "The pen is the tongue of the mind."[6] The byproducts of the act of writing are manifold. One, by moving what is internal to the external, particularly in the case of experiences that trouble us, that diminish the space inside of us, we create more room where new experiences can live. Two, by externalizing our experiences we create literal objects, text on a page, that can then be examined at different angles, as an X-ray can be held up to a light: does this accurately represent my experience or what I wanted to say? Does this look like what I expected, or do I see things here that I am surprised to see? Three, by externalizing we allow others to share in our experiences, not just in the events as they happened but as they *felt*, to us as individuals, through our particular and specific lenses. We also, then, invite others to bring their lenses to our experience, to show us things about ourselves that we did not already know. What do others see in this object that I don't yet see?

My colleague Craig Irvine has written about an experience that is exemplary here. He worked with a student, Ashley, in the second half of her fourth year of medical school, who wrote a story for him about a time she'd been moved by a patient's suffering. Craig writes:

> Ashley's story was about an experience she'd had almost two years earlier, as a third-year medical student, on the first morning of her first inpatient rotation. Early that morning, a patient named Mary was admitted to Ashley's hospital floor. Mary, who was not much older than Ashley, had been hospitalized with sepsis, caused by immune suppression from chemotherapy. Shortly after arriving on the floor, Mary developed Acute Respiratory Distress Syndrome. The entire team ran to her room, and the Chief Resident told Ashley to sit by the bed and encourage Mary to relax. For more than five hours, while residents and attendings ran in and out of the room doing everything

in their power to arrest Mary's respiratory decline, Ashley held Mary's hand, repeating, over and over again, "Just breathe. Relax, it's going to be okay. Breathe. Please try to relax. We're all here for you. Just breathe." When Mary stopped breathing, the Chief Resident pushed Ashley away from the bed, and he and the rest of the team began the code. Death was declared several minutes later. The team abruptly left the room, leaving Ashley alone with Mary's battered body. No one ever spoke to her about Mary's death.

When Ashley finished reading this story to me, she looked up and said, through her tears and without irony, "I just wish I'd been able to do something for Mary, like everyone else. I felt so helpless. Just useless and in the way."[7]

Ashley did not see, until she wrote her story and shared it with others, the centrality of her role with the patient whose death she attended to. It was only by externalizing this narrative and allowing others to peer at it, and tell her what they saw, that she was able to see this troubling experience in a different light than the one she had been carrying around with her. What seemed so obvious to others had been far from obvious to Ashley, in large part because the story had not yet been externalized. And when it only lived inside Ashley, it could not be adequately *seen*. The story needed to leave her, to become an object that could be examined and inspected; she, Ashley, needed to become a *character* in her own portrayal, someone whose story she could see from the outside as others would.

Another dividend to writing and sharing is that almost always, sharing something we have written makes us feel more vulnerable than it does when we tell the same story orally and informally. This tends to be true even if what we are writing and sharing is not particularly personal, or not even true at all. Why is it that sharing what we write makes us feel so vulnerable? I would venture that it is in part because we are forced to commit to something, to one version of the way it was, to one way of telling one thing. You can't as easily "take it back" after it is written down; you have to present it one way, in one form, and then you have to show others this form. This is not at all to say that there only *is* one story or one form for a story—one can go back and go back and tell the same story an infinite number of times, and tell it differently every time. But when we write something down, it becomes calcified in a way and because of this, in the quickly generated form of writing that we work with most commonly in narrative medicine workshops, it is a more raw, less mediated, less comfortable presentation that we are inviting others to see.

It is loss of control, then, that we are wrestling with when we offer up these little pieces of ourselves; not only telling other people a story about our experience but openly asking them to respond to it—inviting them into the space of it. This is both why it is difficult and why it is valuable, for we are often surprised with what we've written and then with the responses to it. In a group of people writing spontaneously, the work of connection is done far more quickly, for the vulnerability that we feel when sharing puts us at each other's mercy—open and available to be heard, misunderstood, judged—and then the responses we receive, often insightful and surprising, build our trust. Quite often in these groups there are disparities of power, privilege, race, and gender, and so this shared vulnerability can be quite delicate and fraught— the byproduct of this, though, is that when connection is forged it is all the more powerful and important to improved practice and communication among the group.

Again, here, we are talking about the uncertainty with which we started this chapter—that feeling of unknowing that is difficult for some health-care providers to accept. Frequently students coming into medical school believe that they can simply learn enough to be certain—that banishing ambiguity and doubt, and thereby remaining less touched by the emotion of the work, is a matter of how much you take in and how hard you work. Surgeon Pauline Chen, in her book *Final Exam: A Surgeon's Reflections on Mortality*, describes this process in terms of the medical student experience in the anatomy lab:

> Aspiring physicians face death directly in the form of the cadaver. And then they tear it apart. Each detail of the cadaver—every bone, nerve, blood vessel, and muscle— passes from the world of the unknown into the realm of the familiar . . . in knowing the cadaver in such intimate detail, we believe that we are acquiring the knowledge to overcome death.[8]

Narrative medicine exercises like the ones discussed above, where students are asked to reveal themselves in a controlled way and are exposed to the views and responses of their peers, can be a helpful tool on the road to accepting the myriad vantage points and possibilities that always surround us and to work-ing through the realities of the work at hand.

Also, not to put too fine a point on it, but this vulnerability mimics in a small, controlled way the vulnerability of a patient asked to put her most deli-cate self in the hands of strangers. Where is trust more essential than among teams of caregivers? This is part of why I believe these exercises to be impor-tant for young clinicians-in-training to get familiar with doing: learning to trust and rely on one another, as well as learning to be open with themselves, are some of the most important skills for them to learn.

The novelist Richard Powers, in an interview with the magazine *The Believer*, said the following: "Story is the mind's way of molding a seeming whole from out of the messiness of the distributed, modular brain. At the same time, shared stories are the only way anyone has for escaping the straight-jacket of self. Good medicine has always depended on listening to histories. So any attempt to comprehend the injured mind naturally inclines toward all the devices of classic storytelling . . . Only inhabiting another's story can deliver us from certainty."[9] This idea, that in inhabiting another's story we are delivered from certainty, is a crucial one and is at the root of everything we do in narrative medicine. It is also, of course, connected to the fear that I touched on above. What happens if we get too far into another's story, the fear says, if we get too invested, too connected? What happens if we get too familiar with uncertainty, so that we realize that the decisions we make are always imperfect?

I suppose I would answer to this: Yes, what happens then? If we follow this fear to its logical conclusions, what is it we are ultimately afraid of? That we will care too much, that our hearts will break? That we will have to face our limits, our mortality, the mortality of those we love? That we won't be able to do the work anymore because the emotional toll will be too great? Again, this is the opening to a larger conversation—but my instinct is that a good healthcare provider will go through all of these things in the course of his/her work, that these things are an intrinsic *part* of the work. What does the avoidance of these things cost the provider? What does the embrace of them cost? I'm not sure there are straight answers to any of these questions, as they are very individually pitched, but I do think it is a conversation worth having.

Forms and Dividends of Creative Writing

There are, of course, many different ways of writing, and many of the dividends of the act change depending on the form, the intent, and the audience. As a fiction writer I have found particular solace and freedom in the act of making things up—changing my own experience so that it looks *and is experienced* other than the way it was for me, which then allows me to see ways that it could have been different. I have also enjoyed the obscuring of what is "true" and untrue, a distinction whose blurriness comes to light easily in the wake of a work of fiction. It is no exaggeration for me to say that writing fiction changed my life, and that my use of craft has been central to my health. This is my particular version of narrative medicine, and I believe strongly in its potential even for people who have no inclination toward writing at all.

When I was young, suffering from a series of tragedies that befell my family, I used writing to process what had happened and what I felt; for me, at that time, writing was a far more comfortable act than speaking. When I was in fifth grade, the oldest of my three brothers became severely mentally ill. Five years later, when I was a sophomore in high school, I lost my father and my youngest brother within six months to brain tumors. I had always been a writer, but in the wake of these tragedies I relied on writing in a new way. For many years I could not speak about what happened because I felt that any words I expressed were inadequate. Writing was the only way I processed any of it for a long time. Finally, 10 years later, it was the writing of my first novel, *The Cure for Grief*, that really allowed me to loosen my hold on the story that was holding me prisoner. I used craft in such a way that it was central to my health.

When attempting to write about my own experiences in a "true" and formal way, I always felt hung up on the fact that no matter what I wrote I could not adequately translate my *exact* experience, my total "truth." Words were inadequate for that, and I couldn't get past that knowledge. Writing fiction, then, and writing about my experiences as if they happened to someone else, allowed me to objectify my "truth" and freed me to triangulate my experience, so that I was not gripping the reality of it quite so tightly. (I put the word "true" in quotes, here, because of the tricky slipperiness of that word—we all often have an expectation that there is a right, straight version of events, but in fact every story is necessarily filtered, narrativized, refracted through many different lenses. The idea that fiction is "untrue" and nonfiction "true" is sometimes a problematic one. More on this below.)

To illustrate this, I'd like to share part of an exercise that I did in graduate school, given to me by the great writer Mark Slouka in a craft seminar. After years of struggling with how to write about my own experiences, it was this exercise that gave me the courage and the voice to do it—an endeavor that became my first novel, *The Cure for Grief*. The assignment was to write a memory as nonfiction and then to write it as fiction—this is an exercise that I now do often on the first day of my writing courses, for I find that it immediately unsettles the students in the best possible way, freeing them to look at their memories, as well as their conceptions of writing, in very different ways.

Here is the nonfiction piece I wrote:

> I don't remember what I did the day my oldest brother came home from college crazy, but I know that after that day, my whole life was different. I don't remember the bus ride to school, if the quadruplets from the up the street were particularly rowdy, if we were on time for homeroom. I don't remember what we were learning in school, if maybe that was when we were doing the Egyptian timelines, or maybe we had sex-ed that day, if we had a spelling bee that day or not. I don't remember if Michael Safran talked to me that day, though I'm pretty sure I wanted him to; I don't remember what we had for lunch though I imagine it was pizza, the rectangle kind, with the option of chocolate milk.

That day, up until the moment that my father approached where I was waiting for the bus after school, was just like any other day before then—a happy, normal, fifth-grade day—and therefore indistinct. It is interesting, then, how vividly I can remember my father that day, in his suit, a bit rumpled from the office, approaching the line where I was waiting for the bus. I don't remember what he said as he held out his hand to me, or whether his face really did look grave, as I imagine it did, or if he made a real effort to hold back his sadness and fear, which I imagine he must have. But I remember the confusion I felt, my father suddenly materializing at my school, a territory he almost never frequented. Did he just want to see me? Did he just get home from work early today? I remember taking his hand and leaving the line.

If I had to pinpoint the moment that my life changed, it would be that moment: taking my father's hand and walking away from that line of children. After that moment, I was not like those kids anymore; suddenly, I was a kid with a secret; I was a kid with a family coping with tragedy; I was a kid with an older brother who was out of his mind.

And then here is the fiction version, which ended up nearly verbatim in the novel:

The day her brother came home from college crazy, Ruby won a spelling bee. The entire fifth grade class had gathered in the auditorium that morning, and Ruby had stayed on stage the whole time, as one by one her classmates misspelled words and Mrs. Henderson, the school secretary, rang the tiny, hand-held bell to signal that they were eliminated from the competition. Ruby's final word, the one that won her the giant trophy that she held in her hand as she made her way out the doors of the school towards the waiting school bus that day, just before her father walked up the long drive toward her, had been profligate, a word she had never even heard before but somehow managed to spell. Prof-li-gate; the word came apart nicely, Ruby's favorite kind of word. It divided itself in front of her, so she could see the letters as she spelled them out. Ruby was in the zone, that morning, the words floating before her, cooperating, dividing themselves into neat little sections she could easily read. Mrs. Butterworth, her teacher, sitting at the front table next to Mrs. Henderson, had a smile on her face whenever Ruby stood before the microphone. Mrs. Henderson would say the word, and Ruby would repeat it back, and she would look at Mrs. Butterworth and Mrs. Butterworth would smile, and nod, and the word would float up before Ruby and divide itself. It was almost effortless.

After the spelling bee, the day was a blur, the trophy burning a hole in the floor next to Ruby's backpack. She couldn't wait to surprise her parents with it; she kept imagining their faces, their mouths like Os, her dad saying "my buttons are popping," her mother making Swedish meatballs for dinner to celebrate. When she thought of the spelling bee, it felt like a dream, and she couldn't quite believe it had been her up there, conquering those words as if she were on horseback, swatting them out of the air with a long sword.

When the day was over, however, and Ruby was making her way to the school bus, walking in the line of children down the walk outside the school, cradling the trophy in her arm like she did her favorite stuffed animal, Bear, whom she had won at a fair, her father was coming up the walk towards her, and the expression on his face was not curious or proud but grave, and he barely looked at the trophy as he took her hand and walked her away. Her friends called out to her—*bye Ruby!*—and she was walking away from them with her father in his suit but this wasn't the way she had pictured it, not at all, and she couldn't remember the last time her father had picked her up from school; had he ever? No, she was pretty sure he never had.

When I wrote the nonfiction version, as you can see, I was hung up on the idea that I couldn't remember it exactly as it was. So much of the piece is the phrase "I don't remember." This bothered me; it made me feel I couldn't possibly do justice to the experience, it brought me very uncomfortably close to understanding the question: *What's the point of writing?* Writing that nonfiction version didn't release or transform the experience for me, it only made me frustrated that I couldn't do it *right*. The fiction version, however, allowed me to externalize the memory, which then allowed me to imagine how it *might have been*, and to accept that as enough. When I gave the moment to my character, Ruby, I could play God in a way; I could declare *this is how it was*, and then it would be so. Interestingly, it is hard for me now to look back on that memory and not think of it the way it was for Ruby—the way that I created it. This is an act of power, of course, of taking hold of an uncomfortable moment that happened to me and making it, rather, a moment that I created, which then puts it under my control.

Of course creating fiction from my experiences does not change any of what actually happened, and what actually happened is central to who I am in a way that the created fiction is not. But by creating a narrative of my experiences, fiction *or* nonfiction, I alter just slightly my *relationship* to these facts, so that I can find in them a different kind of "truth"—not just the truth of facts, but the truth of experience.

Charles Anderson and Marian MacCurdy, in the introduction to their co-edited book *Writing and Healing: Toward an Informed Practice*, write:

> By writing about traumatic experiences, we discover and rediscover them, move them out of the ephemeral flow and space of talk onto the more permanent surface of the page, where they can be considered, reconsidered, left, and taken up again. Through the dual possibilities of permanence and revision, the chief healing effect of writing

is thus to recover and to exert a measure of control over that which we can never control—the past.

As we manipulate words on the page, as we articulate to ourselves and to others the emotional truths of our pasts, we become agents for our own healing, and if those to whom we write receive what we have to say and respond to it as we write and rewrite, we create a community that can accept, contest, gloss, inform, invent, and help us discover, deepen, and change who we have become as a consequence of the trauma we have experienced. . . . [H]ealing is neither a return to some former state of perfection nor the discovery of some mythic autonomous self. Healing, as we understand it, is precisely the opposite. It is change from a singular self, frozen in time by a moment of unspeakable experience, to a more fluid, more narratively able, more socially integrated self.[10]

In his essay in the same volume, Professor T.R. Johnson from the University of New Orleans speaks specifically about how this sort of writing can and should be thought of as creative, while acknowledging that because of the connotations of the word *creative*, using it to describe this trauma writing risks undermining the very serious, very "real world" truth that the work seeks to generate. "If we intend to take the notion of healing seriously," he writes, "we must problematize the easy line between 'creative' writing and writing that purports to be 'factual'; we must understand both more complexly . . ." He writes that if we can learn to see ourselves as moving and changing beings, then we can loosen ourselves from trauma and its consequences, in turn creating a reason to hope. He concludes, "We might thus see writing that heals as writing that . . . helps us to recover the strength to awaken to the flux and flow, the multiplicity of the world."[11] In my experience, this description is exactly right. My own trauma lived quietly and unspeakably within me for many years, and it did a lot of damage. It was only when I allowed it to move outside of me and to change apart from me that I was able to accept it and to accept who I might be without it.

But this same work is valuable for all of us, even with all of our daily disruptions, the traumas that are not so great that they disrupt the flow of our lives. It does not seem a stretch to say that every caregiver, even in training alone, experiences many traumas. And it is not uncommon for traumatic events to come to the surface very quickly in response to a writing prompt—I have never done a workshop with medical professionals where at least one vivid traumatic event has not poured onto the page in the 3-minute window they have to write. I am always amazed at the memories that are called back in response to a writing prompt, decades-old memories leaping to mind and to the page in less than a minute.

In a workshop with pediatricians at Presbyterian Hospital, the prompt we gave was in response to the short story "Axolotl," by Julio Cortázar, where a man becomes so engaged with watching these small creatures at the zoo that by the end of the story he becomes one of them. We asked the participants to write about a time when they were influenced by "another way of seeing." Here was one woman's response:

> I was in the examining room and saw this child unable to talk, to see, with involuntary movements, breathing through a trache and feeding through a tube.
>
> Next to her was an exhausted mother overwhelmed by the care of this child and about to give birth to another one.
>
> I felt full of sorrow, empathy, fear that I could be in her feet.
>
> I offered a respite program. A place where she could place this child for a few days. (A child that should probably not even be alive.)
>
> She looked at me with big eyes and with horrific surprise she said to me: "she is the light of my eyes, my princess. Would never part with her. . . . This is what God gave me."[12]

After she read this, she revealed that this was an event from more than 10 years before, and that she now saw this was a transformative moment for her. "Ever since then," she said, "I have been different with the mothers."

The poet Gregory Orr, author of a book called *Poetry as Survival*, speaks about the sense of order that writing creatively can bring to us: "We often experience the world as confusing and chaotic, especially during crises," he writes. "Our day to day consciousness can be characterized as an endlessly shifting, back-and-forth awareness of the power and presence of disorder in our lives and our desire or need for a sense of order. Most of us live most of our lives more or less comfortably with the daily interplay of these two awarenesses, but in certain existential crises, disorder threatens to overwhelm us entirely."[13] For Orr, survival begins when we "translate" this suffering into language—he writes, "in the act of making of a poem at least two crucial things have taken place that are different from ordinary life. First, we have shifted the crisis to a bearable distance from us: removed it to the symbolic but vivid world of language. Second, we have actively made and shaped this model of our situation rather than passively endured it as a life experience."

* * *

"To me, writing, the writing of literature, is partly an act of protest and defiance, and even rebellion, against . . . the temptation to entrench myself, to set up an almost imperceptible

barrier, one that is friendly and courteous but very effective, between myself and others, and ultimately between me and myself." – David Grossman[14]

Keith Oatley, a professor of cognitive psychology at the University of Toronto, has conducted a number of experiments looking into the effects of reading fiction on the social cognition and emotional perception of adults. In one study published in 2006, he and his research partner found that that "the more fiction people read, the better they were at perceiving emotion in the eyes and, to a lesser extent, correctly interpreting social cues."[15] A year later, his research partner Raymond Mar published evidence showing that a group of adults assigned a piece of fiction to read, as opposed to a group assigned a nonfiction essay, performed better on average on a social reasoning test, suggesting that "even a brief bout of reading fiction can temporarily improve a person's social skills."[16] Oatley writes, "Our accumulating findings are providing increasing support for the hypothesis that reading fiction facilitates the development of social skills because it provides experience thinking about other people. That is, we think the defining characteristic of fiction is not that it is made up but that it is about human, or humanlike, beings and their intentions and interactions. Reading fiction trains people in this domain, just as reading nonfiction books about, say, genetics or history builds expertise in those subject areas."[17]

What I particularly appreciate about Oatley and his colleagues' work is the proof that the value of fiction lies not necessarily in the "made up" aspect of it, in the fantasy, but in the ways that it is always tied to what it means to be human. I often encounter first-time fiction writers who think very seriously that in order to write fiction they must write something wild and fantastical—the breakthroughs come when people explore their fiction with an eye toward expressing something about the human condition. And I believe that everything Oatley and his colleagues have proven and will continue to prove applies just as much to writing fiction as to reading it. The difference may lie only in the frequent truth that when one writes fiction, as opposed to reading it, one learns more about one's own humanity in its relation to others.

A student of ours in the masters program who graduated a few years ago had an inspiring breakthrough along these lines. She is a doctor from Canada who had never in her life written fiction before. Inspired by the nonfiction / fiction exercise in my class, she attempted to write about a memory from her childhood centered around her parents' divorce as fiction and in the second person. She was amazed by the responses to her piece that she received from me and her classmates—the second person worked on more levels than she knew, for it was clear to readers of her piece that she was speaking to herself, and that she had much that she wanted to say to that younger version of her. She said she had only put the piece in second person because she felt the first person was too close and the third person too hard. When she saw the unanticipated dividends of what she had done, she was amazed.

The key here is really about craft—it's about *how* the stories are constructed as much as about their literal content, and beginning to recognize elements of craft in our written narratives can help us begin to recognize the craft in our oral ones as well. Now *craft*, again, is a tricky word—most artists would argue here that craft is always something intentional, worked on, hence *crafted*. I concede this, but I am not quite sure what other word to use to refer to the form and shape of our stories, what we make that is automatic and inherent, not always something purposeful and directed. The graduate student I just mentioned did not put her piece in the second person purposefully, because she thought that would "work" best—she did it unconsciously, because another way of doing it felt too difficult, and her choice there ended up with surprising results. Everything we write is crafted—as soon as we write it down, it takes on a shape, a mode of delivery. This is true for our oral stories as well. Look back at the piece of writing by the pediatrician about the mother with the disabled child that I quoted above: do you see any "craft" there? To me, what is interesting about those few lines of writing is the way the writer manages to turn the child in the piece into a creature much like the Axolotl in the story that she was writing in response to—something otherworldly, not quite human—which then allows her to give the great payoff at the end when the mother reacts to her sentiments with such horror. In just a few lines, dashed off in less than 5 minutes, there is great, and unintentional, craft. This recognition of craft, form, language choice—however it is best referred to—whereby the choice of how the story is told reveals something about its meaning, is the kind of work that can be particularly beneficial to a clinician, who is tasked with hearing stories all day long.

As an element of a month-long elective for fourth-year medical students, I teach a fiction-writing workshop, and at the end of the month I always ask the students to write something about a true medical school experience using the fictional techniques that we have been studying all month long. The very first time I asked the students to do this exercise, a student wrote about a patient experience that had long been troubling her. This patient had been terribly mean to her while he was in the hospital, humiliating her in front of his family and even making her cry. In her piece, she imagined the scenario from the patient's point of view as well as from that of different members of his family. After reading it to the class, she exclaimed with disbelief that she finally felt she understood why the patient had been so rude. Even though what she had written was her invention, the act of attempting to get inside the man had released something for her, she said, and she finally felt capable of letting go of the experience.

Here is the response to the same exercise from one of my more recent students:

> He is a sturgeon pulled onto the fisherman's boat. Flopping, flailing, wrestling to hold onto life while surrounded by a crowd of fisherman, deck hands, first mate. He cannot breathe here, his lungs slowing filling with blood, gasping, coughing, sputtering. The bipap machine, unable to open his airways, was doing no good. It is the pole with hook piercing his cheek, a device to yank him to the deck. He is not meant to be on dry land. He cannot breathe here. When I would pass his ICU bed, I saw him trapped in a web of fishing line, floating to the surface where they are connected to different medications.
>
> They were giving him just enough to sustain him out here, to prevent him from drying out. I saw his bony, armor-like plates along his spine, his scutes, and above his toothless grin a thin moustache, his barbel, which, when he is not here, drag along a river's murky depths. When I entered his room, his tail occasionally flapped under his hospital sheet and blanket when he gasped, reminding me yet again that this is not his natural habitat. He begged us to let him go, to throw him back, that he's not a keeper, but longs to return to the cool independence that water provides him. I prefer the catch and release method when possible, but I am not the captain. I take orders, and so I supported the team's decision for a few more days of high dose steroids. One last effort to transform his lungs into ones compatible with life out here. Then I heard over the loud speaker, "Arrest Stat, CCU, Arrest Stat, CCU", booming ominously. I sprinted down two flights of stairs, knowing it was him, again resisting our interventions against nature.[18]

By inventing an image for the patient she wrote about, this student was able to articulate more clearly the way she felt about his death; by placing him in a creative, imagined context, she could more accurately portray her own true feelings as well as imagine his.

Writing is a way of exploring our particular way of seeing, and of experiencing our thought in real time; as I touched on earlier, it is a way of accessing aspects of our mind and our experiences that we had no access to previously. The fiction writer William Gass writes:

> Language, unlike any other medium, is the very instrument and organ of the mind. It is not the representation of thought, as Plato believed, and hence only an inadequate copy; but it is thought itself. The rationalist philosophers were not right when they supposed that the structure of language mirrored the structure of reality (language and reality bear little resemblance and come from different families); but they were

right when they identified it with thinking itself . . . In reading what the character sees, the reader sees; but what the reader sees, of course, is not the thing but a construction. Since we know that we are witnessing a perception, we are, in effect, seeing an act of seeing, not merely an object, which might be seen in a number of ways, because in the text there are no more ways than are written.[19]

This gets back to what I spoke of before—the act of control inherent in writing of all kinds, and the particular kind that comes in fiction writing. When we write, we present our way of seeing; when we write fiction we dramatize that sight, we create a whole world that represents it. It is as Norman Mailer has written, in an essay called "At the Point of My Pen": "The only time I know the truth is at the point of my pen."[20]

Another reason to write in the clinical context, even if we are not writing fiction, is that writing allows our experiences to become universal, to become simply *human*, which in turn helps us loosen our grip on the sense that they are ours and ours alone. We can share our experiences through writing in various ways, whether it's with someone we invent, with a common image, or with ourselves seen from a different perspective. Sometimes this is in service of the knowledge that we don't have to undergo our experiences alone; in the case of the clinical world, this can be hugely important not only for the writer but for his/her colleagues as well. A written narrative can allow a nurse, doctor, and social worker to recognize their shared experience with a particular patient in a way that might be difficult to do candidly in the everyday context of their lives. Going further, if this mutual recognition occurs and the shared experience is "seen," then the team can hopefully loosen their individual grips on their "ownership" of a particular moment or understanding. This can only result in better care of the patient, for s/he is no longer a battleground for blinding professional concerns.

Writing can also, as another dividend, offer clinicians a safe place to question the way they are taught and the way the medical system encourages them to practice. As an example, I'd like to share with you the recent writing of a second-year medical student who had just finished her Narrative Medicine elective. All medical students at Columbia are required to complete a 6-week narrative medicine selective as part of their "Foundations of Clinical Medicine" course—they choose among a dozen or so different seminars on a wide range of topics including nonfiction and fiction writing, meditation, three different museum courses, a film course, life drawing, philosophy, and graphic art. A few years ago the courses added a final assignment, tailor-made for the particular subject the students were studying, that asked them to apply the skills they had been learning in their Narrative Medicine course to a particular clinical encounter. The results of these assignments were astounding from their very first iteration—they give proof that we are doing something that really has an impact. Here is an excerpt from a piece by one student who took the nonfiction writing seminar:

What I wrote was: "The patient has a prior history of falling when trying to cross the street."

What I wanted to write was: "Ms. W, who is 90, was jaywalking in NYC while returning to her apartment from the liquor store. She "must not have seen an indentation in the road" when she tripped and fell into the street, as her newly purchased bottle of Chardonnay rolled away from her. Ironically, though she endured indurations and scrapes all over her face and arms, the wine bottle remained miraculously intact, untarnished, and ready to drink. Ms. W laughed at the irony of the situation in telling the story, and noted that she had retrieved the bottle before returning to her apartment.

What I wrote was: Patient's MSE was significant for 0/3 objects recalled after 3 minutes.

What happened was: I asked Ms. W if it would be alright to test her memory, given that she'd noticed difficulty finding words over the past year. She replied, "I know, one of them's going to be soldier, right?" "Sure, it can be," I replied, grinning, falling into her infectious rhythm. "Let's make it soldier, apple, and pen." She repeated the three words. She thought hard about them. But when it came time to remember, she could not. "Do you remember that you suggested one of them to me?" I asked, rooting for her. "Soldier!" she said, triumphantly.

What I wrote was the problem list, an assessment, an abbreviated, adulterated, formulaic version of the rich encounter I had had. I was "schooled" numerous times by this waifish, comedic, lovably difficult woman, but here I was leisurely breaking her down to finger, arm, eye, head, from a lofty spot miles away. Deleting the character, leaving the complaints. I know this patient. But who else will?[21]

* * *

Creative Writing and Reflective Writing

Writing, like life itself, is a voyage of discovery. The adventure is a metaphysical one: it is a way of approaching life indirectly, of acquiring a total rather than a partial view of the universe. . . . It is a turning inside out, a voyaging through X dimensions, with the result that somewhere along the way one discovers that what one has to tell is not nearly as important as the telling itself. It is this quality about all art which gives it its metaphysical hue, which lifts it out of time and space and centers or integrates it to the whole cosmic process. It is this about art which is "therapeutic": significance, purposelessness, infinitude.

—Henry Miller, "Reflections on Writing"[22]

I'd like to take a moment to think about the phrases "reflective writing" and "creative writing" and how they are used in the world of healthcare. As I spoke about at the start of this chapter, the reasons for using the word *reflective* rather than *creative* are more complex than a simple definition of terms, and may reflect a certain stigma or discomfort with the vexed concept of creativity. Regardless of what it's being called, more and more medical schools are using writing in their curricula as a tool to get students to explore their complex journeys toward being doctors (many other healthcare professions are also using writing, but for simplicity's sake here I will stick to medical schools).[23] But when the focus is on "reflection" rather than on "creation" some simple but important aspects of the gift of writing are often distorted. Students in schools for health professions are generally in rigorous and regimented curricula, receiving grades and ratings at every turn—it is natural for them to expect that the writing they are asked to do will be assessed in the same ways. Part of the job of the instructors dealing with student writing is to show them this is not the case. Ideally, the writing they do (outside of the regular curriculum, such as papers or statements for applications, etc.) should be offered to them as a place where they can stretch and breathe, a place where they can explore freely what they are experiencing, where they can uncover what they think and feel. To rate or grade a piece of "reflective" or creative writing, as is often done, is to distort the very idea of what writing in these contexts is ultimately for—discovery.[24] How can you rate something as being more or less reflective? If a student brings a memory of his grandfather into a reflection on a patient encounter and another doesn't, does that prove that he was reflecting better or more deeply than the student that didn't include such a memory? If so, why? These kinds of questions seem dangerously subjective to me—one person's judgment of satisfactory reflection may not be someone else's—so in addition to being unhelpful they are potentially inconsistent. The fact that rating rubrics are being developed in this area makes the creative work seem all the more urgent.

One of the complexities here is that these students need readers in order for their work to be seen, heard, validated, and reflected back to them so that they can better see, as we have explored, what there is to be learned. The reader/receiver is crucial. But when the reader is a person in a position of authority to the student, and particularly in an environment where the student is accustomed to being assessed and ranked at every turn, this can be tricky, for the student is then at risk for writing toward what they think their reader wants to hear, aiming for a "right answer" when in fact there is no such thing. It is important that the readers/guiders of the writing do not reward this or feed back into it by upholding rating metrics of any kind in this arena. The only way to prevent this kind of work in students is for us as teachers to encourage them not to write toward any one conclusion but rather to explore their own unknowing, to allow their wrestling with what they are learning to be transparent and often inconclusive.

In many ways this encouragement—the encouraging of what is creative and expansive in student reflection rather than a mere rote recounting of facts—is a radical act in the healthcare environment, and isn't easily done. Readers need to be trained in the techniques of reading and responding to student work, and this can be quite intimidating for those with no background in the humanities or writing (more on this in the following chapter). But it is doable, and it is worth it. Even though this work will not be graded or assessed, through proper introduction and with proper support and guidance students will soon cherish the opportunity to stretch and explore their horizons in a safe and sanctioned way.

For what is reflection, really, but creation? If we are truly reflecting, deeply reflecting, as no doubt all those who ask students to write reflectively are hoping, then we are examining our experiences in a light aimed toward discovery. Creative work is just the same—in fact, you could perhaps equally argue that creative work is reflective work. As the writer Pat Schneider writes: "When we write deeply—that is, *when we write what we know and do not know we know*—we encounter mystery."[25] This sense of mystery may be what the word "creative" adds that "reflective" does not have, at least not in the context of the reflective writing most often done in medical school. "Mystery" may be a frightening word for those in the medical world, as "creativity" tends to be, but both of these words are crucial ones. As Schneider continues,

> Each of us has a private inner life, and in that life there are secrets that drive us to be who we are. Writing is not the only way for a pilgrim to identify, name, and find his or her way through the dark night of the soul. But writing, I suggest, is where we humans most make our own minds visible to ourselves and to others. There, on the faint lines of our pages, we can take down our masks. Ironically, even when we think we are building masks, creating entirely fictional characters, our very mask-making reveals us. In writing, we see, sometimes with fear and trembling, who we have been, who we really are, and we glimpse now and then who we might become.[26]

It should be said that in many ways the terms we use to describe the "voyage of discovery" that is writing are quite irrelevant—it is the spirit with which we use the tool that is most important, and the way that we receive it. Just as form is an automatic byproduct of putting words to paper, creativity is as well, in the sense that something has been born that wasn't there before. This is a fairly magical thing and ought to be treated as such, with respect for the process and for the consequence, which can often be unexpected and exciting and mysterious, no matter the subject being explored. To respect this process entails not only the proper tools to encourage the discovery and exploration, but also the proper training for those who receive it, so that the gifts can be maintained all the way through the process.

The Israeli writer David Grossman gave a talk soon after he lost his son in the second Lebanon–Israeli war. His words say a lot of what I've been trying to in this chapter, speaking directly to many of the reasons to write in the clinical context. I will end with his words:

"When we write, we feel the world in flux, elastic, full of possibilities—unfrozen. Anywhere the human element exists, there is no freezing and no paralysis, and there is no status quo (even if we sometimes mistakenly think there is; even if there are those who would very much like us to think there is).

I write, and the world does not close in on me. It does not grow smaller. It moves in the direction of what is open, future, possible.

I imagine, and the act of imagination revives me. I am not fossilized or paralyzed in the face of predators. I invent characters. Sometimes I feel as if I am digging people out of the ice in which reality has encased them. But perhaps, more than anything, the person I am digging out at the moment is myself.

I write. I feel the many possibilities that exist in every human situation, and I feel my capacity to choose between them. I feel the sweetness of liberty, which I thought I had lost. . . .

I write, and I feel that the correct and accurate use of words acts like a medicine."[27]

Notes

1. May, *Courage to Create*, 11.
2. Montgomery Hunter, *Doctors' Stories*, 5.
3. Blakeslee, "To Advance."
4. Blakeslee, "To Advance."
5. May, *Courage*, 21–22.
6. Cervantes, *Don Quixote*, 568.
7. Irvine, "Ethics of Self Care," 129.
8. Chen, *Final Exam*, 8.
9. Powers, "Richard Powers."
10. Anderson and MacCurdy, "Introduction," 7.
11. Johnson, "Writing as Healing," 86.
12. The writer has granted permission to reprint this text.
13. Orr, *Poetry as Survival*, 3–4.
14. Grossman, "Desire to be Gisella," 36.
15. Oatley, "In the Minds," 2.
16. Oatley, "In the Minds," 2.
17. Oatley, "In the Minds," 3.
18. The writer has granted permission to reprint this text.

19. Gass, *Finding a Form*, 36.
20. Mailer, "At the Point," 4.
21. The student has granted permission to reprint this text.
22. Henry Miller, "Reflections on Writing," 180–1.
23. See Shapiro, Kasman, and Shafer, "Words and Wards"; Wald et al., "Reflections on Reflections"; Wear et al., "Reflection in/and Writing"; Boudreau, Liben, and Fuks, "A Faculty Development Workshop"; Mann, Gordon, and MacLeod, "Reflection and Reflective Practice."
24. See Aronson et al., "A Comparison of Two Methods"; Wald et al., "Fostering and Evaluating."
25. Schneider, *How the Light*, 10.
26. Schneider, *How the Light*, 99.
27. Grossman, "Individual Language," 65.

CHAPTER 10

Can Creativity Be Taught?

Nellie Hermann

Strategies for Writing in the Health Professions

The practice of creativity, as we have seen in the previous chapter, is all around us. Frequently our main job as facilitators or leaders of groups of learners in narrative medicine contexts is to show students the creativity they are capable of and are already using. It is also to support the use of imagination, to show others that there is always more to explore, and that in this exploring is where the discovery lies. Writing, creativity, imagination, exploration—these are not things restricted to people who deem themselves "writers," to people who write professionally or aim for publication. These are tools open to all of us. And part of the way that we teach these tools is to demonstrate them ourselves—to be flexible in our own work, encouraging of explorations as we, too, explore.

Each year at the College of Physicians and Surgeons of Columbia University, the first-year students spend six weeks in required Narrative Medicine selectives, choosing from courses that range far over the humanities spectrum. These courses include meditation, cartooning, fiction and nonfiction writing, philosophy, film studies, and a handful of courses involving the making and/or observing of visual art at local art museums. These courses have been running since 1989 (until the year 2000 they were titled "Humanities and Medicine Seminars"), and until around 2010 they were evaluated in the usual way—students were asked to fill out a questionnaire at the end of their course asking them what they did and did not enjoy about the experience and about what they learned. Over time, however, it became clear that in fact these evaluations could not, because of their very nature, show whether the students were really learning anything in these courses, whether the act of interacting with creativity was doing any good for them in their medical training. In addition, students often complained that we didn't need to draw the lines for them—they understood the connections, they said, between the creative work and their medical school experience; they didn't need to be asked to directly connect the dots.

We decided to revamp the way the courses were evaluated and began asking the students to do tailor-made assignments at the end of each course. These assignments were created by their Narrative Medicine instructors, who asked the students to use the skills they had been working on over the course of the six weeks and apply it to a real medical school experience, preferably a patient encounter. The assignments are themselves creative: the photography course, for example, asks the students to take two self-portraits—one of themselves the way they wish to be seen by the patient, and another the way they think they *are* seen by the patient. One of the museum courses asks the students to write about an encounter with a particular painting; the fiction course asks the students to write a fictional account of a real patient encounter.

Right away, the results of these creative assignments were astounding—a student wrote a description of an in-hospital patient interaction in which she examined the specter of death in the room, reflecting on people she had once known, who were in the room with her in the form of memories and echoes, and the imagined people that the patient had with him. Another student wrote a nonfiction piece about a visit to a local barber, where the interaction was flawed because the student did not speak Spanish. Unable to communicate with the barber, he reflected on a patient encounter he had recently experienced where the tables were turned and the patient was the one unable to understand him. The range of form and content from the start was wide, and it showed the students engaging with their work in many unexpected and interesting ways, coming to conclusions they may not have been able to articulate without the use of the creative permission.

I'd like to share one of these pieces in full, so as to demonstrate most clearly an example of the powerful work being done. The below is by a student who took the film course in 2014:

INT. HOSPITAL ROOM—DAY

An elderly patient, mid-90s, sits reclining in the room bed. He has thin white hair that barely covers his head, but otherwise looks sturdy and healthy. . . . This is EDDIE. Despite the various tubes of blood, saline and blood pressure monitors, he looks comfortable, hands resting behind his head. In a chair at the foot of the bed is JAMES. A medical student, he's a little uncomfortable and nervous. His white coat is too big, his tie is too big and he looks almost like he took them from a real adult to play doctor. . . . He's looking over a list.

JAMES

I think I got all your medications down. So now, um . . . sorry I just forgot what I was going to ask for a second.

He drops his gaze from the patient and looks like he's struggling to remember. It's not hard, he's just too nervous about missing things. Eddie notices and is encouraging.

EDDIE

It's okay, take your time. You're doing great.

JAMES

Oh yeah, do you have any allergies to any medications?

EDDIE

Just penicillin.

JAMES

Okay, I'll just make a note of that real quick.

James picks up his pen and scribbles something. When he puts it back down, he accidentally drops it to the floor. Clumsy too. Everything is bad. We follow his head as he shoots down to pick it up. He grabs the pen but pauses for a moment as he closes his eyes and sighs to himself. It's just a conversation like he has all the time. Why does it feel different with the patient? He sits back up ready for the next mistake.

JAMES (CONT'D)

Sorry, I'm really clumsy today. Those are all the questions I had about medications. Would you mind telling me about your family?

EDDIE

Not at all! What would you like to know?

JAMES

Uh, let's start with do you have any siblings?

EDDIE

I sure do. I have three younger sisters.

(beat)

No wait. I don't.

Eddie brings his hands from behind his head and sets them at his side. He lets his head rest against the pillow, eyes closed, clearly holding back emotion. James looks concerned. Is something wrong? He's unsure how to react. After about 10 seconds, Eddie opens his watering eyes. His voice sounds a little weaker as he speaks again.

EDDIE (CONT'D)

Just two now. My sister passed away just a few months ago. She was 82: the youngest. My baby sister.

SPLITSCREEN. C.U. ON BOTH THEIR FACES—CONTINUOUS

Eddie's eyes still watering, remembering the baby sister. Something in James's eyes now touched, preoccupied. We slow zoom into both eyes. As we do, Eddie's screen transitions to

black-and-white. Now:

SPLITSCREEN. MONTAGE OF BOTH LIVES:

- James, now 12, stands with his two younger brothers around the hospital bed of their newborn sister. / Eddie stands with his two sisters at the wake of their recently deceased sister.

JAMES
(excited whispering)
My baby sister.

EDDIE
(solemn whispering)
My baby sister.

- James watches his sister grow up dancing. She does a string of acrobatic back-tucks and ages a year with each turn. / Eddie walks in a park with his aged youngest sister. She uses a walker. Each time she picks it up and sets it down, she gets a year younger, standing a little straighter each time and walking steadier until the walker is no longer necessary.

- James helping his dancer sister, now 16, recover from a knee surgery. / Eddie helping his sister, early 60s, recover from a hip replacement.

- Scenes start coming faster. James's sister keeps getting older: graduation, dance career, marriage, children, grandchildren. Slowly getting weaker and more frail. / Eddie's sister experiences the same life story but in reverse, becoming younger, stronger, more healthy with each event experienced backwards.

- James, an old man, at the bedside of his now 80 year old sister, greatly ill in bed at home. They're watching her favorite dances together as her eyes droop sleepily. / Eddie, now a young boy, next to his toddler sister in bed. He reads her a bedtime story as her eyes droop sleepily.

- Finally, James stands with his younger brothers, all very old men, at the wake of their sister. / Eddie stands with his sisters at the 1930s crib of their newborn sister.

JAMES
(solemn whispering)
My baby sister.

EDDIE
(excited whispering)
My baby sister.

END OF MONTAGE

INT. HOSPITAL ROOM—CONTINUOUS

Zoom out of James's eyes to return to present. Eddie's eyes still watering and James, though not crying, looks similarly touched. He also strangely seems more relaxed.

JAMES
I'm so sorry to hear that.

EDDIE
She was wonderful. She was always my little sister.

JAMES

They never stop being the baby, do they?

EDDIE

No they don't. I loved her very much.

JAMES

I can tell that you did. I have a younger sister too and I can only imagine. I'm so sorry for your loss.

EDDIE

It's okay. We had a good life together.

A short beat while Eddie collects himself. He puts one hand back behind his head and relaxes.

James looks more comfortable. He sits up straight and more confident. This is just a conversation, with another person just like him.

EDDIE

(smiling)

Okay. What's next?

JAMES

Could you tell me a little bit about your support system? Who do you live with?

As they continue talking inaudibly:

SLOW FADE TO BLACK[1]

What I love most about this piece is the way it literally *shows* us, in a crafted scene that plays out before us in a very particular way, the connection between the patient and medical student and demonstrates the way that this connection palpably brings about a change in the medical student. The entire piece is from the medical student's perspective, despite the fact that the montage includes scenes from Eddie's life as well. It is the medical student who is most changed here, through undergoing the shared experiences of the two men. In this way the writer of the piece *reveals* his experience to us, shares it with us in such a way that it is almost as if we, too, have lived it.

The above piece is an example of what many of these pieces do: they show us, they *enact* for us in a way that no mere check-box evaluation can, the ways that the creative work is operating on the students: creative pathways are being opened and being used, not in order to take them far away from medicine (as, perhaps, an art class on their own time might do) but in fact to help them explore and reflect on their daily lives and what they are learning. These creative activities invite the students to engage and think in multiple directions about the work they are beginning to practice; they perhaps invite them to modes of interrogation that they may not yet have in their arsenal. There is freedom inherent in this; nothing is proscribed, nothing expected except that the students stretch their wings. Perhaps this is why the results are so extraordinary.

We are often asked about how to evaluate the work done in narrative medicine, and whether it makes a difference. Sometimes, using creative means to evaluate this work can be surprisingly successful. What would you think if you were given the above piece of work by the student in the film class? Would you judge that the creative means were helping him to express a difficult encounter? Would you agree that the student was adequately reflecting on his experience? Would you judge that he had synthesized and represented what he had learned? To me, no more words but the ones the student has written are necessary in order for us to understand what he is expressing, and this is the true mark of what he has achieved.

Another example of creative means of evaluation comes from a workshop I led for two years with obstetrics and gynecology residents at New York Presbyterian Hospital. I led this workshop with Abby Winkel, who was herself an Ob/Gyn resident at the time. We started the workshop as Abby's residency research project, which is how we initially were allowed by the department to block off the time for the workshop on the residents' schedule.[2] In the second year of this workshop, in an attempt to better study what we were doing, Abby and I decided to try an experiment. Abby introduced me to the ACGME (Accreditation Council for Graduate Medical Education) competencies—six competencies in which residents are expected to demonstrate proficiency: "Patient Care," "Medical Knowledge," "Practice-Based Learning and Improvement," "Systems-Based Practice," "Professionalism," and "Interpersonal Skills and Communication."

The language of these competencies is often very hard to follow, and Abby felt sure that the residents usually had no understanding of the content of the competencies. So our experiment was to use the competencies as our learning goals. We had six workshops. Each used a competency as our theme, with a text and a writing prompt related to that competency. We wanted to look at whether our reading and writing changed the residents' ideas of what these competencies meant—whether we were actually *teaching* anything by doing this. At the beginning of the hour we asked the residents to write a one-sentence definition of the competency of the day, and then, after we read our text and did our writing, we asked them to write a definition again.

I'd like to share a few of these pieces. These were from our very first workshop of the year, when we focused on "Practice-Based Learning and Improvement." The story we read was a very short story called "Girl" by Jamaica Kincaid. The piece is essentially written as instructions to a young girl from some sort of authority figure—perhaps a mother. I asked the residents, after we had read and discussed the story, to write instructions to themselves in the style of the story.

Here are two of the responses:

1. From a fourth-year resident:

First definition of Practice-Based Learning and Improvement:

"Using experiences in daily care of patients to guide further decision-making."

What she wrote to the prompt:

Don't wear scrubs outside the hospital. If you want to have scrubs your size, you're going to have to bring them home. Make sure to eat breakfast. If you skip breakfast, you'll be grumpy by noon. Don't be grumpy. Nod and smile while I yell at you. I'm not yelling at you. Why did you do that? Present the list at grand rounds. Tell the story so I know what you were thinking. Why did you think that? Do it this way. Wait, I have something else to tell you. Hold on a second, there is something else. Don't be late. Try to move a little more quickly there are a lot of patients on the labor floor right now. You should really check that the junior resident checked that lab. I am going to need you to scrub for this case. Teach your intern to do this another way. Why did you do it that way last Tuesday? Stick around, there's something you should tie up before you go home. Why did you go over your work hours? Change back into your flip flops before you go home.

Second written definition, after reading and writing:

"Incorporating the lessons of the day's work and the experiences around me with the technical and cognitive knowledge I have gained into a more whole image of a doctor."

2. From a third-year resident:

First definition:

Practice-based learning and improvement refers to knowledge gained through patient care and clinical experience, for people in a medical setting.

Prompt:

Don't use your feet to point. Always bow your head when you pass someone older than you. Stand up straight. Use the knife to peel away from you, never toward you. Don't take too much fruit away with the peel. Don't leave too much fruit on the pit. Never use a cutting board for fruit. Finish all of the rice. Don't leave a grain behind.

Cover your knees and shoulders. The neckline of your shirt is too deep. Kneel as you approach the monk. Never point your feet toward the Buddha. Light the left candle first, then the right, then the incense. Monks eat first. People eat later.

Residents don't get to eat.

Second definition:

> Learn by doing. Learn from what you did well, what you did poorly, and think about
> what you would do differently next time around.

Again, this is an example of a simple way to examine what is being done with this kind of creative work. To me, in both of these resident responses the second definitions are exceptionally more clear, more forgiving, more human. The movement between the first definitions and the second, buffered by the writing in the middle, shows that there was a process that took place, a shift, a change that these residents underwent by virtue of doing this creative work in the course of this brief 45-minute session.

It should be noted here that the kind of creative exercises these residents were asked to do (with the exception of the writing of the competency definition) is no different from those I would ask any other population of learners to do. When I teach fiction workshops to medical students, the short stories that I give them to read are no different from what I give students in a liberal arts college class or in our Narrative Medicine master's degree program, and they are asked to write pieces of fiction of their own invention just like in any other class. The content of the class is not at all medicine-focused, and the stories we read do not focus on healthcare. I want to treat them like a group of writers, first and foremost, and by removing the focus on medicine they are likely to be able to see the fictional works that are shared with them more clearly in terms of craft without being distracted by content. They also hopefully may, in the shadow of other published stories and their classmates' work, begin to recognize their own creative work as valuable and as standing up on its own in and among the river of creative writing.

In a workshop like the Ob/Gyn one referenced above, where there is not time to craft a whole syllabus or to carry out a full workshop (where students can respond in depth to one another's work), a slightly different tactic is required. That group met once every six or so weeks, and the time was crammed into an already packed clinical day. In sessions like this, the readings need to be short enough to be read out loud in the group and digested fairly quickly, and then the writing needs to be linked to and inspired by the reading such that the activities will flow easily from one to the next. But still, even when the goal of the session was to teach about an ACGME competency, the readings were not explicitly about medicine, and the writing prompts, while the residents were welcome to write about their hospital lives, were nearly always open to interpretation that could bring the writer to other places. One writing prompt, for example, asked the residents to describe a waiting room—a few wrote about their clinic waiting room, but one described her dentist's office and another her hair salon (where she almost never got to go, anymore, because of her job).

The art of the writing prompt is a fine one, very much dependent on setting, context, goals, and the group of people you are working with; figuring out what makes a good prompt often involves quite a bit of trial and error. A few simple guidelines can be very useful for nearly every context, however: first, the goal for the writing should always be discovery and expansion of mind—the prompt should never provoke a search for a specific answer or encourage narrowing of thinking. Shorter is almost always better; the writing prompt that is convoluted and has multiple bullet points will never be as successful as one that is five words long. Keeping in mind the creative aspect of the work is always helpful when coming up with a writing prompt—one of the prompts we use frequently in narrative medicine, often paired with an excerpt from Michael Ondaatje's novel *The English Patient*, is "Write about a room of care." You can see from this prompt some of why it is successful—nothing about the way it is worded constricts the writer's imagination; the phrase "room of care" is broad enough to bring to mind many different images, not all of them even necessarily involving illness. It also links directly to the excerpted text, which is a description of a woman tending to a badly burned soldier. And this is another guideline that is very important—if the prompt, in its expansiveness, derives from the text that has been read and considered, participants are more likely to jump easily into the creative act than they might be otherwise. Often good prompts can be lines taken directly from the piece of writing shared with the group, or exercises that in some way ask participants to write in an interactive way with the published work (e.g., the above prompt linked to Jamaica Kinkaid's story "Girl")—to write, as we often say, in the shadow of the text. This is why the reading and the writing are so important to do together—a certain mood is created in the examination and discussion of the published work, which then can carry over to the writing, encouraging expansive exploration. It is as if the foundation has been laid, in the close examination of an inspiring piece of writing, for more free-flowing ideas and imagination.

It should also be said that this can absolutely be done with visual art as well, or with music, or with a clip from a film—really with any piece of art that encourages and shapes a supportive creative space for participants to then be inspired to pursue their own explorations.

A Teaching Tool: The Reading Guide for Creative Writing

Writers need readers, and in many instances an act of creation is not complete until it has been witnessed. As is explored elsewhere in this book, the reader's experience of any piece of writing is, in a sense, a co-creation of that piece of writing; and especially in the case of writing done in the clinical context, this co-creation aspect is crucial. This is true, as we have seen, because of how important the recognition of shared experiences can be in the clinical context; also because of what insight can be reflected back to the writer that s/he may not have been able to see without a reader. For a student whose writing is being read by a faculty member, all of this is no less crucial, although the sharing process may be a bit more complicated—when a faculty member recognizes so intimately what a student is going through, it can be harder for him/her to remain fixed to the text and not end up only speaking generally about the content of what has been expressed. It is important to learn through doing this work that in fact, strong sympathy can be demonstrated by the closest attention to what the student has written. In this context, this is the most focused way to listen.

It is also important to stress that the tools of reading and responding to writing can be honed through the act of doing the reading, writing, and responding more and more—you do not necessarily need an advanced degree in English or a writing MFA to make another writer feel heard and responded to. You also don't necessarily need to use advanced literary terms—words like *craft, form,* and *voice* can be intimidating to the lay reader/writer, but these words don't have to be ones you use in your particular situations with colleagues or students or whoever else you may be working with. That said, this work is not easy; reading and responding to writing takes close, attentive and disciplined work, requiring focus and often a reframing of the entire act of listening. These are not skills that are picked up overnight; in many cases they will be best and most easily taught by a writer or someone with a background in the humanities. Later in the chapter I will demonstrate the kind of attention to language that I am speaking about here; for now, it is enough to say that the goal is not praise or commiseration or advice. The goal should be to show how the thing that has been created—the piece of text, language object—reveals itself to the reader, how it is received by the reader by virtue of the way that it is put together. *This is what language does,* in other words, is what you are reflecting to the writer; *this is what you have demonstrated through your use of language.*

Through a grant from the National Institutes of Health that began in 2006, a group of Columbia medical school faculty, all teachers of the "Foundations of Clinical Medicine" course (at other institutions this is called the "Doctoring" course), came together once a week to focus on the teaching of social and behavioral sciences.[3] Under the leadership of Dr. Rita Charon, an important part of what they did each week was read and write together. Most of these faculty members had never done this work before and had no experience with reading and writing in this way. Gradually, close reading and creative writing became an element in many aspects of the Foundations course in both the preclinical and clinical years. In 2012, Columbia inaugurated its Portfolio program for its medical students, an important component of which is a monthly reading and writing exercise done in class, which students then archive in their portfolios. The clinical faculty who facilitate these groups are trained, through their many years of practicing this work, to lead their students through these exercises and respond fully to what they produce.

I want to share a tool that may be useful in the quest to best respond to a piece of writing shared with you in any particular context. Below is a "reading guide" that can hopefully help guide any reader in looking closely at a piece of writing with an eye for reflecting back to its author what has happened in its wake. A few of us at Columbia developed this guide most specifically for helping clinical faculty to look at medical student writing, but some version of this can really be used to look at almost any piece of writing at all.

Reading Guide

1. **Observation:** Signs of perceiving—seeing, hearing, smelling, touching. Details, descriptions, sensory aspects of the scenes.
2. **Perspective:** Were multiple perspectives represented, explored, guessed at? How were these perspectives conveyed?
3. **Form:** Describe the form. What is the genre—story, poem, play, screenplay, parable, cautionary tale, ghost story, black comedy? Notice any use of metaphor or imagery. Describe the temporal structure of the text—are events told in chronological order, in reverse, in chaotic sequence? Are there allusions to other stories or texts? Are there inserted texts (like quotations, letters, sub-stories)? What is the diction—formal, breezy, bureaucratic, scientific?
4. **Voice:** Whose voice tells? Is the narrative told in a first-person, second-person, or third-person voice? Is the teller near or far, intimate or remote, and can you feel its presence as you read? Is the telling self-aware?
5. **Mood:** What is the mood of the text? What mood does reading it leave you in?
6. **Motion:** What does the story *do*? Does the teller seem to move from the beginning to the end? Does the story bring *you* somewhere in its course?[4]

—Nellie Hermann, Rita Charon, Michael Devlin, 2012

I will quickly go over the categories. First—*Observation*. This is really everything that has to do with *perceiving* in the text—all the sensory details that the writer includes. What is *seen* in the text, what is smelled, touched, heard, or tasted? What objects, what physical sensations were included, and what does the choice of details tell us, if anything? Of course there are always details that have been left out, and sometimes these absences can be just as telling as the included presences.

Next is *Perspective*. In a sense, depending on what is being written about, this is a question of empathy: did the writer attempt to imagine what it might be like for anyone aside from his/herself? How did the writer imagine other voices or explore other experiences? Were other people presented only from the outside, or were their internal monologues explored as well?

Third—*Form*. This is about how the piece was put together—I like to say, "how it works." Was it a very straightforward narrative, going from point A to B to C? Was it meandering? Did it jump in time, was there dialogue, was it presented as a scene or a summary? What was the genre? Often new writers are unaware of the forms they are using, and readers or listeners can think more easily about form because they can better see the text as a whole. Sometimes, for example, a medical student's reflection will read like a newspaper article— a simple reporting of facts—and the one moment where the student slips into conjecture is no doubt the moment to focus on. Or maybe a student will write about a mysterious patient and the piece will read like a mystery novel. These are questions of form.

Fourth is *Voice*. What is the voice of the piece—who is telling the story? Is it told in the first person or third, and how might this choice affect other elements of the piece? Is the voice close or far away? How reflective was the teller in the piece, how questioning of his/her self and of what s/he is witnessing as well as of how s/he behaves? This is an especially important element, of course, for clinical students.

Fifth—*Mood*. This is really more about you as a reader: What does the piece make you feel? What is the mood? Is it mournful, exuberant, confused, frantic? What reaction does it engender in you? Very often readers of writing, particularly student writing, feel that they need to keep themselves out of the discussion about the writing, as if admitting personal reactions would compromise the text; but in reality this is impossible. The reader is always involved, for the reader really *co-constructs* the piece of writing, pouring her energy into the text and partially creating it through her reaction. Your personal reaction to a piece of writing can never be removed from your experience of it, and therefore it needs to be part of your response. Keep in mind, though, too, that sometimes the mood of a text can be very different from the mood you are left in after reading it—maybe it is angry, for example, but it makes you feel sad, because you feel you see something in the student's anger that s/he doesn't see. Paying attention to the differences here can be fruitful.

And last is the category of *Motion*—has the writer arrived at a different place at the end than at the beginning? Has the piece taken you anywhere?

Again, this guide is offered here merely as a tool that might help those not used to close reading to look at pieces of writing and see what is there. It is important to note that these are simply elements to look for in a text; these are **not** points of evaluation. In the clinical world we are most often dealing with people who are not overly comfortable with writing and who are often writing about very sensitive topics and experiences. The goal, then, is not to evaluate what they've done and tell them how to do it differently; the goal is *not* to make them better writers. Rather, the goal is to *reflect back to them what their writing shows to their readers*. This is of course much more complicated than "I see something you don't see." It's more that in reflecting back to the writer what *we* see, we invite them to see new dimensions of their own. "I wonder why you've made a jump from this to that," for example, might make a writer see that there's something they skipped because they didn't want to spend time on it.

The Approach to the Writing Student

Below is a piece of writing by a third-year medical student at Columbia P&S, written during his/her Ob/Gyn rotation. This writing, as well as the examples I give later in this chapter, was done as part of a required course for third-year students at Columbia in which they come together once during each clinical clerkship to share prompted writing with one another and a faculty preceptor. Each time they gather they bring responses they have written at home to a particular prompt. These prompts tend to be quite open-ended: for example, the prompt for the Ob/Gyn rotation is "Write about a moment of pain."

> Though the majority of the patients I've encountered on my OBGYN rotation have not been in great pain, there were times where physicians had to be cognizant of the intertwining physical and emotional pain that patients experience. I think this was most notable in the family planning clinic on Saturday where the psychological aspects of procedures weigh heavily on the amount of physical pain the patient experiences. One patient I saw was not at all in conflict about her decision, but she did appear incredibly nervous and reasonably anxious about the procedure. Though I did not get to learn a lot about her and her life during the visit, I imagine that there was some amount of conflict that went into her decision, whether it was moral, religious, interpersonal, intrapersonal, etc., and this conflict had some bearing on her discomfort during the procedure.

The fellow I was with told me after the visit that the patient had been in more pain during the procedure than patients usually are, which made me think that this situation was somewhat reflecting her psychological state rather than solely the physical. The fellow was very good about easing her pain by telling her how to breathe to relieve cramping and giving her the option to tell us when she felt that the pain was too much. I felt that it was important for healthcare providers to recognize and accept that everyone's pain scale is different, particularly in the setting of emotional charged events such as childbirth, surgery, and abortions. I think it is important to remember while physiology, physical exam signs, and medications may be the most salient points to us, patients most saliently feel pain (both physical and psychological) and that is often what is most important aspect to be addressed.

So let's sit with this piece for a minute and look closely at it. Take a minute to read it a few times over. What do you notice here? Using the categories of the Reading Guide, what questions might you ask of this piece of writing regarding details of perception, the perspectives examined or challenged, the form of the piece, or the story being told?

The first thing that jumps out to me is in the first paragraph, with the sentence: "One patient I saw was not at all in conflict with her decision, but she did appear incredibly nervous and reasonably anxious about the procedure." What is the decision in question here? I assume that it refers to the patient's decision to terminate her pregnancy, but this is in fact not said; the fact that the writer does not say explicitly what is the procedure in question interests me. Later in the same paragraph the phrase "her decision" is said again without context. If I were with the writer, I would ask him/her—why not say what the decision was? Does the absence of this detail perhaps reveal some other discomfort with what is being done, either because of the action in the room or as a reflection of some larger cultural or context-based stigma? Perhaps not—perhaps the writer just assumed knowledge on the part of his/her reader—but something tells me that pointing this absence out to the writer would be a fruitful thing to do, perhaps sparking some deeper thoughts about the subject and the experience that s/he may not have yet examined.

I also notice a general lack of perception-based details in the text. In the first paragraph, the procedure is referred to, and we are told that the patient appeared "incredibly nervous and reasonably anxious," but we don't see the evidence that brought the writer to this conclusion. I would ask him/her, what did you see that made you think this? What did the patient look like? Was she wringing her hands, crying, moving around a lot? How could you tell she was "incredibly nervous"? I'd like to see the room and see the patient and the doctor, and even the writer too. Again, purely a hypothesis, but I wonder if the lack of specific detail reflects a larger discomfort with what went on in the room. The above-quoted sentence begs further examining—if the patient is content with her decision, why is she also "incredibly nervous"? Is she worried that the procedure may not be safe, or is she in fact not as confident in her decision as she might be trying to be? I would like to see the writer pursue this further, as this is a dichotomy that s/he is raising **perhaps without even knowing it**. Being asked to further describe the room **rather** than being asked directly to explore the deeper questions at work here might allow the writer to come to the exploration of the deeper issues on his/her own.

Finally, I'd like to spend a minute on this sentence: "The fellow I was with told me after the visit that the patient had been in more pain during the procedure than patients usually are, which made me think that this situation was somewhat reflecting her psychological state rather than solely the physical." This is a fascinating sentence, and a compelling conclusion—full of insight and keen observation, though it is all beneath the surface. Why would an expression of "more" pain lead the student to conclude the patient was in emotional distress? We don't have any hard evidence of the patient's emotional distress in the piece—if anything we are told that she feels "content about her decision"—so I'm all the more curious about the conclusion that the student draws here. What is his/her evidence for this conclusion? I don't doubt that s/he has the evidence, but I want it to be shown to me. My guess is, in the attempt to put it down on paper, to justify the conclusion almost like a mathematical proof, the writer will discover more about how s/he came to this conclusion than s/he might already understand.

Now, one of the frequent questions I am asked when looking closely at a piece of student writing like this is about time—what if we don't have time to sit with each student and talk in depth with them about their writing, what if we don't have time to ask them to go home and write something else or to clarify what they've done? My answer to this is similar to the answer we give to the same type of question, which is asked frequently, about narrative medicine work in general: "How can we do this work if we don't have more time to spend with patients?" My answer is that this all takes less time than it seems, and if done properly in the long run it actually **saves** time rather than costing it. When it comes to writing, the fact of having a reader can go a long way—even if you don't have time to sit and follow up with the student, you can write your thoughts and queries on the piece so that the student can follow up on his/her own time. Chances are, if a student feels that someone else is interested in what they are doing, that s/he has sparked something in someone else, then the student is more likely to go home and revisit the writing, or even simply to think a little differently about the experience on their subway ride home. This alone can be a change in perspective that is worth the work.

Let's look at a few more examples of student writing. Below are two pieces that students wrote about their neurology clerkship. The prompt for neurology is, "Write about a time of hope or despair."

What do you notice about these two pieces when placed side by side?

1. Ms. D was lying peacefully in bed, lights low, sun slowly rising in the background behind the huge clear windows. Though she appeared so comfortable, so rested, so at ease within the ambience of the dim lit room, a war was waging inside of her brain. It was the mighty neurons versus. . . . the other mighty neurons, firing at each other, firing again, dead comrades resting in peace, others taking their place. Ms. D had been in status epilepticus for 5 days without relief, four high dose anti-seizure meds given to her twice per day, yet failing to bring peace to the battleground occurring in her head. As I watched Ms. D lying in the bed with her daughter on her side, we reminisced about the good old days, videos of Ms. D singing in the church, laughing and carrying on a conversation, though even at that point she herself knew of her eventually fatal condition, metastatic adenocarcinoma to the brain. Her daughters explained they were saddened not by the news, but by the absence of their mother's voice, lost within her epilepsy, the fear of never hearing it again. By the sixth day things looked up. It turned out adding a fifth drug to the concoction was all she needed to finally quell the war within her brain. By the seventh day she opened her eyes and said "Hello!", her gaze steady as she followed you around the bed. Though she couldn't yet follow many commands, she looked out the window and yelled "Sunny Day!", her daughter laughing in the background. Day 8 was different. She continued to improve, though by now some human characteristics had returned with her speech, the power to have insight. As if truly awakening from all her drugs and becoming more aware of her situation, after finally realizing that it was no longer an easy task to read her own on the page, only then was she finally back, only then did she start to cry.

2. The nature of neurological disorders seems to present particular challenges to both the patient and provider. Despite its central role in who we are and how we interact with the world, the nervous system represents a significant conceptual challenge for patients. Unlike the common illnesses of internal medicine, which often lend themselves to fairly accurate and comprehensible analogies of broken pumps and filters, neurological illnesses lack such easily accessible real world points of reference. While comparisons to computers and cables may help illustrate the basic functions of the CNS and PNS, they merely introduce another complex and widely misunderstood system that brings the patient no closer to an understanding of his illness. Patient understanding is often further complicated by the limited insight

offered by neurology in terms of prognosis. Faced with conceptual barriers, prognostic statements of limited certainty and varying religious/ethical values, patients and families are prone to conflict in the setting of a devastating neurological injury. While even the most seasoned clinician may experience frustration with the resulting conflict and indecision, it may be helpful to consider these issues and offer appropriate understanding and guidance.

To me, these two pieces side by side illustrate some very important writerly points. Perhaps most obvious is how the first piece so clearly tells a story—with a full arc, ending with the patient crying, giving a kind of resolution—where the second piece is almost totally abstract, exploring no one perspective and giving nearly no sensory details at all. How does the experience of reading these two pieces differ? I am pulled into the scene of the first one from the first sentence— "lights low, sun slowly rising . . . behind the huge clear windows"—I can **see** where we are and feel invited into the room, witness and co-inhabitant of the scene. In the second piece there is no scene—from the first sentence we are in the space of abstraction, with no real ground to stand on. "The nature of neurological disorders seems to present particular challenges for both patient and provider." Look at that word, *seems*, and how it removes what little certainty there is from this statement. It "seems" to present challenges—does that mean it doesn't really present them? It only seems to? And is it the "nature" of neurological disorders that seems to present the challenges, or is it the disorders themselves? You can see what I'm getting at here—even within this one sentence we can see the lack of firm ground that is the readerly experience of this whole piece. That said, it is clear to me that this student is writing this vague reflection **because of** real interactions and experiences that s/he must have had—phrases like "patients and families are prone to conflict in the setting of a devastating neurological injury" tells me that this writer was witness to any number of such conflicts, certainly more than one. So why is s/he not writing the story of one or more of these? Why is the writer choosing to abstract the situation so severely that we see not even one clear person in this piece, neither patient nor physician? Perhaps the notion of representing one of the scenes that the writer was privy to is a bit daunting to him/her. If I were responding to this student, I would ask this directly, saying that I'd like to understand what incidents made the student draw these conclusions, asking for actual scenes and details. It's the old writerly edict "show don't tell," and we can see in this piece why it is important.

I think this need for detail—for **narrative**—is such an important lesson, one that is illustrated by this exercise but applies far beyond it. Even though they are not about exactly the same things, in a way the first piece can be seen as an illustration of some of what the second piece is wrestling with. And what do we gain, with the narrative first piece; what do we gain with the full presentation of the scene and its characters? We gain understanding; we gain insight. We see a single patient in her current environment—we are so present with her that we even see the sun, rising—and we glimpse her, too, in her element outside the hospital. We see the conflicts she, and by extension her family and the doctor, are wrestling with. We gain proof, in other words, of the kind of "conflicts" that patients with neurological disorders struggle with, perhaps related to the kinds of conflicts referred to in the second, abstracted piece. When the story is told, its nuances can be explored. I would be very curious to ask both of these students what their experiences were like in writing these pieces, whether they gained any insight or felt any relief after writing them. My guess is that the answer for the first student would be yes, while the second student might say that s/he was still struggling to articulate what the piece was trying to get at.

One more piece of student writing, this one written during a student's Medicine rotation:

> My experience on the wards could be best described as a sort of cultural immersion. Like any traveler in a foreign land, I've felt an ever-present tension between the excitement of taking part in new experiences and the fear of revealing my otherness. While my over-stuffed, short white coat undermines any attempt to truly avoid detection, I've tried to soften my foreign appearance by taking on the language and practices of the locals. This has involved both learning new terms/practices and refining my understanding of others. Initially, I was most challenged by the disconnect between my concept of the doctor–patient relationship and the reality of a physician's role in the hospital. My previously held vision was colored, in large part, by the commonly encountered phrase "at the bedside." Expecting to spend a significant portion of my day interacting with patients, I was of course surprised by the reality of hospital life in which other health care providers attend to most immediate patient needs. While I quickly gained appreciation for the division of labor, in that it allows physicians more time to orchestrate care, it seems that even the most frequently hospitalized patients still expect a more significant physician presence at the bedside. This disconnect seems to create tension between the patient, who feels neglected, and the physician, who feels under-appreciated for his efforts away from the bedside. While both positions are understandable, it is important to appreciate the patient's status as a refugee of sorts, who finds himself in a foreign land with concerns far more pressing than assimilation. Perhaps greater efforts to actively inform patients of the physician's role away from the bedside would help alleviate the consequences of this cross-cultural misunderstanding.

The first thing that jumps out at me here is the student's wonderful use of metaphor—using the reading guide, I would say the genre here is almost an allegory. The comparison between the medical student as traveler/foreigner, whose foremost desire is assimilation, and the patient as refugee "with concerns far more pressing," is fascinating, and I'd love to ask the writer here how this metaphor came to him/her. I wonder if the writer had the metaphor fully thought through at the beginning of the piece, or whether it became further fleshed out as the writing went on—in other words, was the metaphor a vehicle for any discovery? I would also like to see the writer push the metaphor even further—if the patient is a refugee and the student a foreigner, what is the doctor? It is curious to me that the physician is not assigned a clear character role in this place, although the physician's presence is much discussed and we know the physician feels "under-appreciated for his efforts away from the bedside." Though the student concludes with the wish that the patient be better informed about what the physician does away from the bedside, I wonder how this conclusion might be expanded if a bit more time were spent on the metaphor itself, and the physician were given a clear character role as the other players are. What further insight might the writer gain into this "foreign land" if s/he were really to push the metaphor here and imagine this place in its full foreign-ness, its true allegorical nature? Perhaps we could even see a scene that illustrates the "cross-cultural misunderstanding" that is at play here? This piece is full of possibilities and my hunch is that if the writer spent just a bit more time on what has already been put into motion here, the payoff for insight could be enormous.

Finally: Focus on the Creative Spark

I hope that even these few examples of student writing in the clinical context are enough to illustrate the ways that the reading guide can possibly be used to help look at a piece of writing, and also the ways that any writing and any writer can be read with the same eye—toward creativity, excavation, insight. What are these students being asked to do, in the end, except to illustrate what they've been through, to think critically and creatively about their experiences? In the excavation of what they've already done, in the reflection back to them of what their writing is showing, they will inevitably gain even more insight. Some version of the Reading Guide categories can be applied to every piece of writing that we encounter, as can some version of this same process whereby we expose what the writing shows to us, and can then reflect this back to the writer to help him/her think more deeply about what s/he may not be seeing. Of course the demands of this encounter change depending on the setting in which we are doing this, whether we are performing this act in the role of teacher, facilitator, colleague, or participant. The more we respond to others' writing the more comfortable we get reading these different situations and understanding what the writer may need in response to his or her writing. I hope this illustrates not only how a piece of writing can be read but also how crucial these readings are for the completion of the exercise—without a reader, the exploration is incomplete.

In all of this work, it is a good guideline to remember to keep the focus always on the spark of creativity. If you ask yourself, when putting together workshops or exercises or writing prompts, or even when giving feedback to learners, whether what you are proposing will spark creativity in them, you will be led in a better direction than you otherwise might be. The goal should always be expansion rather than constriction. As you do it more, you will become more adept and comfortable with this kind of work, and it will begin to flow more easily.

One day in the spring of 2014, a student in my Narrative Medicine master's class brought a dead bird into the classroom. The bird, apparently, had fallen from the sky near where she was sitting waiting for class to begin—she had picked it up with a newspaper. The bird was perfectly intact, and looked just like it was sleeping; she lay it on the table next to her. Now, how should a teacher react to a student bringing a dead bird into class? We had read the poetry of Mark Doty for class that week—loving evocations of nature, meditations on death sparked by interactions with landscapes of the sea. It felt somehow fitting for there to be a messenger from the natural world in the room with us. The student said she wanted to keep the bird, to bring it home with her after class and bury it—strange as it was, it didn't feel right to tell her she had to bring it back outside. It also didn't feel right to proceed as we normally would, the recently deceased bird just lying there on the table. This was narrative medicine after all, where looking squarely at death is one of the things we try to do.

So I asked the students to get up and come around to where the bird was lying on the table, and to spend a few minutes just looking at it. Someone knew the type of bird that it was—a Northern Flicker—and confirmed it on the Internet. Then, once everyone was back in their seats, I asked them to write a five- to ten-line poem about the bird. That done, we went around the room and shared the results. The poems were wonderful—varied, deep, complicated, personal. I will share here the openings of just a few, and the shortest one in its entirety, just to exhibit the variety in the work:

> Do birds have eyelids, I
> wonder. How can we draw
> the shades on that pained squint, the streak
> of red, not blood, that smears
> his crown? He seems to have torn

a seam—down bursting through like the sides
of an old teddy bear, the kind
retired to a box in the attic.

* * *

My cat kills birds regularly
I try to stop him
Many times pulling a bird
from his jaws.
Sometimes they live,
mostly they die.
I console myself by saying
"they're only sparrows"

* * *

"Look me in the eye when I'm hurting you." Dead eye, reptilian
eye Scales beading along the lash line. "I want to see you
cry." Wetness lingering, flattening already Feathered eyelids
angled in.

* * *

Here is this thing, this living breathing bird
beautiful doesn't quite capture
all of its dead essence, now does it? his blood is pooling to the bottom
and body is now
stiff.

* * *

Dead Woodpecker

> the northern flicker
> wants to be buried
> to fall further from the sky
> push down through the earth
> drip from the bones
> leak color into the soil
> yellow running through
> the veins of the feathers
> blood fixed in the body
> a tuft of white
> escapes the stiffened bird
> release

Each one of the poems from the class reflected the students' individual voices—and to hear them all together after such a strange and unexpected turn of events was a truly revelatory experience. It reminded me once again that flexibility in the classroom and in the teaching of creativity is absolutely essential—and that the students I had the pleasure to work with were capable of beautiful spontaneous creative work, no matter what they might have thought about their own abilities (many of them never having written creatively before). It proved to me, again, again, that so much of this thing we call creativity is within us, just waiting for the invitation to express itself.

Notes

1. Each student/writer quoted in this chapter has granted explicit permission to reprint his or her text in this chapter.
2. See Winkel et al., "No Time to Think."
3. The grant is entitled "Human Experience and Behavior in Health and Illness," NIH NHLBI 5K07HL082628.
4. Charon, Hermann, and Devlin, "Close Reading and Creative Writing."

QUALITATIVE WAYS
OF KNOWING

From Fire Escapes to Qualitative Data: Pedagogical Urging, Embodied Research, and Narrative Medicine's Ear of the Heart

Edgar Rivera Colón

Narrative Prelude

What informs a life's work, whether it is community-centered ethnographic practice or the clinical care of patients in crisis-ridden urban health centers bereft of resources, oftentimes strikes me as the stuff of memories and dreamscapes. For example, I grew up during the 1970s in a northern New Jersey ghetto community. The sounds, smells, sights, tastes, and scattered affective landscapes of those days are in my embodied thoughts every semester as I teach a new cohort of narrative medicine students the ins and outs of qualitative research methods. I often imagine my pedagogical tasks would be easier if I could borrow a time machine from some twenty-fourth-century physics department colleague and go back in time with my students to that little strip of no more than ten blocks that was my world as a child of Puerto Rican migrants in 1970s downtown Jersey City.

But where would I take them to learn something of the experiences that led me to become an ethnographer and a teacher of qualitative research methods many decades later? First and foremost, I would take them to my cilantro-green fire escape—my part of it anyway—jutting out from the third floor of my aunt's building. I remember how the green paint glistened against the flesh-colored bricks that encased our two-room apartment on Wayne Street. The fire escape was my favorite place to be as a child: a breezy "betwixt and between" realm where the heat and manic activity in my mother's kitchen and on the

street below could be observed, discerned, and attended to from a porous distance. In this way I could interact with, but not be consumed by, the warp and
woof of domestic social reproduction or, upon the jet-black tar of my native
block, fights over stickball rules or the nuances of double-dutch. There I would
sit with my students in the day's heat and explore what was happening in my
mother's kitchen and down on Wayne Street: both expanses would be available for us to observe, write field notes, and discuss.

What would they see and notice? With whom would they converse? What
meanings would they cull from the interplay of conversations, observations,
and the sublime messiness of getting into *being with folks*? What stories would
they tell as a consequence of our time-travel exercise? How might a given student's sensorium be reassembled by this ethnographic field? Would they note
the differences in ethnicity, race, gender, and age in this working-class neighborhood and home-world that the forces of time and ruthless gentrification
have evaporated decades ago? If they stretched their bodies and eyes a bit, they
could see the place where my uncle worked: the massive buildings of the Dixon
Ticonderoga pencil factory, home of the dreaded No. 2 pencil of standardized
testing lore. Like the pencils, the factory is ribboned by a green and yellow line
that announces the kingdom of No. 2 production.

Beyond just observing from a distance, we would have to go inside and interact with a much younger version of my mother, and down into the street to
jump rope, eavesdrop on the older residents' gossip, and play some stickball
while avoiding the sneaker-sucking gum spots on the steamy tar streets. My
little green fire escape would function as a launching pad, a trans-temporal
comfort zone, from which to immerse my students in the social life of Wayne
Street during one of the many blazing hot summers of my 1970s childhood.
That steel perch allowed me for countless hours to become a keen observer
of social interactions and escape my status as younger son, bookworm, and
spoiled nephew, even when blustery autumnal winds announced winter's
advent. My ghetto fire escape was the hard, somewhat rusty, metal scaffold that
allowed me to climb up and enter into qualitative research's many mansions.

Alas, borrowing time machines as easily as one might request books from
a university's interlibrary loan services is a long way off, and certainly beyond
the likely lifetimes allotted for my students and me, even if we are all lucky
enough to live into a splendid old age. So I remand my imaginary trans-
temporal comfort zone to future generations of ethnographers and, as our
neighborhood Italian basement wine craftsman Old Man Marcela would tell
us to do on Wayne Street and in life, "Work with what ya' got, kids." *Work with
what ya' got*. But what do I have when I begin to introduce narrative medicine's
newest generation of thought leaders and practitioners to qualitative research
methods? Every semester I am blessed to have an eager and motivated group of

students, many of whom have training in the quantitative methods of the natural sciences and/or clinical experience from the healthcare field, or even pastoral work as ministers and chaplains. Admittedly, it is not my beloved green fire escape—but it is a good start.

Demystifying Qualitative Research Methods

The first item on the agenda is demystifying qualitative research methods. I assure my students that it really isn't rocket science, but it is layered and subtle; in truth, the only sound entry to this particular royal road to social scientific knowledge is constant and disciplined practice, reflection on that practice, and the invaluable return to the fluid materiality of practice but at a higher level of comprehension and rearticulation. I remind them that we are all lay social scientists of one kind or another, constantly scrutinizing and, more importantly, interpreting our own social actions, the actions of those who immediately surround us, and even social actors and contexts we will never know in the flesh. In this demystifying process, it is key to remind students how immersed we all are in social scientific ideas and speculations. We are social beings and thinkers *tout court*. And that is fertile field for sowing and reaping at the end of a semester's work.

One of the better turns in public health literatures and practice in the last two decades has been the push toward an assets-based approach to public health challenges, as opposed to a deficits-based and pathology-replicating paradigm. To wit: assume that people are already doing the work of self and community care, and build on the insights and strengths culled from such efforts. This novel approach has been described as *intravention* in contradistinction to an *intervention*. Sociologist Samuel Friedman and his colleagues use the term *intravention* to describe the insights that come from many years of fieldwork among poor, IV-drug using populations in New York City. Their work has demonstrated "that most residents of an impoverished New York City neighbourhood actively urge other people, including both drug users and non-users, to engage in certain behaviours that decrease the HIV-related and other risks of drug use and sex. These 'urgers' include users of drugs and of alcohol as well as other residents . . . We called such urging 'intravention'. Intravention is prevention activities that are conducted by community members."[1]

The pedagogy I deploy in class with my narrative medicine students is one of *intravention* or *instructional urging,* to help students discover and reframe the inchoate qualitative research skills in the social tool kit with which they, and all of us, traverse the world in our constant quest to meet our pressing needs and changing desires. In line with this approach to qualitative methods instruction is a very clear and simple *desideratum*: we sort of know this stuff already. The trick is to explicate that implicit knowledge and mobilize students' practical and affective energies to make known what is still under their respective cognitive radars. Moreover, pedagogies of intravention are most efficacious when students locate themselves in the practice of social research by not forgetting their embodied stories, which animate the research questions they choose to pursue and the methods they use to practice qualitative methods.

The next step is to clarify for students that qualitative research methods do not fall from the sky or emerge from personal revelation, but arise from the give and take of ordinary social life itself, even from *their* daily comings and goings as graduate or medical students and busy people living in a manic, global hub like New York City. In short, the material basis for qualitative research methods are the social practices that structure the intersubjective work and pleasures of everyday life. For example, the deep and long conversation with a friend or even a stranger on a specific topic or set of topics is transformed, via the standards of social scientific collective scrutiny, debate, peer review, and validation, into the in-depth interviews practiced by ethnographers. Likewise, consider those vibrant and contentious group discussions among friends or colleagues in a busy Manhattan diner about the pressing social problems of the day being distilled over time into focus group methods. If we attend closely and with care to the ways in which we interact and observe people we may know—and the many we do not know but might wish to know—at a loud night club or a ritual-based gathering, we begin to recognize the social-kinetic rubrics that participant observation or "structured hanging out" entail.

The goal of qualitative research is to understand the vital and concrete manifestations of social life and the meanings that emerge from, structure, and inform these phenomena. Marx, one of the founders of Euro-American social research and theory, writes in *Grundrisse*: "The concrete is concrete because it is a concentration [or synthesis] of many determinations, hence a unity of the diverse."[2] It is this synthesis of the ordinary and varied forms of communication and interaction, in which we all participate, that over time and with practice have developed into qualitative research methods.

An Embodied, Reflexive Practice

Denzin and Lincoln define qualitative research in the following manner: "Qualitative research is a situated activity that locates the observer in the world. It consists of a set of interpretive, material practices that make the world visible . . . qualitative research involves an interpretive, naturalistic approach to the world. This means that qualitative researchers study things in their natural settings, attempting to make sense of, or to interpret, phenomena in terms of the meanings people bring to them."[3] *Situated activity . . .* how do students get situated? By returning to their bodies and re-situating those bodies in culture—but not a folkloric sense of culture, or the facile and truncated multiculturalism of twenty-first century corporate-managed diversity. Rather, a grounded and robust sense of culture embedded in history, the uses and abuses of political power, and the increasingly stratified economics which have typified the American polity these last four decades.

At root, students must come to grips with the reality that their bodies are the primary tools of observation and data collection in qualitative research. Much like the novice Trappist monk—who enters the monastery to escape the world but finds the world has become ever-present in his memories, dreams, and desires—to enter into qualitative research practice is to inhabit one's body in another way. The monastic path is not a leaving of the world but an intensification of being immersed in it via an unusual and distinct register. So, too, with qualitative research practice for the narrative medicine initiate, and even the seasoned ethnographer, the body's manifest sensoria are intensified and rerouted in new, unexpected, and at times even disturbing ways. Along with a return to embodied life via an alternate route, students must begin to appropriate, cognitively and in practice, the idea that the kinds of epistemological and ontological object–subject cuts that the quantitative sciences make are simply not easily translatable into qualitative practice. The main problem is that any distinction between the subject and the object is always already nestled in human experience and perception. There is no higher extra-experiential, epistemological court to which one can appeal. *What we decide to be objective and subjective realities are irrevocably enfolded in experience and the social worlds that allow those actions to unfold, flourish, and fade in order to emerge in other forms.* I like to imagine that when students begin to wrestle with and unevenly appropriate this fundamental insight, they begin to cross a kind of epistemological rubicon. After that crossing, the real battle is joined on the field of practice.

However, a word of caution has to be inserted in this discussion: the demand that qualitative research practice makes on students to re-assume their embodied selves for the sake of qualitative knowledge production can be a ruse if their bodies are accounted for abstractly and not in their unique concrete historicity. The danger is that the students will assume their embodied practice but in a universalizing way, which may inadvertently usher in the proverbial Hegelian conceptual night in which all cows are black and distinctions are impossible. In becoming re-embodied in qualitative research practice, the particularity of each student's relationship to power, privilege, and social penalty is indispensable. The methodological requirement that ethnographers be self-reflexive is about staking out the investigator's social positioning in this society as it is, and how she fits into and/or is askance to the fairly stable, but always evolving, manner in which economic and symbolic resources are asymmetrically distributed in the United States.

Therefore, I usually remind students of my social positionality as a light-skinned, cisgender son of working-class Puerto Rican migrants who identifies as queer and was educated in mostly white-dominated, bourgeois educational institutions. This reminder is not an invitation to an exercise in self-gratifying displays of identity politics per se, but rather a way of comprehending the multiple vectors or differential axes (e.g., race, class, sexuality, gender, etc.) of material and symbolic privileges and penalties, which traverse and produce my sense of self as well as my biases and ideological commitments. I then ask students to locate their specific social positionalities and consider that they bring all of those elements—with good, bad, neutral, and ambivalent effects—into their qualitative research efforts. *Reflexivity is about accounting for oneself within the structuring dynamics of an American society that ideologically insists on the political equivalence between people as citizen-subjects/consumers while constantly producing life-crushing material stratifications across institutions, especially in our corporatized, time-squeezed, and beleaguered healthcare system.*

Summing up lessons learned after her 30 years of practice in an entirely different realm, a gestalt therapist colleague told me that the most difficult thing to do in life is simply to show up to one's own life and problems, given that it is so much safer to show up to everyone else's lives and problems. Likewise, the self-reflexive stance in qualitative research is showing up honestly to a research project with no place to hide, especially that oft-sought-after epistemic *cordon sanitaire*: the cool stance of scientific objectivity and emotional non-entanglement. The validity of qualitative data is not arrived at by denying one's biases. Quite the opposite is closer to the truth: one accounts for those biases and ideological blocks by locating the enabling structural material conditions for their production and reproduction, and how they might affect the research process from beginning to end.

Making the World Visible

Qualitative research makes the world visible in new and compelling ways. Narrative medicine students know from their exposure to European phenomenology that the self is a bloom-like nexus where self and world interarticulate. As a material and intersubjective social scientific knowledge-producing practice, qualitative work engages practitioners' bodies as entry and exit points through which the meaning-worlds of social actors embedded in particular places and times come to light for analysis and interpretation. If we can imagine researchers and research subjects as embodied condensation and articulation matrixes/carnal points of collective histories, economic forces, and culturally felt knowledges, among many other things, then we can grasp how the world can flower from the data culled from these apparently discrete individuals. Narrative medicine students are trained to conduct in-depth individual and group interviews and do participant observation because these methods produce data that reveal the layered panoply of meaning-worlds that live in dialectical tension with systemic inequality and structural violence.

Marxist literary theorist Raymond Williams, in an essay discussing art objects, talks about "structures of feeling." Williams writes: "We are talking about characteristic elements of impulse, restraint, and tone; specifically affective elements of consciousness and relationships; not feeling against thought, but thought as felt and feeling as thought: practical consciousness of a present kind, in a living and interrelating continuity. We are then defining these elements as a 'structure' . . . Yet, we are also defining a social experience which is still *in process*, often indeed not yet recognized as social but taken to be private, idiosyncratic, and even isolating, but which in analysis (though rarely otherwise) has its emergent, connecting, and dominant characteristics, indeed its specific hierarchies."[4]

Williams captures in the realm of aesthetic objects what a good qualitative researcher is seeking to harvest as her data, via the methods of interviewing and participant observation: the imbrication of feeling and thought, the liveliness of the social that is still in the process of formation (i.e., the social-emergent), and, crucially, social phenomena as they appear to inhere in the register of unique autonomous individuality when, in point of fact, they live and breathe in overarching structures which circulate dominant ideologies and reproduce robust and enduring hierarchies. If one takes seriously the insight that language has its own register of materiality, and ideas become social forces, then words as forms of doing need to be connected to the predictable patterns of relationality and power that structure work over and through institutional and community settings.

My students learn to watch and listen to the constant humming of the social machinery and ask very basic questions: Who and/or what forces am I hearing and seeing at this moment? What do these sounds and interactions tell me about the house of the social, of which we are all denizens even in our most private or public instances? Is there an outside to all this humming and cacophony? What new sounds and doings am I witnessing as an ethnographically informed interviewer and observer? These questions generate data, but they also became heuristic levers that produce other spaces for new questions and findings.

Narrative medicine is a distinctively new sound in healthcare and medical education. It hums and rhymes akimbo to the pervading hegemonic sounds of the machinery of the healthcare-industrial complex. Many narrative medicine students come to our program precisely to develop an ear to listen to such cutting-edge soundscapes and acquire a new vocabulary to act in ever more efficacious and humane ways as clinicians, artists, teachers, researchers, writers, and activists of all stripes. Narrative medicine was born from the crises engendered by the new market commandism (i.e., the neoliberal fix) that economic and political elites across the Global North adopted in the wake of the mass protracted struggles for economic redress and social inclusion that the 1960s and 1970s ushered in and that still resound to this day. Beginning in the late 1970s, on one side of the Atlantic Margaret Thatcher and her Tory colleagues rolled back the social gains of ordinary Britons, while on the other side the telegenic and avuncular Ronald Reagan and a newly invigorated Republican Party set out to whittle away and ultimately decimate the social safety net and labor gains accrued through popular struggles during the New Deal, the Great Society programs, and the Civil Rights Movement—the grandmother to this day of so many efforts to right the historical exclusion of women, LGBTQ communities, the disabled, Native Americans, Latinos, Asian Americans, and other communities of identity and affiliation. This war on the social gains of the many by the few has been so effective that the political lingua franca across the Global North's centers of capital and power is inflected in Reaganite and Thatcherite terms, even by well-intentioned, erstwhile reformers. What proffers itself as economic and political common sense is a result of these revanchist policies enacted during the last four decades in the service of greater concentrations of wealth and ideological dominance.

In the United States, during the last four decades, there is almost no institution that has been spared the costs of this redistribution of wealth upwards. Healthcare has suffered enormously from these cutbacks and givebacks. From a purely labor standpoint, clinicians from various disciplinary formations have suffered the fate of craftspeople and artisans of old: their medical art and craft has been stripped, albeit partially at this stage, of the professional independence and humane work pacing that doctors of prior generations depended upon to deliver quality care to their patients. To paraphrase Marx, all that was medically solid in the craft of healing has been subjected to the fires of metrics and a labor speed-up familiar to any auto worker on an assembly line, but may be confusing to those who have donned the white coat as an external sign of their vocation as healers and teachers of the healing arts.

Amid this specific twenty-first-century American institutional and social context, narrative medicine began its work of imagining something different: a new and progressive assemblage of work, clinical care, and hope in landscapes that at first blush seemed hostile to these kinds of changes. My colleagues in narrative medicine asked a very direct and layer-revealing question: *Is this all we can do?* Moreover, they asked the right question in a mode and tempo that ran counter to the temporal logic of the historical moments we are all living. They saw and understood the crisis that healthcare was living—enduring, really—and instead of speeding up they deliberately slowed down. On the face of it, this slowing down appears counterintuitive and impractical. Yet—as popular educators and sound artists Robert Sember and Dont Rhine like to tell their students and audiences—the most effective way to enter and reshape a crisis is by refusing its logic of speedy alacrity and manic fetishizing of commodified newness. Rather, the critical and humane response is to slow down, take stock, and go deeper into the limits and possibilities within the contradictory social and cultural forms inherent in the wide institutional contours and interstices of the crisis at hand. In essence, the forces that are antagonistic, even lethal, to the full flourishing of human freedom depend on all of us ordinary people, professionally credentialed or not, speeding up and going along with the time-squeeze and work overload. To unlearn and untangle this imposed mania is definitely part of the work of narrative medicine, as well as qualitative research learning and practice.

As another way to consider this point about slowing down our eyes, ears, and minds in the service of better learning and care, take the following line of thought: the Marxist tradition sees as its *telos* the abolition of all classes as the last step in the realization of human freedom outside the strictures of economic necessity. For Marx and his followers, all human history is really a pre-history moving toward that moment where the line between human freedom and material necessity is dissolved by way of collective transformative praxis. In contradistinction, one strand of feminism does not see the goal of women's liberation as the abolition of gender, but its multiplication beyond the binary logic of male/female that structures patriarchy. This particular strain of feminism asked a potent question: what kind of bodies, desires, and worlds might be forged when there are many genders to embody and not just a paltry two?

In one sense, narrative medicine aligns with the logic of liberatory multiplicity found in the feminism I just adumbrated above. This logic of expansion of embodied worlds is quite distinct from the logic of abolition that I underlined in Marxist theory. Narrative medicine is countercultural and institution-reformatting inasmuch as it labors to produce an expansion of time, paradoxically, by slowing down. The logic at play is expansive, meaning-stretching, and life-world extending. Clearly, this is not the métier of speed-ups, multitasking as productivity strategy, and quantitative healthcare metrics as the only assessment coin of the realm.

The Ethnographic Witness

I proffer these insights to bring up a key question: what is the motion at the heart of narrative medicine? Or, to put it more sharply in the context of this essay, how do the respective motions of narrative medicine and qualitative research practices converge and cross-fertilize each other? Charon describes the motions or movements of narrative medicine as "the triad of attention, representation, and affiliation."[5] The clinician attends to the patient's illness story, represents that story to the patient in various forms, and affiliates with the patient through the dialectic of listening and response that constructs an ethos of care that hails both of them as human beings searching for meaning and healing. Clearly, to figure this movement in a strictly linear fashion would do an injustice to the iterative and recursive nature of the patient–clinician relationship that, in its best moments, is multidirectional and layered.

Similarly, qualitative researchers listen with their ears, eyes, minds, and hearts. In collecting data they begin the work of representing via textual, visual, and oral means the life-worlds and meaning landscapes of those whose stories are rarely visible in the halls of power and decision making. In this instance, the qualitative practitioner becomes an "ethnographic witness" to the exclusions that are the enabling material conditions of elite institutional privilege and ethical indifference. The practitioner of qualitative methods also constructs affiliation, not only by establishing rapport for entering those other spaces but also building a form of care-laden solidarity by getting the research subject's life, work, challenges, loves, and social sufferings "right," such that when she is presented with the drafts of a write-up she can recognize herself and her worlds in these distillations of a whole way of life. Qualitative research- ers use all the tools at their disposal (e.g., structured observation, participation observation, in-depth interviews, focus groups, community archives, material cultures, etc.) to learn by heart and mind what is at stake when we ask individu- als and whole communities to tell us their stories: the ones that build bridges between the exigencies of the present, the lessons of the past, and the potential horizons for development and progress that the ever-receding and expanding future may hold.

It is an extraordinary privilege to be able to attend to, listen, record, repre- sent, circulate, and return those stories to one's research subjects. During my dissertation fieldwork I shared a chapter with one of my main informants that focused largely on him and his community activism and work. His immediate response to my draft chapter caused me to pause and realize how much an act of care crafting another's story can be. He simply said: "No one has ever writ- ten about my life. It makes me feel good and affirms the community work I've done all these years." He appreciated that I had listened to his words and ways and given him a form of it that he could critique and appreciate.

Narrative medicine and qualitative research allows for ordinary folks and their stories to be listened to in a disciplined and attentive manner. I often ask my students if they have ever been really listened to in a caring and open way. I'm regularly dismayed at how few of them have had that experience. The activist lawyer and theologian William Stringfellow went to the root of why listening is transformative: "Listening is a rare habit among human beings. You cannot listen to the word another is speaking if you are preoccupied with your appearance or impressing the other, or if you are trying to decide what you are going to say when the other stops talking, or if you are debating about whether the word being spoken is true or relevant or agreeable. Such matters have their place, but only after listening to the word as the word is being uttered. Listening in other words is a primitive act of love, in which a person gives himself to another's word, making himself accessible and vulnerable to that word."[6] When this type of listening—an attending entangled in the suturing dynamics of love—begins via the tools of qualitative research, our course ends and the students refiguring the world in all its sadness and hope begins anew.

Notes

1. Mateu-Gelabert et al., "For the Common Good," 144.
2. Marx, *Grundrisse*, 101.
3. Denzin and Lincoln, *Handbook of Qualitative Research*, 3.
4. Williams, *Marxism and Literature*, 132. Emphasis in the original.
5. Charon, *Narrative Medicine: Honoring*, xi.
6. Stringfellow, *Count It All Joy*, 16.

PART

VII

CLINICAL PRACTICE

CHAPTER 12

A Narrative Transformation of Health and Healthcare

Rita Charon and Eric R. Marcus

RC Tells the Clinical Story

A patient whom I have known and taken care of for decades made an urgent appointment to see me.[1] (I will call her Ms. N.) She had been told in an emergency room that she has diabetes. This news was intolerable to her, for complex reasons that I only partly understood. We talked for some time, I examined her, and we made some plans for what to do in the face of this news.

I found myself writing about the encounter the next day as I sat on a plane, and after writing a couple of pages I felt that I understood much more clearly what had happened. But that was my perspective, and I wanted to learn the patient's point of view. So I mailed the two pages to her once I returned home. When she next came into the office for her follow-up visit, she held my letter in her hands and said, "Every time I read this, I cry." I had come close, in her mind as well, to what had happened between us.

> February 10, 20xx
>
> Two middle-aged women sit in a cramped clinic office in upper Manhattan. They have known one another for decades, one of them moving through a series of health reversals and accomplishments and the other, as her doctor, accompanying her through them.
>
> The patient's health has been robust—a history of severe asthma and allergies in childhood; some minor skin ailments; osteoarthritis; eventually a total knee replacement through which she sailed. A stalwart Upper West Sider, an activist and progressive, a wife and mother, a university professor, a force of nature, the patient bicycles the river, eats sensibly, helps the planet and her spot on it to be as safe for life as it can

be. The women had both been part of the movement to end the Vietnam War. They had taken to the streets with Our Bodies, Our Selves. They staked their own lives and careers on ideals of fairness and freedom. Neither had become rich or famous, and yet both felt somehow that they had been dutiful to their commitments to the good and the right.

Today, the patient is in crisis. [A doctor in a local Urgicare Center told her that] she has diabetes, started her on daily medication, and told her to check her blood for sugar daily. Terrified, the patient felt some iron door on her health slamming shut. Diabetics get heart attacks, strokes, lose limbs, go blind, need dialysis. Had she not been taking care of herself? Had she not been doing *enough* to care for herself? Should she have worked harder to lose the weight that kept creeping up? Was it so grave to have a bagel with cream cheese now and then? Did the ice cream cone on those sweltering August afternoons consign her to this? She savaged herself, flagellating herself for impulses given in to, pleasures happily indulged in. She must have had a death wish all this time, and all this time she thought she was doing okay. How much more can one do? How could she have done this to herself?

Now, as she sits across the desk from this doctor who knew her as a young mother, she sees herself not in freshness but in demise. This diagnosis of diabetes, such as it was, catapulted her into an unadulterated face-off with aging and death. . . .

Even though her hair has turned white and her movements have become deliberate, she doesn't ever feel old. She works 150% time teaching at two different universities. She insists on cycling, doing all her own heavy housework, lugging groceries from Fairway, walking through the park to the Met instead of grabbing a cab. She sees right now, in this horrible epiphany, how she has been trying to prove something. She has been in a fruitless effort to prove her youth, her strength, her everlastingness. But now, with this sudden news of a new dread disease, she recognizes the subterfuge. She has been fooling herself. She has indulged in a stupid fantasy of health while, within her cells, damage is already underway.

They sit at the desk staring at one another, saying little, taking one another in. Slowly, the doctor wonders aloud about what this epiphany signifies. They ease from talk about blood sugar to talk about love and meaning. They wonder, together, how growing old can *happen* with clarity and truth. Must we lie to ourselves in order to endure? Can we accept our limited time on earth and still enjoy it? Not technical but personal, their conversation deepens the contact between them so that they both, now, as they speak, are discovering why they do what they do, what the deep strata of desire and meaning might be. They come together to expose the ground floor of self—its stark realizations of the limits of a life and, maybe, at the depth of that starkness, also a gratitude and awe that the life has been given to begin with.

The doctor examines the patient, listens to the clear lungs, tracks the regular heart beat, finds no place that hurts. They meet in this odd intimacy, not of love or friendship but of ongoingness. Perhaps, the doctor ventures, the elevated sugar was caused by this bad viral infection. That happens regularly. Perhaps we might first let you fully recover from the viral illness and then see if the sugar levels off. Maybe we can find a way to understand this situation that doesn't condemn you to such self-blame and dread. Maybe we might see within this ordeal some thirst for life, some appetite for life. Maybe we can find ourselves on the side of life.

They both feel that they've found solid ground. The patient will continue to be elementally shaken by this sudden forced confrontation with her mortality. This confrontation takes its toll. And yet, it gives her something strong. It corrects an illusion. It rectifies slipshod trains of thought that overlook the finitude of this life of ours. Not with disillusionment but with truth can these women proceed. They both resume their days, having together undergone a powerful experience. They see now, both, the implacable passage of time and, in the shadow of that merciless knowledge, their grasp on the beauty of this life, its shy worth.

This story is not the conventional kind of clinical reporting that would be found in a medical record. Instead, I adopted methods, approaches, genres, and formal structures of creative writing in my efforts to see what it is that had occurred between my patient and me that day. Like any creative writing it was unpredictable, not forethought, coming out of darkness. I knew some of the features of my patient's early life and, as I wrote, these details came to me as well. I recalled that she had been ill as a child. Her mother had treated her as a sick child, prohibiting her from climbing trees and doing vigorous exercise. There was a good deal of resentment even now about the ways she felt she had been stunted by being assigned the sick role in the family. So the appearance of this acute illness now seemed to reawaken the voice of her mother, as if she were now being scolded by the now-dead mother for not having followed the orders to be still and slow and careful.

I had certainly not made a decision on the plane to write about myself in the third person. It is simply how it came out. The story sought to emphasize the connections between my patient and me, and I realized only afterwards that writing it with a first-person "I" would have enforced a difference between the "I" and the "she." The third-person narration avoided this formal split, letting me represent the two women similarly and yet independently. The act of writing, especially in the third person, about what had happened in my office shifted my own subject position from that of an agent to that of a witness. I was able to "see" my patient and myself from the same distance and angle as two different human beings. By pushing myself outside of the narrative driving seat, where the first-person narrator invariably sits, my writing gave me a position from which to see both of us in separate but equal light.

But it was not I who chose this form; it was the story itself. This is one of the dividends of narrative medicine techniques in clinical practice. That which exists in one's "unthougtht known" has a chance to surface into awareness.[2] The work of the encounter was accomplished by the two women sitting in that clinic room as they choreographed their roles in view of their histories individually and together, and as they triangulated on this illness from its opposite sides. The work was also done on the plane as I, hands on laptop, let the story seek its own form from sources quite out of my awareness, having percolated over the day and night since that clinical encounter.

My writing exposed more clearly than had my memory what had happened during this visit. It also showed me what it had exposed me to. Even working in a hospital as I do, I do not daily, actively confront the limits of my own life. But through the agency of my patient's merciless honesty about her mortality, I too underwent a graphic face-off with my not-too-far-off death. So as we sat together at my desk we looked at one another with recognition, a reciprocal recognition in which we became mirrors for one another at the same time that we were still doctor and patient. The fact that we shared some actual features of life as politically active women professors in our sixties living in Manhattan may have quickened this process of reciprocal recognition but, along with encounters with other patients around that same time, it opened to me a powerful new realization about the clinical life. By accepting, consciously, that I share with patients the status of living-toward-death, we, together, somehow, see in the inevitability of a death to come the wordless worth of the life to come.

I see even now as I write this representation of the event, some years later, that this reciprocal recognition might help clinicians to face the existential dilemma of mortality. How does one live one's life around sick and dying people without being paralyzed by the resultant and realistic fear of death? One strategy that doctors and nurses may unconsciously adopt early, in a life saturated with illness and death, is to assume that their nearness to disease and death confers personal immunity from it. In a simmering fantasy we exclude ourselves from the ranks of humans who will sicken and die as a strategy to get through the shock of our close contact with all the tragedies we witness (see Chapter 5's discussion of spaceship ethics). Perhaps the reciprocal recognition that I underwent with Ms. N. could, if developed mindfully, encourage an awareness of the universal fate of living creatures and minimize the objectifying forces that separate and protect the doctor from the patient. We meet in the shocking universals of the human fate, a fate shared. Zeus, in John Banville's novel *The Infinities*, envies humans their mortality. As he gazes down at us hapless mortals from atop Mount Olympus, he says:

> This is the mortal world. It is a world where nothing is lost, where all is accounted for while yet the mystery of things is preserved; a world where they may live, however

briefly, however tenuously, in the failing evening of the self, solitary and at the same time together somehow here in this place, dying as they may be and yet fixed forever in a luminous, unending instant.[3]

This, perhaps, is the work of healthcare—to make clearings where we mortals, solitary and at the same time together. can envision what awaits us and can gather courage and acceptance from one another as we move toward our ends. That some are afflicted with disease and some spared makes all the more collective the inevitable end that awaits each one. Perhaps within the cone of light shed by illness onto the void of mortality, all who undergo or witness illness can maybe *see* together more clearly the shape of our human fate, the tempo of gain and loss, and the harmonies of the sounds of life and death. Only then, perhaps, can we enjoy each luminous, unending instant.

EM: Concepts—Transference and Transitional Space

Transference: As I learn about Rita's and her patient's experiences, I see aspects familiar to the psychoanalyst and, although this is an internal medicine and not an analytic encounter, I offer some thoughts from my field that may deepen our appreciation of what Ms. N. has taught us. In illness a person is faced with a version of herself, we can call it the *ill self.* The patient in this account experienced the shocking tension between what she knows herself to be—a physically strong and intellectually vital university professor, activist, committed wife and mother—and what this acute illness forced her to see as herself: guilty, indulgent, doomed to an early death. Her rage perhaps stemmed from the deletion of the healthy, or at least usual, self by her experience of her ill self, as if the ill self trumped all that she had come to know about who she is.

I are using the word *healthy* here to refer not to a biomedically measured, normed health status but to the person's experience of what constitutes his or her personhood. This ill self differs from the actual bodily illness, which in this case is a body with a higher than normal level of glucose. The experienced ill self includes not just reality but memory, fantasy, and emotion. The self-blame, the savaging, the assessment of herself as having held stupid fantasies of immortality, were all manifestations of the sudden emergence of this alternative to the self imposed by the actual illness events of her body.

In the office, it was as if the doctor were faced with these two selves—there was the healthy self whom Rita had accompanied for decades through illnesses and difficulties and triumphs, and there was the ill self who was the self-scorning butt of scathing judgments about the most fundamental aspects of self. The doctor had the chance to illuminate the healthy self and minimize the ill self, as if to redress the skewed balance between the two.

Psychoanalytic concepts can illuminate some of the startling things that occur in a narrative practice of medicine, and certainly in this particular account of a medical encounter. The concept of transference—that the psychoanalyst replicates the role of a significant other in the patient's life—helps us to think through this situation. In psychoanalytic treatment, gradually the patient may transfer onto the doctor past feelings or patterns of behavior toward a parent or other important person in his or her life. This double life of treatment allows the patient to recognize the feelings, benign or noxious, aroused by the person transferred onto the analyst, thereby allowing the patient to work through feelings that could not be worked through in ordinary life.

In the situation of physical illness, however, another dynamic seems to prevail. The illness, not the doctor, becomes the location onto which feelings or behavior patterns toward a significant person can be transferred. In cases of serious physical illness, the transference to the physician is replaced by a transference to the illness. The ill self becomes an autonomous self-representation at odds with the healthy self. If, through transference, this ill self-representation becomes occupied by a significant other in the patient's life, the patient is doubly cursed by the reality of the illness and the metaphor of the illness.

That there was an echo in all this of her mother's I-told-you-so voice intensified the effect of the events on her sense of self. Ms. N. had a maternal transference to her illness, meaning that her mother, in memory, influenced or inhabited this illness. Other forms of transference are possible in states of illness. Instead of a transfer of a significant person onto the illness, some patients may transfer neurotic fantasies or specific fears. But in this case we can speculate that this construct, the ill self, became a locus for the patient's blaming, scolding mother. We can almost hear the mother's voice ventriloquized by the patient: "This illness is your fault, it is punishment, you brought this on yourself. You are a bad daughter. If only you had listened to me."

Other crises—bankruptcy, divorce, or being fired from a job—do not attack the body in the way that health reversals do, for these other crises do not cross the boundary around the actual, physical body-self as illness does. When physical illness strikes, it alters the real body. This alters the experience of the real self, for they are of course united in the person. When the real body calls forth emotional meanings, then the emotional meaning of the real physical illness may invade the experience of the real self or person. One feels the emotional significance to be real. Ms. N.'s emotional experience of being ill, influenced by the fantasy of her mother's punitive voice, spilled over into her experience of herself in her life. Then, how one fears one is, as a person, becomes felt as reality.[4] The real self and the emotional self have merged because the real body and the ill body have merged.

In the face of threat to the body in particular, all the more necessary are maneuvers that support the patient's confidence in the ongoingness of the self. It is exactly when the body is felt to be untrustworthy by the self who lives with it that some external stabilizers can appreciably maintain health. The internist subdues the illness in the body so that the patient can once again feel her usual self rather than her ill self. The psychoanalyst strengthens the healthy self to better fight against the ill self and the ill body. The narratively trained clinician does both; strengthens both the body and the self.

Transitional space: From early childhood on, human beings have the capacity for symbolic experience. Pediatrician and child psychoanalyst D.W. Winnicott describes this experience as halfway between reality and fantasy. Our patient's body is reality. The meanings she transfers to it are fantasy. Her experience of her illness is therefore a mixture of fantasy and reality. Winnicott called this experience *transitional experience.* He pointed out that this mixture of fantasy and reality can be experienced through a real object or a real person—in this case a real illness—and can be used as a transition for psychological development and a reorganization of meaning. It can function as a new internalization of meaning and therefore develop a new relationship to reality. However, in illness the transitional experience has different outcomes. The patient's illness becomes a transitional object, but instead of being a developmentally useful experience it becomes a noxious one.

The doctor—and in this case the doctor's writing—opens a transitional space, in Winnicott's terms, between Ms. N.'s ill self and her healthy self. This has the potential to rescue the patient from her use of the real bodily illness as a noxious transitional object. Having known the patient prior to this acute crisis, the doctor can keep alive the picture of that earlier, healthier self while the turmoil of facing illness proceeds.[5] In effect, the doctor in this situation says, "Listen, let me join you with this, please. Let me join you with this not only as an observer, but as a participant. And once you do that, we will then be able to help you separate out your real self—which happens now to be ill but is many other things, too—from your self-representation, now, as your ill self." If this comes about, the patient has another resource to use in recruiting her underlying strengths to help her face the crisis. The narrative physician offers herself and the narrative technique as a temporary transitional space for the purpose of separating a noxious reality from emotional fantasies about it, and catalyzing a healthier transitional relationship to the doctor to help with emotional growth and a new adaptation.

This transitional space gives the patient an option to free herself from the engulfing and terrifying self-representation as ill, weak, guilty, and doomed, and to accept again a self-experience of integration and health. Within the transitional space, the patient's dark and terrorizing fantasies about the existential dilemmas of the illness can be held at bay from contaminating the space of identity. That is what we help her with. Now the illness can become merely an illness, to be dealt with in practical ways, and not as a representative of a terrorizing, depressive experience of a scolding mother.

Rita's awareness of the patient's life and power and abilities and desire to be well and her writing about it for the patient functioned as a tactile reminder to the patient that, in addition to currently having a new illness problem, she was still all those healthy things that she has been all her life. In Winnicott's terms, this is the development of a *facilitating environment* or a *holding environment*, whereby a patient is recognized by the therapist in a stable, trustworthy, dependable space of safety.[6] An ongoing process in effective psychotherapy, this environment allows a patient facing an acute crisis to remain in contact with the more organized self that existed prior to the crisis. Once the self shifts to a more stable, organized self-representation and away from the current ill self, health has a chance. Growth and development have a chance. Otherwise, health and self remain captive to illness.

Developing this facilitative environment takes action on the part of the doctor. Unlike the neutral, effaced practice of the classical analyst, the doctor here is active not only in listening for the patient's words and nonlanguage communications but also in imagining the patient's world and freely expressing to the patient what is seen. In psychoanalyst Milton Viederman's words:

> Activity resides in imaginative, ongoing formulations in the consultant's mind of the patient's presentation and experience and the appropriate communication of such inferences to the patient. To accomplish this end, the consultant must enter the patient's world; develop a picture of him, of his experience with the people in his surround, and to communicate appropriately this awareness to him in a language that is familiar to him. In so doing, a climate develops in which the patient feels recognized and understood. The consultant is reciprocally recognized and becomes a "presence."[7]

Narrative medicine's practices of listening as a reader and writing down for the patient what is heard is precisely what Viederman means by activity in the consultation room. The concept is a strong one—it proposes to use the full resources of the doctor's person to benefit the patient. There is a sanctified space there in our clinical heads if we build it. It is waiting to receive what we experience with patients. It does not have to do with the feeling of pity or wanting to help. It is the cognitive and emotional ability and wish to connect with another human being. An ill human being who is suffering. It requires motivation and the ability to receive another human being. What this can do is to allow patients a new experience of themselves with their illness. The new experience is one where the experience of the real self is of a strengthened real self and not a weakened real self.

How, though, do we protect ourselves from suffering along with the patient? How do we practice without being engulfed in sadness? I think we protect ourselves from it by building an object-representation of our patients' experience, uncontaminated by our own self-representation. So, when we feel for them and with them, we are feeling what they feel about them, not what we feel about ourselves. The terror and withdrawal and burnout occur when we start to feel about ourselves what the patients feel about themselves; we ourselves despair as we sense their despair. Then the boundaries are blurred, and no good work can occur. We can be deeply moved and we ourselves grow when we experience the other in his or her otherness.

RC: Concepts—Creativity, Reflexivity, Reciprocity

Creativity: Years ago, I recognized the triangle of practice whereby I talk sequentially with what I first thought of as the "self" of the patient and the "body" of the patient.[8] It is as if I somehow become an interpreter between the patient's body and self, those two entities that, *in times of illness*, cannot on their own communicate. They speak different languages.[9] I experienced this odd split but did not understand what it meant.

I see now, through my tutelage with Craig Irvine on dualism and with Eric in psychoanalytic theory, that when I translate between the patient's "self" and "body" I might function as an intermediary between them, forming what Eric calls a transitional space, working to preserve the unity of their lived experience as not one or the other but both body and self and both ill and well. It may be, Eric suggests, that the salient split is not the dualism of body/self but a tension between the ill self and the healthy self.

Not a static quality, health is always in dialectic with its opposite, perhaps not quite illness but fragmentation or discord or disunity. Health conceptualized in this way resembles the biological concept of homeostasis, a state of integration in which the disparate organs and tissues are in harmony, each doing its part with unseen distinction and each in constant feedback with the others via hormonal and neural signaling, initiation of genetic activity, and triggering of protein synthesis. Disease, according to this definition of health, would be understood as rupture, alienation of one part from the other, incoherence.

"Health is life lived in the silence of the organs." These words were written by French surgeon René Leriche in 1936 and brought to contemporary attention by the work of physician and philosopher Georges Canguilhem.[10]

Canguilhem developed a series of revolutionary propositions for an anti-positivist and egalitarian consideration of health and disease, associated with a radically altered conception of the relation between clinician and patient. Canguilhem—perhaps echoed by George Engel in his biopsychosocial model for healthcare—reaches beyond the precincts of biological states to consider the homeostatic balance of a person with social and cultural forces and elements outside of the boundaries of the skin.[11]

Perceiving the clinical encounter as if it were a meeting with two different entities who do not speak one another's language —ill self and healthy self— makes sense on the background of Canguilhem's and Leriche's sense of health. The development of disease does not negate the healthy aspects of the person, despite his or her fear that it might. However, the enduring unity, whether the organs are silent or not, may be undetectable to the person at the time disease arises. The enduring unity may be undetectable to the clinician as well. Both these undetectabilities are consequential.

The enduring unities of ill self and healthy self can be brought back into view, for both patient and clinician, through creative acts. Creativity—the use of the imagination, curiosity, permitting one's mind to travel, resonating to affective signals from self and others, associative thought—within routine clinical practice promises to be a mode of reintegrating the self of the patient that is fragmented by illness or threat of illness. Simultaneously, creative acts in clinical routines might reintegrate the clinician's cognitively, professionally, and emotionally split subjectivity.[12]

Clinical practice can be experienced as a hemmed-in set of algorithms, standard practices, evidence-based decision making. Sometimes it feels as if there are few degrees of freedom in diagnosing or managing patients' health conditions. The low-density lipoprotein portion of total cholesterol must be under 100 unless there is a history of or risk factors for coronary disease, in which case it must be under 70. A hemoglobin A1C, a diagnostic test for diabetes, of greater than 7 dictates that pills or insulin or at least substantial dietary change is warranted. That these guidelines change over time and, like the LDL targets, are sometimes abandoned, reduces confidence in them but does not reduce anxiety about the risk of disease.

At the same time, or in times alternating with the hemmed-in times, we can feel the tremendous sensation of freedom, letting our minds travel, relying on what feels like intuition or second-sight in choosing what to do in clinical moments. Not a defiance of external standards—the algorithms are there for a reason—the creativity of practice can be experienced as a departure from the routine, a sense of buoyancy, a lift of insight that comes unbidden. I saw for the first time a 44-year-old woman with brittle diabetes who had had too many hospitalizations to count for either perilously low or perilously high glucose levels and who had abandoned several of the endocrine clinics in the city out of frustration.[13] I remember not interrupting her as she told me the long story of her disease. She was furious—angry at her body, angry at the doctors who had not helped her, angry that because of her poor health she had not been able to fulfill her dreams of starting her own business. At one point in what felt to me like an existential tirade, she stopped talking. I too remained silent. Holding back tears, she broke our silence to say, "The only thing I want now is a new set of teeth." Diabetics can develop intractable infectious gum disease, and she had already lost all her top teeth. Medicaid had paid for a denture, but it was ill-fitting and she could not wear it. Medicaid would not pay for a second set. So she hid her mouth when she talked. She couldn't laugh in public. She did not have a sex life. She was furious. We decided to concentrate only on getting her a new denture. I cashed in favors with my friends in the dental clinic, wrote letters to Medicaid that her life was at stake without the new teeth, and in three months she came into my office beaming and beautiful. Now, what gave me the permission to spend that first three months not even checking her glucose or fine-tuning her insulin? It was a stroke of recognition that *this* was the way to proceed. I recognized a path that might lead to some solid ground between us, and it certainly did, with her glucose achieving better control than it had in years and her confidence in her personal agency spilling over from caring for her diabetes to starting her business and developing new intimate relationships.

A creative clinical practice releases the unthought known for consideration. In a situation with patient and clinician, the creativity "belongs" to both and to both together—both individuals can be free from constraints to see things as they are not always seen. Winnicott, who started his professional career as a pediatrician, writes:

> [C]ertain conditions are necessary if success is to be achieved in this search [for the self]. These conditions are associated with what is usually called creativity. It is in playing and only in playing that the individual child or adult is able to be creative and to use the whole personality, and it is only in being creative that the individual discovers the self. . . . The general principle seems to me to be valid that *psychotherapy is done in the overlap of the two play areas, that of the patient and that of the therapist.*"[14]

Narrative medicine's emphasis on close reading and creative writing results in clinical dividends by bringing creativity into routine healthcare practice. We have moved even beyond the kind of active listening encouraged by Winnicott and Viederman in our rigorous practice of illuminating knowledge of the patient with the lights available through creative writing. Such writing, either by the patient or by the clinician, can be done not because the writer *knows* something but because the writer is *seeking* to see clearly what is perceived. It is hypothesis-generating, not hypothesis-testing. It follows the well-established aesthetic precept that representation is necessary for perception. In the words of philosopher of art Nelson Goodman, "[T]he object as we look upon or conceive it [is] a version or construal of the object. In representing an object, we do not copy such a construal or interpretation—we *achieve* it."[15]

I would not have achieved my view of Ms. N. by simply listening to her and thinking about our conversation. I do not believe my writing in the electronic medical record would have achieved the clarity I found while writing on the airplane the next day. By giving her what I wrote in a narrative form that allowed for temporal disjunction and metaphorical movement, I took a chance: I offered her the hypotheses I generated about her situation and, indeed, our situation. The test of the hypotheses would occur upon her reading and responding to them. Psychoanalyst Hans Loewald describes this phenomenon in psychotherapy:

> Language, in its most specific function in analysis, as interpretation, is thus a creative act similar to that in poetry, where language is found for phenomena, contexts, connexions, experiences not previously known and speakable. New phenomena and new experience are made available as a result of reorganization of material according to hitherto unknown principles, context and connexions.[16]

I discovered several months later what our narrative actions had accomplished, and I see in retrospect that Eric's formulation of what occurred during that first visit seems accurate. In the interim, my patient's blood glucose had gradually come under control. But she had developed a new health problem that required diagnostic tests and medication. This time, she did not reexperience the existential terror that had accompanied the new diagnosis of diabetes. At the close of an office visit with me when we dealt with the new problem, I wrote a note in the electronic chart summarizing our conversation, the findings, and outlining our plans.

After I finished writing my note, I turned the monitor toward her and asked her to read it and tell me what I had gotten wrong or what she thought did not belong in a chart that could be read by other clinicians. I then gave her the keyboard and asked her to complete the story of our visit.[17] I gave her a few minutes in my office to do this. When I returned, she said, "You might have to fix the pronouns, because I started with 'she' but ended with 'I'." Here is part of what she wrote:

> Feel empowered by making choices which have contributed to weight loss and a general feeling of who is in charge here. Need to make more of a concerted effort to walk

... at one time walking was both physically satisfying but also added to feeling less depressed. Thinking of myself as an old person is not as good as thinking of myself as a person who is old. My students think I am great, my co-workers appreciate the role I play in my students' lives, and that is my greatest sense of satisfaction and it allows me to appreciate the years of experience which lends itself to my teaching. My mother's voice does not have to be silenced but certainly toned down to a low murmur.

The creativity of our writing—and then of reading what one another had written in a spirit of co-discovery—resulted in a feeling of resonance between us. We had "between us" formed something of value in our relationship, in the continuing management of her medical conditions, and in her growing awareness of her own strength and health. That she "heard" her mother's voice in the terror of those early months with diabetes and that she could now tone it down to a low murmur seems to validate Eric's hypothesis about the transferential qualities of physical illness. More importantly, it shows that Ms. N. was able to emerge from two situations of illness with an increased self-regard, complex psychodynamic insight, and a sense of the beauty and worth of this life.

Reflexivity: A core dimension of the creative process is reflexivity, conceptualized as the capacity of an individual to observe the self with the same methods with which that individual studies phenomena. The concept of reflexivity is most often used by social scientists, oral historians, or psychotherapists to suggest that the clinician or scientist or anthropologist must recognize the role that he or she plays in the phenomenon under study.[18] The early roots of theorizing on reflexive practice arose in the work of Jürgen Habermas, Paulo Freire, and Donald Schön in works that emphasized not only the individual's self-reflection but also insisted on the reflexive capacity to interrogate and critique the social world in which any individual's practice exists.[19] Prodded by the prodigious and pathbreaking theorizing of anthropologist Pierre Bourdieu, social sciences and the humanities have learned both to attend to the reflexive capacity of the individual researcher and to enlarge the scope of reflexive practice to encompass the societal sources of meaning-attribution and positional power, and to never forget the embeddedness in an individual's worldview of the very products of that world he or she is viewing.[20]

One dimension of reflexivity corresponds with physics' observer principle that states that the act of observing or measuring something alters it. But the social scientist or clinician goes beyond the observer principle to also recognize the similarities between what the observer and the observed *do*. For example, the social scientist studying scientific laboratory life realizes that he or she is, in a manner of speaking, doing to the scientists being observed what the scientists are doing to the mice or chemicals that they study, and that the social scientist shares with the scientists a governing culture, disposition, blind spots, unexamined assumptions, and the like.[21]

The reflexive practitioner takes account of multiple contradictory perspectives, sees himself or herself from outside the self, critiques not only his/her actions also but his/her stance, and acknowledges the co-creating role he or she plays in the study of the object as it unfolds.[22] Transcending the reflective stance, the reflexive stance requires not only the capacity to examine one's own actions and motives in retrospect but also to undertake "real time" narrative awareness of self and other in the midst of complex relational practice. In this way, the practice as it occurs is informed by a simultaneous awareness of its impact on self and other. Reflexivity doubles life: one experiences an event while simultaneously experiencing one's experience. It insists on a social inquiry of the individual's actions in the world as well as a critique of the social and political dimensions of that world that, by necessity, determine the actions of individuals within it.[23]

Finally, it includes the partner in the process. Sociologist Elliot Mishler describes the process of co-creation of the meaning of a research interview:

> [T]he discourse of the interview is jointly constructed by interviewer and respondent. . . . [B]oth questions and responses are formulated in, developed through, and shaped by the discourse between interviewers and respondents. . . . [A]n adequate understanding of interviews depends on recognizing how interviewers reformulate questions and how respondents frame answers in terms of their reciprocal understanding as meanings emerge during the course of an interview.[24]

The reflexive stance has come to be seen as a freeing stance, a position from which all individuals who participate in the practice have the power and resources to create the self in dialogue with, and not just in answer to, the social and built environment into which they were jettisoned by birth.[25] Reflexivity has become a standard-bearer for those within constructivist social sciences and humanities who place ultimate value on the personal freedoms of a self in dynamic dialogue with his or her surround.

Creative teachers or psychotherapists practice reflexively in appreciating the dynamic interplay of their work with their students' or clients' work.[26] Novelists and painters rely on reflexivity to read or behold their own autobiographical contribution to the meaning of their work. Poet Mark Strand reviewed the 2013 exhibit of Edward Hopper's drawings at the Whitney Museum:

> [W]hen we look at the painting of a building or an office or a gas station, we say it's a Hopper. We don't say it's a gas station. By the time the gas station appears on canvas in

its final form it has ceased being just a gas station. It has become Hopperized. It possesses something it never had before Hopper saw it as a possible subject for his painting. And for the artist, the painting exists, in part, as a mode of encountering himself.[27]

A most generative use of the concept of reflexivity for narrative medicine, including its pedagogy and its clinical practice, is the recognition of dynamic feedback within a system—a classroom, a clinic office, a psychoanalytic session—whereby what occurs influences both what will occur next and what has already occurred; what occurs influences what each participant might think the other is doing; what occurs influences the very conception of what the work *is*. Cause is effect, and effect is cause. It is an awareness of the fluid, multidimensional and multitemporal mutual influences on a phenomenon. What happens in the narrative medicine seminar room feeds back to the teacher to alter his or her conception of what is being taught and hence what is to be taught next, so that the ideas and content of the class spiral to an always new location in response to what happens in the classroom. Likewise, in the clinical office the agenda of care is in constant redefinition as aspects of clinical situations gradually become perceivable. Through narrative practices of clinical relationships, the problem list written for the patient is in constant flux in response to what is experienced, learned, and gradually illuminated by the very process of care underway. In narrative medicine clinical practice, the care informs itself.

Reciprocity: Two persons undergo an experience—a surgical operation, a boxing match, a research interview, the act of making love. Both are agents; both are influenced by the other's agency. Neither alone determines what happens (despite the assumptions of the inexperienced surgeon, who learns better after a while). In the alchemy between them a singular event occurs, achieved by their intersection in action. In the presence of reciprocity, both participants achieve a combination of instrumental gains, personal reward, and mutual recognition. Both participants both learn and teach, comfort and receive comfort, and grow in self-knowledge and knowledge of the other by virtue of what has occurred.

The concept of reciprocity has a vast train. In studies in anthropology,[28] law,[29] philosophy,[30] social psychology,[31] international relations,[32] economics,[33] even biological sciences,[34] investigators have studied the structures and practices of mutual giving. Reciprocity can be individual, organizational, singular, or shared. Reciprocators may "give back to" the one who gave to them or they may, in serial reciprocity, repay someone far afield from the initiator of the gift.[35]

The concept of reciprocity helps the narrative medicine clinician to recognize the intimate intersubjective processes that unfold between their clients or patients and themselves.[36] Recent research studies in a variety of healthcare professions—nursing,[37] midwifery,[38] general medical practice,[39] mental health care[40]—single out reciprocity as a variable that predicts satisfaction on the parts of both providers and clients. Although different definitions are used for reciprocity in these studies, the underlying concepts of mutual recognition and a shared sense of reward from the clinical relationship are common to them all:

> Reciprocity is therefore not constituted by the care given but rather manifests itself in the shared meanings between nurse and client that their encounter creates. Where those shared meanings are positive ones, genuine caring has occurred, and the reciprocity created generates therapeutic outcomes for both the nurse and client. . . . The client gains efficacy in coping with the concerns underlying help seeking, and the nurse experiences efficacy in the provision of care that genuinely helps. A mutual effort in which each party brings to the situation what they are authentically able to give creates meanings that change the outcome for the better.[41]

Narrativity confers a particularly reciprocal stamp on anything it touches. Without rehearsing the transhistorical and transdisciplinary development of the concepts of narrative reciprocity, I will comment on aspects of contemporary thought that illuminate the urgency and mutual benefits to healthcare of a commitment to a narrative reciprocity.[42] At the core of the concepts of narrative medicine, as demonstrated in earlier chapters of this book, is our framing principle that the central events of healthcare are the giving and receiving of accounts of self. The literary and narratological frameworks we cite are valuable to narrative medicine precisely by helping us to examine and articulate the processes and consequences of those reciprocal tellings and listenings.[43]

In any form of telling of the self, as has been articulated in Parts I and II of this volume, the teller requires a listener to register that a story has been told. The process through which one comes to *know* the story of one's life is, perhaps, that life's task.[44] Many aspects of the life story are either obscured by emotional trauma or are out of the reach of infancy memory. One certainly seeks confirmation and additional knowledge outside of one's ken, but factual confirmable evidence is not all the teller of a life-story seeks. Says William Maxwell in his novel *So Long, See You Tomorrow*, which is itself a retelling of events of his own life:

> What we, or at any rate what I, refer to confidently as memory . . . is really a form of storytelling that goes on continually in the mind and often changes with the telling. Too many conflicting emotional interests are involved for life ever to be wholly acceptable, and possibly it is the work of the storyteller to rearrange things so that they conform to this end. In any case, in talking about the past we lie with every breath we draw.[45]

The teller may seek an "acceptable" story, as Maxwell notes. Alternatively, the teller may seek recuperation of a past, reliving of some past events, absolution for what he or has committed in that past, or putting something to rest by having it witnessed. In my role as attending physician, I have the occasion to observe and comment on medical students' interviews of patients in the hospital. This time, the patient was a man in his late 50s with end-stage liver cancer, a result of hepatitis C infection. My role was to witness the conversation between my student and his patient. I listened with awe as this gentleman told the young student about his life as a heroin user, about the street fights in which he had gotten the scars on his abdomen and back, about his wrecked marriages and lost children. And then, having told these parts of his life to my student, he felt able to tell the student what it was like to be dying. Once he had given an account of that which had brought him to the point of dying, he could represent forcefully, unsparingly, unforgettably to the student and me the existential pain and vision he now experienced. This he felt was his duty, in reparation for that which he regretted having done, and he appreciated the student's visit as an opportunity to share what he had learned at such great cost to himself and others. The student knew to not interrupt this man's monologue except for softly spoken thanks at the end. Instead, we both offered our silent and alive attention as witnesses to his heroic tale of self. Afterwards we did not know which of the two of them had derived more from the telling, but we knew it was transformative.

Philosopher Adriana Cavarero offers a framework with which to understand these scenes of telling. "The category of personal identity postulates *another* as necessary . . . Identity is an in-born exposure."[46] Exposure, requiring the one to whom one exposes, is the mode of coming to "hear told" the story of identity. Hannah Arendt writes in *The Life of the Mind* that "the 'sensation' of reality, of sheer thereness relates to the *context* in which single objects appear as well as the context in which we ourselves as appearances exist among other appearing creatures. The context qua context never appears entirely; it is elusive, almost like Being."[47] Locating the human being within the context of objects and other appearing creatures intensifies Arendt's message: *we exist in a reality so as to appear, so as to be exposed, perhaps so as to be recognized.* Perhaps our very reality is a product of the exposure afforded by the presence of others in our contexts, those to whom we choose to appear.

This is what happens in routine narrative practice. The doings of healthcare—diagnosing the hepatitis C, documenting the hepatocellular carcinoma that can occur as a result of the viral illness, offering all treatments possible to the patient—are accompanied by this duty to witness and the willingness to let another be heard. This is not an unusual aspect of routine healthcare. The opportunity declares itself with regularity. As reported by the community midwives and nurses and mental health professionals I have cited above, the reciprocity that arises when one registers the appearance of another and when one assents to the role of witness can shift a practice of healthcare from instrumental custodianship to intersubjective contact.

Beyond individual clinical practice, the consideration of reciprocity opens up critical social inquiry regarding balances of power and balances of resources. The dominating social and organizational structures of healthcare, including the steep status hierarchies between professionals and patients, are called into question when healthcare is conceptualized as, potentially, a reciprocal endeavor. Patients are neither the objects nor the "human subjects" of the healthcare procedures. Rather, those who seek care are in reality the drivers—and payers—for the entire undertaking of healthcare.

Ultimately the value of the concept of reciprocity is to remind the listener to consider the mutual rewards of listening. When others challenge us that no doctor or nurse or social worker has the time, today, to listen in the way that we describe, we often ask if we have the time *not* to. Without the attention, the affiliation between teller and listener—and therefore the clinical partnership and shared decision making—does not develop. And without giving the attention, the listener does not receive his or her own reward from the encounter—the confirming recognition of oneself *as* a witness, *as* a person with the courage to be Cavarero's and Arendt's occasion of exposure and identity. We learn, through such encounters, that our being-in-the-world—today, now, here, with this person—matters at the level of another's identity. Our skill and devotion have made possible an articulation and an exposure of the teller's self that would not have happened without us. The difficulties in fulfilling the duties incurred in the listening do not exceed the pleasures of having accomplished it.

Coda

Psychotherapist and literary scholar Kathlyn Conway writes about the split patients experience between their ongoing self and their ill self, and suggests that writing about the illness may help the patient to lessen the split:

> Those who write about their illness and disability are often caught between two characterizations of the self. On the one hand they want to represent a devastated, broken or interrupted self, the more complicated self discussed by contemporary theorists of autobiography. On the other, even while proclaiming their old self is gone, they set out to reclaim, in the act of writing, parts of that old self. In this sense they use writing

much as traditional writers of autobiography have—to bestow coherence. They talk about their old self, review what has happened to them, and place themselves once again in their own familial or literary ancestry.[48]

If the processes of healthcare are creative and reflexive, then the insights that patients gain from writing about their illness and disability may be also available to clinicians as they write about the events of practice. If indeed the processes of healthcare are reciprocal, these insights may be routinely available to both patients and clinicians by each reading what the other writes about their shared experiences, together developing insight, shared awareness, and equally powered affiliation.

Ms. N. read this chapter in its entirety. Over two years had passed since the encounter and the events described here. We sat together in my office. She was overcome by the extent to which Eric and I had contemplated her situation, and she was grateful for it. She had read the chapter, closely, twice, remembering the events, seeing things as she read that she had not seen before. She said, and I paraphrase: "I had not known myself before as well as I did after reading this chapter."

Perhaps the organs will not always be silent. Perhaps the capacity for creativity and play will be subdued in the face of serious illness. Canguilhem's focus on the singularity of each person reminds us nonetheless of a unity never absent from the self:

> The singular individual is perceivable because of the difference from everyone else; the singular individual is alone because separate from all others. It is the concept of a being with no concept, being foreclosed from any attributions except that of being himself . . . unclassifiable, just about unique in the entire humankind.[49]

We trust that the balance and integrity of being and of care are within our grasp, if we seek them, if we can envision them, not altogether out of reach but, there, as we strive to improve this care we give and receive. In the end, says Canguilhem:

> It is not the doctor but the health that cures the sick.[50]

Notes

1. The patient has been an active partner in the work I report here and has given enthusiastic permission to me to describe in print our reciprocal work. She has read this chapter in its entirety and gives permission for its publication in this volume.
2. Bollas, *Shadow of the Object*.
3. Banville, *Infinities*, 272.

4. Marcus, *Psychosis*, 42.
5. See Viederman, "A Model for Interpretative Supportive Dynamic Psychotherapy" and "The Induction of Noninterpreted Benevolent Transference."
6. Winnicott, *Maturational Processes*.
7. Viederman, "Therapeutic Consultation," 153.
8. Charon, "The Patient, the Body, the Self."
9. Charon, "Narrative Medicine as Witness."
10. Canguilhem, *Normal and Pathological*, 91. See also Canguilhem, *Writings on Medicine*; Fantuzzi, "Sound of Health."
11. Engel, "Need for a New Medical Model."
12. See the wide-ranging "How Creativity Works in the Brain," a report produced by the National Endowment for the Arts on a colloquium among neuroscientists and artists about the nature and source, within the brain, of creativity and creative acts.
13. The patient gave me enthusiastic permission to write about or to discuss our partnership.
14. Winnicott, *Playing and Reality*, 73, 72.
15. Goodman, *Languages of Art*, 9.
16. Loewald, "Therapeutic Action," 26.
17. More and more electronic health records allow patients access to their medical records, and some invite patients to add their perspectives to the record. There are means of inviting patients to contribute to their records, as long as their authorship of the contributed text is made clear in the record. See Delbanco, "Inviting Patients."
18. See Stoller, *Sensuous Scholarship*.
19. For background see Habermas, *Knowledge and Human Interests*; Freire, *Pedagogy of the Oppressed*; and Schön, *Reflective Practitioner*.
20. Bourdieu, *Outline of a Theory*; Bourdieu and Wacquant, *Invitation to Reflexive Sociology*.
21. Bloor, *Knowledge and Social Imagery*; Latour, *Laboratory Life*.
22. Lieberman et al., "Reflexion and Reflection."
23. See Ng et al., "Reclaiming a Theoretical Orientation" for an incisive discussion of the growing interest in reflection within health professions education, calling for an emphasis on critical social inquiry and proposing that the reflection movement does not going far enough in challenging dominant practices and structures within mainstream healthcare that determine the plights of both patients and professionals in contemporary healthcare.
24. Mishler, *Research Interviewing*, 52.
25. Riach, "Participant-centered Reflexivity."
26. Allen, "Reflexivity in Teaching."
27. Strand, "Mark Strand on Edward Hopper," 40.
28. MacCormack, "Reciprocity."
29. Hale and Hale, "Reciprocity under the Antitrust Laws."
30. Von Tevenar, "Gratitude."
31. Molm, "Structure of Reciprocity."
32. Keohane, "Reciprocity in International Relations."
33. Fon and Parisi, "Reciprocity-Induced Cooperation."
34. Nowak and Roch, "Upstream Reciprocity."
35. Moody, "Serial Reciprocity."
36. See Launer, *Narrative-Based Primary Care*, chapters 14 and 16, for a discussion of the synchronized elements of a narrative primary care, focusing on the symmetry of giving and receiving in routine clinical interactions.
37. Marck, "Therapeutic Reciprocity."
38. Billie Hunter, "Importance of Reciprocity."
39. Street, Gordon, and Haidet, "Physicians' Communication."
40. Sandhu et al., "Reciprocity in Therapeutic Relationships."
41. Marck, "Therapeutic Reciprocity," 51, 52.

42. Among the great thinkers whose work probes intersubjective reciprocity through narrative acts, see Arendt, *The Human Condition* and *Life of the Mind*; Nancy, *The Inoperative Community*; Ricoeur, *Oneself as Another*; Taylor, *Sources of the Self*; Benjamin, "The Storyteller"; Butler, *Giving an Account*.
43. Charon, "Narrative Reciprocity."
44. Butler, *Giving an Account*; Schafer, *Retelling a Life*.
45. Maxwell, *So Long*, 27.
46. Cavarero, *Relating Narratives*.
47. Arendt, *Life of the Mind*, 51.
48. Conway, *Beyond Words*, 59.
49. Canguilhem, "Fragments," 93. Translation by RC.
50. Canguilhem, "Fragments," 95. Translation by RC.

CHAPTER 13

Clinical Contributions of Narrative Medicine

Rita Charon

Health is life lived in the silence of the organs.
—Réne Leriche, 1936[1]

The clinical consequences of narrative medicine are the measure of the promise of our work. Although the conceptual and pedagogic dimensions of our work continue to grow, the North Star guiding narrative medicine has been, from the start, to improve health care. We have the benefit of on-going discerning dialogue about the contributions of narrative medicine to the clinical enterprise, as both critique[2] and confirmation of the dividends of narrative rigor in routine clinical practice.[3] Our experience and the experience of others have demonstrated the potential of narrative practices to transform healthcare. Emergency medicine physician and fiction-writer Frank Huyler proposes the following reasons for providing narrative training in healthcare:

> Studying the humanities ... [helps us] ... become more aware, more insightful, more reflective, and—ultimately—more influential in shaping the trajectory of healthcare. It's about encouraging the facility, willingness and ability to enter into the larger public debate in these cacophonous times, when collective silence will not serve.... And, finally, it is about providing an outlet for both emotional engagement and self-reflection in a culture that typically denies both, looks outward rather than inward, and too often ignores not only the personal costs but the personal rewards of medical work.[4]

This chapter gives examples of several forms of clinical narrative medicine practice that have developed since the 2000 emergence of narrative medicine, catalogued into (1) interview/relationship techniques with individual patients, (2) clinician and healthcare team development, and (3) deployment of novel narrative practices in routine clinical care. This is not to be taken as an exhaustive list of procedures but rather as an invitation to conceive of, together, the affiliative road ahead.

Individual Interview/Relationship Techniques

An Open Beginning: We have learned through practice in many clinical disciplines and specialties to open a conversation with a patient with a broad, non-directive invitation to speak. The wider the first question posed to a patient the better the conversation ensues, the more one can learn about the patient, and the greater are the number of things the patient and clinician can do together. Many interview technique manuals endorse the "open-ended question" as a cardinal feature of a patient-centered interview; we have come to consider that openness as a feature not of the end of a question but rather as the beginning of the very posing of it.

In my own internal medicine practice, I often begin an encounter with a new patient with this invitation: "I will be your doctor, and so I need to know a great deal about your body, your health, and your life. Please tell me what you think I should know about your situation." In beginning a conversation with patients I know well, I have learned to signal a similar openness to begin wherever the patient chooses to begin. Such linguistic practices invite the patient to frame the problems that require our attention and to include in our gaze whatever events or situations might be related to the present concern. The triad of body, health, and life seems wide enough not to exclude many things that might be on that patient's mind.

I have trained myself to listen to the answer to this question without writing, typing, scanning the computer monitor—hands in lap, listening. The rolling of the office chair away from the computer monitor toward the patient as he or she sits in the other office chair is itself a meaningful physical action. Attentive listening is the core of the practice, far more important than exactly what words are used. It is here in the reception of the patient's response that the narrative aspects of the healthcare encounter occur and that all the skills of narrative medicine are put into practice. Philosopher and activist Simone Weil writes, "The capacity to give one's attention to a sufferer is a very rare and difficult thing; it is almost a miracle; it *is* a miracle."[5] Never fully achieved, this state of attention is, nonetheless, what the nurse or social worker or chaplain or physician seeks to attain. Weil continues:

A quarter of an hour of attention is better than a great many good works. Attention consists of suspending our thought, leaving it detached, empty, and ready to be penetrated
by the object; it means holding in our minds, within reach of this thought, but on a
lower level and not in contact with it, the diverse knowledge we have acquired which
we are forced to make use of . . . as a man on a mountain who, as he looks forward, sees
also below him, without actually looking at them, a great many forests and plains. . . .
Love for our neighbor, being made of creative attention, is analogous to genius."[6]

An open beginning, met with however pure an attention one can achieve,
lets the listener hear the patient uninterruptedly speak. This close listener,
this reflexive listener, notices how he or she feels while listening, senses the
shifts in mood like shifts in the weather, notices the questions generated in
himself or herself by the listening, generates hypotheses while listening about
what it all might mean. Here is where the rigorous training in close reading
enters the clinical practice. The attentive listener who has learned how to
get the news from stories, who has learned to pay attention, while reading,
to both content and form, to be aware of genre, diction, metaphor, time and
space, tone, and mood, can learn to follow complicated stories as they are
being told. This "close listener" can hold in the mind all details, paradoxes,
ruptures, feeling along with the teller as the account is being given. He or she
rides the patient's account in real time, curious—why this now, where might
this be going?

Exhausting and replenishing, achieving this state of attention is perhaps the
igniting act of humane healthcare. Attentive reception of the patient's account
of self then permits or even requires action taken on behalf of the patient,
always within sight of the personal context that frames the clinical concern.
As a result of the careful and creative attention, the listener can begin to understand what matters to the patient and even, over time, to learn something
about how the patient's mind works. When this encounter occurs within a setting of healthcare, it takes its direction toward the physical or mental concern
that occasioned the visit. Once the clinician learns how the patient frames the
problem that has brought him or her to seek healthcare, that clinician then fills
in the narrative history with the more standard clinical interviewing questions
about past health, family history, specific symptoms, and current conditions.
As I reflect on my own experience with individual patients, I realize how pivotal and meaningful were those very first things I learned about a person as he
or she exposed the "sounds of the organs" to a stranger.

Open-ended and nondirectional clinical conversations are by no means
unique to narrative medicine and are recommended by many of the clinical interviewing textbooks.[7] What becomes possible with narrative medicine training is to know what to do with the open-ended answers. When the listening

is accompanied by subtle awareness of narrative forms, temporal structures, invocations of space, and figural language in what the teller says, the listener squanders nothing that is said or that is even left unsaid.

Such listening routines have been adopted by persons trained in narrative medicine practicing in a variety of specialties. Malgorzata Nowaczyk, a medical geneticist who studied with us in narrative medicine workshops, recognized the subtlety and power of the stories she was hearing from her patients, her patients' terror, and the sense of rage at the cosmic unfairness that sent their families an unearned rare genetic disorder. She published an essay in the medical genetics literature introducing a form of attentive listening that acknowledges this terror in patients while exposing the listening clinician to its dread: "Many published first-person illness narratives contain elements of chaos; if we listen closely to our patients in clinic we may find chaos there as well."[8] Sarah Chambers and Julie Glickstein, pediatric cardiologists at Columbia who worked closely with the narrative medicine team in our faculty development seminar for physicians, recognized the narrative complexities involved in first performing echocardiograms for fetuses thought to have serious cardiac abnormalities, then translating to the parents what the fetus wordlessly told them in the gray images, and then listening to the responses of the families while the doctors helped them to make decisions.[9]

These two studies are examples of recent publications using narrative medicine principles and methods in clinical encounters with individual patients. Narrative interviewing techniques have been adopted by others in multiple settings and specific clinical situations, including in caring for patients with Ehlers-Danlos hypermobility syndromes,[10] assessing decision-making capacity for inpatients,[11] caring for women who get pregnant after receiving liver transplants,[12] and developing therapeutic relationships with chronically ill hospitalized patients.[13] In all these settings, the development and deployment of attention and the capacity to capture and act on the evidence of patients' narrative accounts promise more informed care for patients and, for clinicians, a heightened sense of having been of service.

Clinician and Healthcare Team Development

Clinicians Write As reflective and creative writing methods are adopted in health professions schools, clinician/educators themselves are exposed to the fruits of narrative work. As a dividend of Columbia's inclusion of creative writing for students in its curriculum, the faculty members engaged in this narrative pedagogy have learned to use the same methods in their educational and clinical practices.[14] Their adoption of narrative methods in their own practice and teaching outside of the medical student course has functioned as powerful role-modeling for their students, who witness their teachers using what they preach as serious components of their professional lives.[15]

Once the Program in Narrative Medicine was launched in 2000, groups of clinicians at Columbia requested some training in writing for themselves. As one example, the general pediatricians who teach courses including creative writing exercises formed a "Narrative Pediatrics" group, meeting once a month with a narrative medicine facilitator, sometimes with the residents and students, to join in close reading and creative writing. Over the course of the seminar's few years perhaps 100 pediatricians have attended at least a few sessions, and a core group has attended each session religiously. Participants have reported that the seminar gives them perspective on their practice, increases their curiosity about patients, increases their readiness to "take the next chart out of the box," and lets them see more of the world around them.[16] Such narrative medicine seminars are underway with regularly scheduled meetings for fellows in palliative care, pediatric cardiology, and child psychiatry; for residents in obstetrics and gynecology, primary care medicine, family medicine, and radiology; for social workers; for chaplains; and for faculty from a variety of departments combined.

Similar narrative training is underway in a variety of clinical sites for physicians of many specialties, nurses, physical therapists, social workers, chaplains, and even prisoners and wardens at a maximum security prison, all facilitated by narrative medicine faculty and Master's Program graduates in New York. The pilot study for a novel narrative medicine training program at a nursing home facility in New York has completed a feasibility study of narrative training among staff nurses and recreation therapists who work with long-term residents. Leaders of these groundbreaking efforts are now launched on the process of outcomes research with a range of variables chosen for testing and study.

In all these settings, clinicians learn the skills of close reading as participants together read complex texts of poetry, prose, visual art images and objects, or performance arts. Through their own deliberations on the workings of the text, each participant comes to locate his or her own sense of what the text means. They are then invited to write to an expansive prompt in the shadow of the text, getting the chance to represent their own emerging perceptions aroused by it. Finally, when they each read aloud what they've written, their listeners/readers can join them in seeing what has been created.[17]

Parallel efforts in narrative faculty development are ongoing in a growing number of institutions in the United States and abroad in a range of departments and faculty teaching academies.[18] Triangulating evidence for the utility in practice of the teaching of these skills is available from the development of narrative training for practices other than healthcare. Judith Moran, a family lawyer and graduate of the Master of Science in Narrative Medicine graduate program, has replicated our practice at the University of Baltimore School of Law, on whose faculty she is appointed; the conceptual framework, pedagogy, and goals of improving practice and professional care for clients are identical in the two professions.[19]

Interprofessional Education and Practice: Since the mid-1980s, health professionals and national and international bodies advising them have called for improvements in the effectiveness of the healthcare team.[20] Although there are yet to be strong bodies of evidence supporting the hypothesis that strengthening healthcare teams improves the quality of the care, health education certifying boards and public and private providers of health insurance are requiring that students and clinicians be trained for interprofessional education and practice.[21] Beginning in 2014 with a gradual roll-out, the health professions schools of dental, medical, and nursing schools are being required to provide interprofessional education for their students as a condition of certification by their licensing boards.

There are many reasons that healthcare teams are less than effective. As specialization in healthcare has accelerated and as healthcare roles have proliferated, an industrial assembly-line model hove into view, each member of a team completing his or her small part of the action with little appreciation of the whole. More sinisterly, the implacable hierarchy of healthcare, in which white male physicians continue to occupy the positions of power, replicates and even intensifies the biases and patterns of domination of its wider culture. An academic medical center stages drama after drama in which persons from many professions fight among themselves for small gains—classroom space, internal resources of money or time, influence on institutional policy, seats at tables of authority—while decisions are typically made in board rooms in which physicians predominate. Inevitably, the hierarchical divides widen and stiffen even among the ranks far from the power pinnacles. Within community hospitals or clinics, these patterns can be broken; it is from such places that models of effective healthcare teamwork are likely to arise.

In the face of such overdetermined dysfunction, many approaches to improve the healthcare team have arisen.[22] One approach to improving the function of healthcare teams is a practical, task-based framework.[23] Typically, members of a team charged with accomplishing a particular healthcare task—in an operating room, emergency room, labor and delivery room, or general medical hospital ward—are gathered to practice the tasks they must together do. These training sessions use role-play scenarios, clinical vignettes, or simulations using dummies or actors portraying patients to demonstrate the task in question. Behavioral learning objectives are drawn up prior to the exercise.

In keeping with the mainstream educational methods used in health education, these objectives must be stated as observable behaviors. Checklists of the
team-supportive behaviors on the agenda are used to assess the success of the
individuals in the team and the team itself, sometimes as self-report by learners and sometimes completed by trained observers who attend the session with
the learners.[24]

More nuanced approaches to collaborative team development arise from
social scientists, particularly in the fields of gerontology and end-of-life care—
specialties in which effective teams of members of multiple disciplines are
critical for effective care of patients. The field of Narrative Gerontology arose
at the millennial turn to connect narrative theorists with clinicians and social
scientists committed to improving care for the elderly.[25] Their scholarship and
research have expanded to contribute to the conceptual and pedagogical work
of healthcare teams in general.[26]

The conceptual frameworks that guide their development and evaluation of interprofessional education include social science and psychology-
derived relational theories, social identity theories, self-presentation theories, sociology of professions, and the discourse and power analysis of
Michel Foucault.[27] Such factors as early professionalism into role, hierarchical status differences between professions, structural silos that divide professions from one another, and organizational structures that may permit or
prohibit change are relevant to the fate of efforts to instill teamwork among
healthcare professionals.

Narrative medicine brings contrasting and complementing conceptual
frameworks to bear on these models to improve healthcare team effectiveness. Narrative training and practice guide members of interprofessional
teams to find their common ground. This ground can be found *under* the distinctions that separate them, for they have all chosen their careers, at least
in part, because of a commitment to patients and in answer to a calling to
work with the sick.[28] Rather than focusing on the contrasts among professional identities of members of a team, narrative medicine methods illuminate the common values and desires of persons prior to their becoming
members of a profession or in excess of their membership in a health profession. The expansiveness, creativity, and reflexivity of narrative medicine
learning makes room for interprofessional groups of students or clinicians
to see one another in fresh light, not in terms of turf or traditional roles but
as colleagues facing always-new problems and opportunities in joining with
patients in their care.

In practice, narrative medicine brings to interprofessional education and
practice its signature methods of close reading, creative writing, and attention

to telling and listening as co-creators of narratives. Creativity, reflexivity, and reciprocity are as present in interprofessional pedagogy as they are in the clinical practice. In addition to the narrative theoretical frameworks from the social and behavioral sciences, we include the literary and aesthetic ways of knowing and doing. Through the intersubjective contact that can occur in narrative medicine teaching, participants from various professions meet as *themselves*—themselves as tellers and listeners, readers and writers—in the process exposing their own perspectives, imaginations, memories, and values. All that happens in the descriptions of seminar practice in earlier chapters of this volume can occur among these interprofessional learners. Participants are present not as healthcare team members with a particular task to do; they are present in their full, daring subjectivity.

In a 4-year project funded by the Josiah Macy, Jr. Foundation, the Program in Narrative Medicine at Columbia brought together first faculty and then students in Columbia's dental, medical, nursing, and public health schools to join in intensive narrative work. As is typical of our work anywhere, we introduced the group members to one another through creative acts. We read great texts, watched movies, wrote creatively, interviewed one another about complex questions. The texts and movies and interviews usually had little to do with healthcare, and we members of the group were not present as representatives of our professions. Instead, we had a chance to be present ontologically, epistemologically, and morally. In a matter of months, the groups of faculty or students came to know one another deeply and to be committed to improving the teamwork in our institution.

Our evaluation of the courses has included qualitative methods of focus groups, ethnographic interviews, and attention to emergent phenomena. The results of our evaluations point to deepening knowledge of one another and of each profession's concerns and perspectives in healthcare. The students learned what they do *not* know but can rely on their team members to know for them. Developing sustained contact with colleagues from the other schools was itself an accomplishment that led to loosening of the strictly professional lenses through which we all see our work. In effect, the narrative medicine work released individuals from their profession's restricted epistemologies and practice frameworks. Not just for the sake of improving the safety and quality of patient care, our interprofessional work sprung us from the inevitable traps of professional identity.

Whether in the classroom prior to joining healthcare teams in the hospital and clinic or on the site of the work itself, narrative medicine methods bring unique value to healthcare team development. Amid the dramatic changes in the structures and values of American healthcare that are driven by economic and commodification priorities, concerns and worries mount. Clinic staff members rebel against the 12- or 15-minute office visit, wondering how anyone can deliver effective healthcare to persons with hosts of physical and social/economic threats to good health in so short a time. Hospital routines are governed by needs to document all activities (in large part by the economic need to bill for them), usually on remote computer terminals, taking the nurses and doctors and residents and therapists away from actual sustained contact with patients. Hospitals make major decisions about spending and saving without transparency, so that healthcare workers are surprised and saddened to see their units closed to make room for new money-making enterprises. The competition among major health systems for business, the greed of some of those who work among us, the health gaps between poor and well-off patients that are intensified by our stratified healthcare dishearten us, make us worry that we cannot deliver acceptably good care, drain our sense of community and self-regard.

In the face of these challenges, committed healthcare professionals are organizing—through interprofessional groups, professional societies, groups engaged in humanizing healthcare, political collaboratives for primary care, and issue-based associations—to build processes of egalitarianism and diversity into the power structures and organizational patterns of clinical work. As the drive to improve healthcare teams continues, we can envision growing roles for those equipped with narrative skills in clinical practice and clinical teaching. Despite the disillusionment engendered by the contemporary bureaucratic climate of major health centers, our narrative capacities can let us perceive the value of our work, can inspire us with means to counter the depersonalization of our institutions, and can guide us toward means to improve, always, the care of the sick.

In these settings, all the more necessary are the clearings that narrative medicine can open. Not only do these clearings accomplish intensive personal and small-group work. They are also the crucibles for social activism as peers and colleagues discover in one another—and then perhaps more forcefully within the self—rage, protest, and idealism silenced. This is the beginning of a critical inquiry; this is the birth of consequential social action toward change.

A unique and inspiring experiment in narrative healthcare team development is taking place in Göteberg, Sweden, and we include it here as an exemplar of the consequences of full narrative consciousness on healthcare team development in mainstream healthcare institutions. Inspired by the concepts of narrative medicine and patient-centered care, the nurses, nurses' assistants, and physicians in a large community hospital in Sweden instituted patient-centered and team-based work rounds. No longer does a patient being admitted to hospital meet sequentially with the different members of the professional team. Instead, the patient is invited into the team's comfortable office to sit and speak with all members of the team at once. As the guest of honor, the patient is heard carefully by all members of the team. The patient, in turn, is assured that all professionals caring for him or her will hear the same story and agree among themselves on a plan of action.

Nurses, physicians, and nursing assistants describe the improvement in the care they can provide since they began team-based rounds.[29] Their work proceeds more quickly and smoothly, they feel more satisfied with the quality of their work, and they experience a closer relationship among themselves and with the patients. They experience new joy among themselves and with their patients thanks to this experiment.

Novel Narrative Practices

Clinical Charts: The emphasis narrative medicine places on representation extends to the institutional and legal records kept of healthcare work. The rise of the electronic health record has transformed the reporting routines in the United States and elsewhere. While promising gains in patient safety and integration of clinical information, use of the computerized record often leads to faceless care, patients greeted not by the faces but the backs of their now-typing clinicians.[30] Because the electronic health records were tailored from platforms used in patient accounts and billing, they do not allow the writer to "think like a clinician." Instead, the electronic records are geared primarily toward diagnostic and procedural coding, in part to enable optimal billing.[31] Formats of most electronic health records require writers to register data by choosing items from drop-down menus or placing check-marks in boxes. As a result, clinicians lose the opportunity to think systematically through a clinical situation as they do by writing the note sequentially and organically. .However, despite many of the mechanized aspects of the current electronic medical record, clinicians maintain the opportunity, in most electronic platforms, to write freely within the chart, although time to do so is usually extremely limited.

The quest to restore the narrative to the medical record has become a rallying cry for many clinicians committed to their own narrative practices, while the time constraints of an increasingly economically driven healthcare system raise a barrier against the full use of writing as discovery of one's own clinical thoughts and one's awareness of the patient's situation. To restore the narrative will require not only a rigorous justification of the importance of writing in clinical decision making and in developing therapeutic alliances. It will also require solid evidence that the time devoted to narrative practices of writing, on the part of both clinicians and patients, is repaid in improvement of the clinical outcomes of our practices. Such research is now beginning to get underway in ambulatory care settings, end-of-life settings, and clinical training settings. This research imperative is one of the most urgent commitments of narrative medicine today.

One way to preserve the value of the health record is to invite the patient into it. An ambitious project called "Open Notes," arising from the Beth Israel Deaconess Hospital in Boston, has studied the consequences of allowing patients to read their physicians' notes.[32] Although there was reticence on the part of physicians at the outset, there were beneficial outcomes when patients read what their doctors wrote about them, including an increased sense of control for patients, increased knowledge about their health situation, and increased fidelity to taking prescribed medicines. Around a third of the patients had privacy concerns, and a very small percentage felt worry or confusion upon reading what their doctors wrote. At the end of this ambitious outcomes research, all patients and physicians opted to continue using Open Notes. This exploratory study heralds important shifts in the written communication in healthcare, suggesting the power of the written narratives of even routine primary care.

Increasingly, patients are given access to portions of their electronic health records by their healthcare institutions. Through patient-accessible portals, patients can retrieve test results, diagnostic imaging interpretations, and reports generated at visits with clinicians anywhere in the institution. Still in its testing phase, patients' access to clinical electronic charts raises new and sometimes troubling questions about the lack of agreement among clinicians on the meaning of diagnostic testing results, and diagnostic suspicions held by the clinician but unspoken to the patient. Patients' access to their own records necessitates a new level of attention for both accuracy and discretion among those who write in the chart—which, in retrospect, will likely be seen as an improvement in the documentation and in the care itself.

More and more clinicians routinely give the patient a copy of what they have written after the encounter. The simple practice of giving the patient a copy of what one has written is consequential. With the paper copy of what the nurse or therapist or physician has written in hand, the patient can more easily recall events of the clinical encounter, can show the note to others for help in understanding the proceeding, and can identify questions that escaped asking. Patients keep track of these notes and consider them valuable aspects of their health work. I have been in the habit of providing my patients with a plastic binder with the name of our hospital and the legend, "Patient-Held

Medical Record" on its face as a reminder that the patient "holds" the history of care himself or herself. Knowing that the patient will read what the writer writes also acts as a potent reminder to write in words and not numbers and acronyms, and to write in a style that the patient will be able to read and comprehend. More powerfully, the practice reminds the clinician that the office or hospital visit contains not only what the clinician values but also what the patient might value. The summary of the visit needs to include all that was discussed, not only the things the clinician considers salient to the care. Hence, this simple practice of giving the patient a copy of the note helps to emphasize that *all* that transpires in a health encounter matters—not only the test results and medication dosages but also the conversation about the death in the family, the worry about a child, or the triumph of landing the job or graduating from college—and contributes to the creation of the book of care.

The practice of asking the patient to contribute to the medical record, as described in Chapter 12 in this volume, is one component of the next stage in this work. The boundaries between clinician and patient are, perhaps, becoming more permeable as we develop increasing awareness of the damaging divides between us. A vision of the future of narrative medicine includes movement toward equalizing the power of voices within the care and the representation of that care. A talisman as well as a reality in healthcare, the clinical chart occupies a pivotal space in the always evolving processes of care. Despite its being embroiled in—some would say highjacked by—the electronicization of healthcare, we can seize the power of writing and use it for the sake of equality, justice, and truth within the work we do.

Bearing Witness in Healthcare: Narrative medicine has developed a practice of witnessing in clinical settings. Before describing this clinical method, a summary review of bearing witness in contexts of health and social justice seems called for.

Enormous events and events of enormity require witness. Acts that surpass reason, whether they be acts of nature or faith or good or evil, demand formal acknowledgment even while they may exceed the observer's capacity to acknowledge them. That which requires witness is, by definition, that which cannot be subsumed within an explanation. Beyond fact, beyond history, that which requires witness remands the participant and the observer into the hermeneutics of presence. Lyric poetry, music, dance, and works of visual art are some of the means that have been used to mark the witnessing or memorializing of a grave event that cannot be represented in ordinary language.

The chorus of classical Greek drama fulfills the role of the witness to events that the protagonists in the drama cannot fully perceive for themselves. Not only, "This *happened*," say the members of the Chorus in Euripides's *The Trojan Women* but "This matters":

> The sacrifice is gone and the sound of joy,
>> The dancing under the stars and the night-long prayer:
> The Golden Images and the Moons of Troy,
>> The Twelve Moons and the mighty names they bear:
> My heart, my heart crieth, O Lord Zeus on high,
> Were they all to thee as nothing, thou thronèd in the sky,
> Thronèd in the fire-cloud, where a City, near to die,
>> Passeth in the wind and the flare?[33]

Here the Chorus functions as the collective voice of Troy from outside the action. The Chorus is present in the play as witness to the sacrifice of Troy, lamenting—in the name of the whole city—to the gods who allowed the destruction and despairing at the passing of their beloved city into "the wind and the flare."

We can distinguish between the eyewitness of an event and the one who bears witness to it.[34] This double meaning of the act of witnessing alerts us to its conceptual complexity, underlining the tension between fact and meaning. The eyewitness might testify at a court proceeding as a provider of historical fact—he or she might deliver a presumably verifiable account of a crime in a trial or identify a perpetrator in a police line-up. The one who bears witness—as a participant, observer, or marker of an event—is charged with the more significant duty to stand, personally, as one who recognizes the meaning of the event. The Quaker practice of collective silent standing for peace in public places, displaying signs declaring the subject of concern, accomplishes the complex task of both attesting to the standers' own commitment to peace and bringing to the attention of passers-by *their* need to concern themselves with the war in the Middle East, the threat of nuclear war, or the dying of the planet. The mothers and grandmothers of children disappeared in South America's dictatorships reversed decades of indifference and denial by their risky and permanent state of personal physical witnessing—not to a set of facts they could assert but to the state of "factlessness" surrounding the loss of their children.

Warning against the too-facile acceptance of either the reliability of witnessing or the impossibility of it, historian Hayden White notes that "we must not take the naturalness of seeing for granted."[35] White studies the records of the Holocaust written by Primo Levi, both a survivor of Auschwitz and the documenter of its atrocities. A chemist who asserted that he used his scientific skills of observation and analysis to document life in the camps, Levi in fact transmutes his report of the Final Solution in poetic texts of paradox:

"It is us again, grey and identical, small as ants, yet so huge as to reach up to the stars, bound one against the other, countless, covering the plain as far as the horizon; sometimes melting into a single substance, a sorrowful turmoil in which we all feel ourselves trapped and suffocated; sometimes marching in a circle, without beginning or end."[36]

White points out that "[t]he most vivid scenes of the horrors of life in the camps produced by Levi consist less of the delineation of 'facts' as conventionally conceived than of the sequences of figures he creates by which to endow the facts with passion, his own feelings about and the value he therefore attaches to them," suggesting that even the eyewitness requires representational forms that can handle both fact and meaning.[37]

Literary scholar Geoffrey Hartman and psychoanalyst Dori Laub founded the Fortunoff Video Archive for Holocaust Testimony at Yale University, giving survivors of the camps the opportunity to add their testimonies to the archive of the atrocities. The videotaped interviews are spare close-ups of survivors recounting their memories, gently and unobtrusively guided by the interviewer's perceptive comments. These interviews are not held as historically verifiable fact but as the means by which those who lived through the Holocaust are afforded a setting in which to express and therefore to know what they underwent.[38] The authentic report—not the same as the verifiable factual report—is described by Hartman as both a witnessing to what happened and a witnessing of the person to whom it happened: "If authenticity is to prevail, the survivor as witness to the traumatic event will be at once a first person and a second person: one who is able, despite everything, to say 'you' to the self that has remained, one who seeks an 'I-Thou' relationship with a disappeared or damaged self."[39]

Bearing witness is a powerful dimension of religious life, offering the self as one-who-testifies, sometimes at one's own risk, to the truths and values of a faith. Religious witnessing may be accomplished wordlessly with garb, ritual, or ordinary daily habits that mark the person as a person of faith. Widespread political traumas and injustices can be faced with collective bearing of witness to atrocities not in trials of blame but in search of futures. Truth and Reconciliation rituals, most powerfully achieved in South Africa as apartheid was challenged, provide public opportunities for the wrongs to be exposed toward the strengthening of the post-trauma society.[40]

Acts of witness occur not only in the face of large historical events of terror and war but also in the intimacy of personal relationships. The acts of recognition that transpire between mother and infant are, some assert, foundational for the lifelong capacity for address and response in the intersubjective relations with others that lead directly to personhood.[41] Therapeutic relationships provide powerful scenes of witness, where the witnessing indeed constitutes the therapy. Psychoanalyst Warren Poland describes witnessing in analytic treatment as a reciprocal state with transferential engagement:

> By witnessing, I refer to an analyst's activity, that of "getting" what the patient is saying without doing anything more active about it. . . . It is the analyst's functioning as a patient's other who maintains an actively observing presence, who recognizes and grasps the emotional activity in the mind of the patient at work. . . . Witnessing as an analytic function refers to the analyst as beholder, grasping and respecting both the patient's meanings and the meaningfulness of those meanings from a position of separated otherness.[42]

In the innovative form of family therapy they have named narrative therapy, Michael White and David Epson have introduced "outsider witnesses" to attend therapy sessions with a client and his or her family. The outsider witnesses are chosen on the grounds of some similarity with the client so that the client's story will in some way resonate with their own experience. The witnesses can then, in conversation with the therapist while the client is present, demonstrate how listening to the story has aided or inspired them in their own lives.[43] Not unlike the members of a Greek chorus who contextualize the events being enacted, the outside witnesses' presence nests the situation of this family within wider spheres of social or interior experience, reducing the isolation of the suffering family while offering company and affirmation as they struggle toward health.

Narrative medicine has developed a tradition of witnessing within practices of individual patient care. A combination of the eyewitness and the bearing of witness, narrative medicine witnesses attend clinical encounters in order to give to their participants a finely perceived written representation of the events of their meeting.[44] With permission from both patient and clinician, the witness attends a visit, takes field notes as would an anthropologist, and writes from those notes a portrait of what occurred during the contact. Because the witness is not participating directly in the encounter, he or she can view and register much that, being embroiled in the event, neither participant can see. Clinicians have been grateful for the added dimensions of knowledge, available in the witness notes, about the encounter and about themselves, often including the witness notes in their own private files about patients. The Witness Notes are at times offered to patients as well, not as a transcript but as a portrait of their efforts toward their health.

Narrative medicine's form of witnessing achieves several simultaneous goals. The gravity of the clinical encounter is recognized and perhaps heightened by the formal act of witnessing it and by producing the resultant document capturing the event. Even routine clinical encounters spent largely in discussion of symptoms, maneuvers of the physical examination, review of laboratory test and imaging results, and decisions about treatment can be recognized as complex subtle social events saturated with powerful emotion and bespeaking power relations, agreement or conflict regarding beliefs about health and illness, efforts to exhort or appease, evidence of attachment or indifference. Both participants in the encounter are witnessed. The observer pays attention to the patient's situation and the clinician's situation, silently asserting the reciprocity of effort, the potential for contact, the shared awareness of the importance of what they do together. The witness himself or herself, often unused to clinical settings, has the opportunity to contribute to the gravity of the proceedings, saying through his or her silent amanuensis that this event happened and this event matters.

Clinicians See

Beyond the dividends of narrative work and skills development, narrative capacities let individual clinicians see. I close this chapter by returning to Frank Huyler's testimony to the world of perception and activism aroused by the narrative skills of attention and representation.

Huyler describes a middle-of-the-night encounter with a woman in the midst of a large and perilous heart attack. She was homeless, living on the streets, and schizophrenic, and this combination of social factors had made it impossible for her to keep up with needed treatments for her heart disease, leading to this big MI. Huyler realizes that the $7,000 spent on the coronary artery stent placed in the woman's circulation could have been better spent on housing, pills, and a bus pass (and why do stents cost $7000 apiece anyway?, he asks). In defense of giving clinicians the narrative gifts of the humanities, Huyler writes:

> I can hardly remember any of the thousands of lectures I've attended. . . . What I do remember are the patients I've seen over the years; the many moments, dramatic and small alike; the many colleagues and residents and students and nurses I've worked with; . . . the pleasure of coming home to clean sheets after a night shift; the flash of dread when the trauma pagers go off; the black, excoriating feeling of making a big mistake; the distinct aesthetic satisfaction of suturing a laceration; the intense stillness when a code is called and everyone stops; the occasional, silent glory of being right; the grief of the consultation room and the relief of the consultation room; the sounds and lights; the radio, the sirens; the screaming drunks and the quiet drunks; the brave and the cowardly. . . . Somewhere in the impossible mix is the sense that all of us in [healthcare] are doing work, however imperfectly and at times despite ourselves, that counts.

It is precisely this sense of significance, of stakes that actually matter, of work with larger meaning, that drives the rigor and discipline of medical culture, the physical exhaustion, the endless phone calls in the middle of the night, all those pages both read and written, and all those lectures both given and received. . . . So much of medicine is . . . anonymous, thankless, faceless, and uncertain but necessary nonetheless. This necessity bears reminding, in part because it affirms our better natures, the good we sometimes do despite our indifferences.[45]

The practices described in this chapter can add up to a deepening of the realization of the sublime in healthcare. Narrative skills enable one to fully perceive and to represent what occurs in healthcare. Through rigorous routines of capturing in words and text that which occurs in care settings, narrative medicine moves clinical practice toward its ideals of creativity, reflexivity, and reciprocity. Whether inviting a patient to co-construct the clinical record or bearing witness in the clinic, these routines establish the singularity and gravity of clinical events. They donate a sense of the high stakes of healthcare, letting both patient and clinician acknowledge the moment of what they together do.

Notes

1. Leriche, cited in Canguilhem, *Normal and Pathological*, 91.
2. See O'Mahoney, "Against Narrative Medicine"; Woods, "The Limits of Narrative."
3. See Lewis, "Narrative Medicine and Healthcare"; McKechnie, "Anxieties of Communication"; Vannatta and Vannatta, "Functional Realism"; Gold, "Narrative Medicine"; Launer, *Narrative-Based Primary Care*; Greenhalgh and Hurwitz, *Narrative Based Medicine*.
4. Huyler, "Woman in the Mirror," 919.
5. Weil, *Waiting for God* (2001), 64, as quoted by Schweizer, *Waiting*, 88.
6. Weil, *Waiting for God* (1973), 111–12, 149.
7. See Lipkin, Putnam, and Lazare, *Medical Interviewing*; Fortin et al., *Smith's Patient-Centered Interviewing*; Newell, *Interviewing Skills for Nurses*; Coulehan and Block, *Medical Interview*.
8. Nowaczyk, "Narrative Medicine in Clinical Genetics," 1946.
9. Sarah Chambers and Glickstein, "Making a Case."
10. See Knight, "Role of Narrative Medicine."
11. See Mahr, "Narrative Medicine and Decision-making."
12. See Donzelli, "Role of Narrative Medicine in Pregnancy."
13. See Rian and Hammer, "Practical Application of Narrative Medicine."
14. Amiel et al., "Narrative Medicine."
15. Devlin et al., "Where Does the Circle End?"
16. Martinez, "Feeding the Soul."
17. Winkel et al., "No Time to Think"; Charon, "Our Heads Touch"; Charon, "Why Read and Write?"; Olson, "Narrative Medicine."
18. For examples of faculty and resident development training in narrative medicine, see Branch et al., "Good Clinician"; Singer et al., "Four Resident's Narratives"; and Liben et al., "Assessing a Faculty Development Workshop."

19. Moran, "Families, Law, and Literature."
20. World Health Organization, *Learning Together*; World Health Organization, *Framework for Action*; Institute of Medicine, *Crossing the Quality Chasm*; Josiah Macy, Jr. Foundation, *Annual Report 2012*.
21. Reeves et al., "Interprofessional Education"; Interprofessional Education Collaborative Expert Panel, "Core Competencies."
22. Greer, "Status of Interprofessional Education"; Ho et al., "Making Interprofessional Education Work."
23. Weaver et al., "Anatomy of Health Care Team."
24. West et al., "Tools to Investigate"; Graham, West, and Bauer, "Faculty Development."
25. Kenyon, de Vries, and Clark, *Narrative Gerontology*; Kenyon, Bohlmeijer, and Randall, *Storying*.
26. Clark, "Narrative in Interprofessional"; Clark, "Emerging Themes."
27. Thistlewaite, "Interprofessional Education"; Reeves et al., *Interprofessional Teamwork*.
28. Sands, Stanley, and Charon, "Pediatric Narrative Oncology"; Charon, "Writing in the Clinic."
29. Lövtrup, "Here Is the Patient"; Baathe et al., "Physician Experiences" http://wardround.net/research/.
30. Reis, Visser, and Frankel, "Health Information and Communication"; Bates and Gawande, "Improving Safety."
31. Cimino, "Improving the EHR."
32. Delbanco, "Inviting Patients to Read."
33. Euripides, *Trojan Women*, 65.
34. Oliver, "Witnessing," 80.
35. Hayden White, "Figural Realism," 113.
36. Levi, *Survival in Auschwitz*, 62.
37. Hayden White, "Figural Realism," 119.
38. Laub, "Bearing Witness"; Hartman, *Scars*.
39. Hartman, *Scars*, 19.
40. Ross, *Bearing Witness*.
41. Cavarero, *Relating*; Butler, *Giving an Account*; Arendt, *Human Condition*.
42. Poland, "Analyst's Witnessing," 21.
43. Michael White, *Working with People*.
44. Charon, "Narrative Medicine as Witness."
45. Huyler, "Woman in the Mirror," 920.

AUTHOR BIOGRAPHIES

Rita Charon is a general internist and literary scholar at Columbia University. She is founder and Executive Director of the Program in Narrative Medicine at Columbia, which oversees the required Narrative Medicine curriculum for Columbia medical students and the Master of Science in Narrative Medicine graduate program at Columbia. Her research in narrative dimensions of clinical practice and education has been funded by the National Institutes of Health, National Endowment for the Humanities, and several private foundations. She publishes and lectures internationally on narrative medicine, narrative ethics, and the teaching of close reading and creative writing in clinical settings. She is author of *Narrative Medicine: Honoring the Stories of Illness* and co-editor of *Stories Matter: The Role of Narrative in Medical Ethics* and *Psychoanalysis and Narrative Medicine.*

Originally trained in pediatrics and public health, **Sayantani DasGupta** is a faculty member in the Masters Program in Narrative Medicine, The Institute for Comparative Literature, and the Center for the Study of Ethnicity and Race, all at Columbia University. She is the co-chair of the Columbia University seminar in Narrative, Health and Social Justice, and on the editorial board of the journal *Literature and Medicine.* Sayantani is the author or co-editor of four books, including *Stories of Illness and Healing: Women Write their Bodies* (Kent State, 2007) and *Globalization and Transnational Surrogacy in India: Outsourcing Life* (Lexington, 2014). Her writing on narrative medicine, pedagogy, race, gender, and social justice has been published widely including in *The Health Humanities Reader* (RUP, 2014) and *Keeping Reflection Fresh* (KSUP, 2016). More on her work can be found at at www.sayantanidasgupta. com.

Nellie Hermann is a graduate of Brown University and the MFA program at Columbia University. She is author of novels *The Cure for Grief*

(Scribner: 2008) and *The Season of Migration* (FSG: 2015), which was a *New York Times'* Editor's Choice. She is a recipient of a 2016 NEA literature fellowship, teaches writing at Barnard College, and is the Creative Director of the Narrative Medicine program at Columbia University's College of Physicians and Surgeons.

Craig Irvine is the Program Director of the Masters Program in Narrative Medicine and Director of Education of the Program in Narrative Medicine at Columbia University. Dr. Irvine holds a PhD in Philosophy. For almost 20 years he has been designing and teaching narrative medicine curricula for residents, medical students, physicians, nurses, social workers, chaplains, dentists, and other health professionals. He has 30 years of experience researching and teaching the history of philosophy, phenomenology, ethics, humanities, and narrative medicine. He has published articles in the areas of ethics, residency education, and narrative medicine, and has presented at numerous national and international conferences on these and other topics.

Eric R. Marcus, MD is Director of the Columbia University Center for Psychoanalytic Training and Research and professor of clinical psychiatry at the Columbia University College of Physicians and Surgeons, and he is also a founding faculty of the Narrative Medicine Program. He is a distinguished life fellow of the American Psychiatric Association; a fellow of the New York Academy of Medicine and of the American College of Psychoanalysts, and past president of the New York County district branch of the American Psychiatric Association as well as the Association for Psychoanalytic Medicine. His areas of research involve symbolic alterations of reality in psychotic and near-psychotic phenomena and in psychoanalytic social science research using medical student dreams to study the effect of medical pedagogy and the stages of development of the capacity for medical empathy. His latest book is *Psychosis and Near Psychosis: Ego Function, Symbol Structure, Treatment*, revised third edition, forthcoming in 2017 by International Universities Press.

Edgar Rivera Colón is faculty at Columbia University's Narrative Medicine program, where he teaches qualitative research methods. He is also Assistant Professor of Sociology and Urban Studies at Saint Peter's University, The Jesuit University of New Jersey. Dr. Rivera Colón, a medical anthropologist, does ethnographic research on New York City's House Ball community. He is an expert on Latino gay and bisexual male sexual cultures and HIV, and regularly trains public health professionals in cultural and structural competency in working with Latino/a LGBTQ communities. He is working on a co-edited volume entitled *Queer Latino/a Theologies and the Churches*.

Danielle Spencer is a faculty member of the Program in Narrative Medicine at Columbia University as well as the Einstein-Cardozo Master of Science in Bioethics program. Her research interests include the personal essay, clinician memoirs, and visual culture, and she is working on a book about the phenomenon of "discovering" a dormant cognitive or perceptual difference from the norm. Spencer presents regularly at medical humanities and bioethics conferences, and her work has appeared in *The Lancet, Creative Nonfiction, Esopus, The Hungarian Review, WIRED,* and *The Routledge Companion to the Philosophy of Medicine.* She was artist/musician David Byrne's art director for many years and collaborated with Byrne on a range of exhibitions and projects, and also worked with photographer Nan Goldin.

Maura Spiegel is a professor of English who has been teaching fiction and film at Columbia University and Barnard College for the past 20 years. She is a founding member of the Program in Narrative Medicine at Columbia University College of Physicians and Surgeons, where she teaches in the MS Program and offers film courses to first-year medical students. With Rita Charon, she was the co-editor-in-chief of the journal *Literature and Medicine* (Hopkins UP) for seven years. She co-authored *The Grim Reader: Writings on Death, Dying and Living On* (Anchor/Doubleday) and *The Breast Book: An Intimate and Curious History* (Workman). She writes on numerous topics related to narrative, and her book on the life and movies of Sidney Lumet is forthcoming from St. Martin's Press.

BIBLIOGRAPHY

Academy of Achievement. "Elie Wiesel Interview—Academy of Achievement." June 29, 1996. http://www.achievement.org/autodoc/page/wie0int-2.

Ahbel-Rappe, Sara. "Plato's Influence of on Jewish, Christian, and Islamic Philosophy." In *A Companion to Plato*, edited by H. H. Benson, 434–50. West Sussex: Blackwell, 2009.

Allen, Katherine R., and Elizabeth B. Farnsworth. "Reflexivity in Teaching about Families." *Family Relations* 42 (1993): 351–56.

Altieri, Charles. "Affect, Intentionality, and Cognition: A Response to Ruth Leys." *Critical Inquiry* 38, no. 4 (2012): 878–81.

Amiel, Jonathan, Anne Armstrong-Coben, Melanie Bernitz, Julie Glickstein, Deepthiman Gowda, Gillian Graham, Nellie Hermann, Constance Park, Delphine Taylor, and Rita Charon. "Narrative Medicine in Education and Practice." In *Behavioral Medicine: A Guide for Clinical Practice*, 4th ed., edited by Mitchell Feldman, John Christiansen, and Jason Satterfield, 505–13. New York: McGraw Hill Education, 2014.

Anderson, Charles, and Marian MacCurdy. "Introduction." *Writing and Healing: Toward an Informed Practice*. Urbana, IL: National Council of Teachers of English, 2000.

Arendt, Hannah. *The Human Condition*. Chicago: University of Chicago Press, 1958.

Arendt, Hannah. *The Life of the Mind*. New York: Harcourt and Brace, 1971.

Arntfield, Shannon, Kris Slesar, Jennifer Dickson, and Rita Charon. "Narrative Medicine as a Means of Training Medical School Students toward Residency Competencies." *Patient Education and Counseling* 91 (2013): 280–86.

Aronson, Louise, Brian Niehaus, Laura Hill-Sakurai, Cindy Lai, and Patricia S. O'Sullivan. "A Comparison of Two Methods of Teaching Reflective Ability in Year 3 Medical Students." *Medical Education* 46 (2012): 807–14.

Attridge, Derek. "Innovation, Literature, Ethics: Relating to the Other." *PMLA* 114, no. 1 (1999): 20–31.

Attridge, Derek. "Performing Metaphors: The Singularity of Literary Figuration." *Paragraph: A Journal of Modern Critical Theory* 28, no. 2 (2005): 18–34.

Augustine. *The Confessions of Saint Augustine*. Translated by Edward B. Pusey. New York: The Modern Library, 1949.

Aull, Felice, and Bradley Lewis. "Medical Intellectuals: Resisting Medical Orientalism." *Journal of Medical Humanities* 25, no. 2 (2004): 87–108.

Baathe, Fredrik, Gunnar Ahlborg, Annica Lagstrom, Lars Edgren, and Kerstin Nilsson. *Journal of Hospital Administration* 3, no. 6 (2014): 127–42. Published online October 27, 2014. doi:10.5430/jha.v3n6p127.

Bachelard, Gaston. *The Poetics of Space*. Translated by Maria Jolas. Boston: Beacon Press, 1994.

Bakhtin, Mikhail. "Forms of Time and of the Chronotope in the Novel: Notes toward a Historical Poetics." In *The Dialogic Imagination: Four Essays*, edited by Michael Holquist, translated by Caryl Emerson and Michael Holquist, 84–258. Austin: University of Texas Press, 1981.

Bakhtin, Mikhail. *Problems of Dostoevsky's Poetics*. Edited and translated by Caryl Emerson. Minneapolis: University of Minnesota Press, 1984.

Baldwin, Clive. "Narrative Ethics for Narrative Care." *Journal of Aging Studies* 34 (2015): 183–89.

Banfield, Ann. "Time Passes: Virginia Woolf, Post-Impressionism, and Cambridge Time." *Poetics Today* 24, no. 3 (Fall 2003): 471–516.

Banville, John. *The Infinities*. New York: Alfred A. Knopf, 2010.

Baron, Richard J. "An Introduction to Medical Phenomenology: I Can't Hear You While I'm Listening." *Annals of Internal Medicine* 103, no. 4 (1985): 606–11.

Barthes, Roland. *The Pleasure of the Text*. Translated by Richard Miller. New York: Hill and Wang, 1975.

Barthes, Roland. *The Rustle of Language*. Translated by Richard Howard. Berkeley: University of California Press, 1989.

Barthes, Roland. *S/Z: An Essay*. Translated by Richard Miller. New York: Hill and Wang, 1974.

Bates, David W., and Atul A. Gawande. "Improving Safety with Information Technology." *New England Journal of Medicine* 348, no. 25 (2003): 2526–34.

Beauchamp, Tom L. "Principlism and Its Alleged Competitors." *Kennedy Institute of Ethics Journal* 5, no. 3 (1995): 181–98.

Beauchamp, Tom L., and James F. Childress. *Principles of Biomedical Ethics*. New York: Oxford, 1979.

Beauvoir, Simone de. *The Ethics of Ambiguity*. Translated by Bernard Frechtman. New York: Citadel Press, 1948.

Bechdel, Alison. *Fun Home: A Family Tragicomic*. New York: Houghton Mifflin, 2006.

Benjamin, Walter. "The Storyteller." In *Illuminations: Essays and Reflections*, edited by Hannah Arendt and translated by Harry Zohn, 83–109. New York: Schocken Books, 1969.

Bennett, Jane. *The Enchantment of Modern Life: Attachments, Crossings, and Ethics*. Princeton, NJ: Princeton University Press, 2002.

Berger, John. "One or Two Pages about Vigilance." *Brick: A Literary Journal* 95 (Summer 2015), 126–29.

Bergson, Henri. *Time and Free Will: An Essay on the Immediate Data of Consciousness*. Translated by F. L. Pogson. New York: Harper, 1960.

Berthoff, Ann E. "Learning the Uses of Chaos." In *The Making of Meaning: Metaphor, Models, and Maxims for Writing Teachers*, 68–72. Upper Montclair, NJ: Boynton/Cook, 1981.

Best, Stephen, and Sharon Marcus. "Surface Reading: An Introduction." *Representations* 108, no. 1 (Fall 2009): 1–21.

Bhabha, Homi K. "The World and the Home." *Social Text* 31–32 (1992): 141–53.

Bialostosky, Don. "Should College English Be Close Reading?" *College English* 69, no. 2 (2006): 111–16.

Blakeslee, Sandra. "To Advance, Search for a Black Cat in a Dark Room." *The New York Times*, June 18, 2012. http://www.nytimes.com/2012/06/19/science/ignorance-book-review-scientists-dont-care-for-facts.html.

Bleich, David. *Subjective Criticism*. Baltimore: Johns Hopkins University Press, 1978.

Bloor, David. *Knowledge and Social Imagery*. London: Routledge and Kegan Paul, 1976.

Bollas, Christopher. *The Shadow of the Object: Psychoanalysis of the Unthought Known*. New York: Columbia University Press, 1987.

Booth, Wayne C. *The Rhetoric of Fiction*. 2nd ed. Chicago: University of Chicago Press, 1983.

Booth, Wayne C. *The Company We Keep: An Ethics of Fiction*. Berkeley: University of California Press, 1988.

Borges, Jorge Luis. "A New Refutation of Time." In *Labyrinths: Selected Stories and Other Writings*, translated by James E. Irby, 217–37. New York: New Directions, 1964.

Bosk, Charles L. *All God's Mistakes: Genetic Counseling in a Pediatric Hospital.* Chicago: University of Chicago Press, 1992.

Boudreau, J. Donald, Stephen Liben, and Abraham Fuks. "A Faculty Development Workshop in Narrative-based Reflective Writing." *Perspectives in Medical Education* 1 (2012): 143–54.

Bourdieu, Pierre. *Outline of a Theory of Practice.* Translated by Richard Nice. Cambridge, UK: Cambridge University Press, 1977.

Bourdieu, Pierre, and Loïc J. D. Wacquant. *An Invitation to Reflexive Sociology.* Chicago: University of Chicago Press, 1992.

Brain, Peter, trans. "Galen on the Ideal of the Physician." (Opt. Med.). *South African Medical Journal* 52 (1977): 936–38. Translation of *Claudii Galeni Opera Omnia*, vol. 1, 53–63, edited by C. G. Kühn (Leipzig, Cnobloch), 1821–33.

Branch, William T., Jr., Richard Frankel, Catherine F. Gracey, Paul M. Haidet, Peter F. Weissmann, Paul Cantey, Gary A. Mitchell, and Thomas S. Inui. "A Good Clinician and a Caring Person: Longitudinal Faculty Development and the Enhancement of the Human Dimensions of Care." *Academic Medicine* 84, no. 1 (2009): 117–26.

Branch, William T., Jr. "The Ethics of Patient Care." *JAMA* 313, no. 14 (2015): 1421–2.

Brockmeier, Jens. *Beyond the Archive: Memory, Narrative, and the Autobiographical Process.* New York: Oxford University Press, 2015.

Brockmeier, Jens, and Donal Carbaugh, eds. *Narrative and Identity: Studies in Autobiography, Self and Culture.* Amsterdam: John Benjamins Publishing Company, 2001.

Brockmeier, Jens, and Hanna Meretoja. "Understanding Narrative Hermeneutics." *Storyworlds* 6, no. 2 (2014): 1–27.

Brockmeier, Jens, and Rom Harré. "Narrative: Problems and Promises of an Alternative Paradigm." In *Narrative and Identity: Studies in Autobiography, Self and Culture*, edited by Jens Brockmeier and Donal Carbaugh. Amsterdam: John Benjamins Publishing Company, 2001.

Brody, Howard. *Stories of Sickness.* New Haven, CT: Yale University Press, 1987.

Brooks, Cleanth. *The Well Wrought Urn: Studies in the Structure of Poetry.* New York: Harcourt, Brace and World, 1947.

Brooks, Cleanth, and Robert Penn Warren. *Understanding Poetry.* 3rd ed. New York: Holt, Rinehart and Winston, 1960.

Brooks, Peter. *Reading for the Plot: Design and Intention in Narrative.* New York: Alfred A. Knopf, 1984.

Brown, T. *The Mechanical Philosophy and the "Animal Oeconomy."* New York: Arno, 1981.

Broyard, Anatole. "The Patient Examines the Doctor." In *Intoxicated By My Illness and Other Writings on Life and Death*, edited by Alexandra Broyard, 33–58. New York: Fawcett Columbine, 1993.

Bruner, Jerome. *Acts of Meaning.* Cambridge, MA: Harvard University Press, 1990.

Butler, Judith. *Giving an Account of Oneself.* New York: Fordham University Press, 2005.

Butler, Judith. *Precarious Life: The Powers of Mourning and Violence.* New York: Verso, 2006.

Butler, Judith. *Undoing Gender.* New York: Routledge, 2004.

Butler, Judith. "Your Behavior Creates Your Gender." *Bigthink Video.* Recorded January 13, 2011. http://bigthink.com/videos/your-behavior-creates-your-gender.

Canguilhem, Georges. "Fragments." *Revue de Métaphysique et de Morale* 90, no. 1 (January–March, 1985): 93–98.

Canguilhem, Georges. *The Normal and the Pathological.* Translated by Carolyn R. Fawcett. New York: Zone Books, 1991.

Canguilhem, Georges. *Writings on Medicine / Georges Canguilhem.* Edited and translated by Stephanos Geroulanos and Todd Meyers. New York: Fordham University Press, 2012.

Carel, Havi. *Illness: The Cry of the Flesh.* Durham, UK: Acumen, 2008.

Carrese, Joseph A., Erin L. McDonald, Margaret Moon, Holly A. Taylor, Kiran Khaira, Mary Catherine Beach, and Mark T. Hughes. "Everyday Ethics in Internal Medicine Resident Clinic: An Opportunity to Teach." *Medical Education* 45 (2011): 712–21.

Carson, Ronald. "Interpretive Bioethics: The Way of Discernment." *Theoretical Medicine* 11 (1990): 51–59.

Cassell, Eric. *Talking with Patients*. Vols. 1 and 2. Cambridge, MA: MIT Press, 1985.

Cassell, Eric J. "The Nature of Suffering and the Goals of Medicine." *New England Journal of Medicine* 306, no. 11 (1982): 639–45.

Cavarero, Adriana. *Relating Narratives: Storytelling and Selfhood*. Translated by Paul A. Kottman. London: Routledge, 2000.

Certeau, Michel de. *The Practice of Everyday Life*. Translated by Steven Rendell. Berkeley: University of California Press, 1984.

Saavedra, Miguel de Cervantes. *Don Quixote De La Mancha (Oxford World's Classics)*. Translated by Charles Jarvis. New York: Oxford University Press, 2008.

Chalmers, David J. *The Conscious Mind: In Search of a Fundamental Theory*. New York: Oxford University Press, 1996.

Chambers, Sarah, and Julie Glickstein. "Making a Case for Narrative Competency in the Field of Fetal Cardiology." *Literature and Medicine* 29, no. 2 (Fall 2011): 376–95.

Chambers, Tod S. *The Fiction of Bioethics: Cases as Literary Texts*. New York: Routledge, 1999.

Charon, Rita. "At the Membranes of Care: Stories in Narrative Medicine." *Academic Medicine* 87, no. 3 (2012): 342–47.

Charon, Rita. "The Ecstatic Witness." In *Clinical Ethics and the Necessity of Stories: Essays in Honor of Richard M. Zaner*, edited by Osborne P. Wiggins and Annette C. Allen, 165–83. New York: Springer, 2011.

Charon, Rita. *Narrative Medicine: Honoring the Stories of Illness*. New York: Oxford University Press, 2006.

Charon, Rita. "Narrative Medicine as Witness for the Self-Telling Body." *Journal of Applied Communication Research* 37, no. 2 (2009): 118–31.

Charon, Rita. "Narrative Reciprocity." *Hastings Center Report* 44, no. 1 (2014): S21–S24.

Charon, Rita. "Our Heads Touch—Telling and Listening to Stories of Self." *Academic Medicine* 87 (2012): 1154–56.

Charon, Rita. "The Patient, the Body, and the Self." In *Narrative Medicine: Honoring the Stories of Illness*, 85–104. New York: Oxford University Press, 2006.

Charon, Rita. "Why Read and Write in the Clinic? The Contributions of Narrative Medicine to Health Care." In *Routledge Handbook of Language and Health Communication*, edited by Heidi Hamilton and Wen-Ying Sylvia Chou, 245–58. New York: Routledge, 2014.

Charon, Rita. "Writing in the Clinic, or What Might Be Expressed?" In *The Future of Scholarly Writing: Critical Interventions*, edited by Angelika Bammer and Ruth-Ellen Boetcher Joeres, 87–99. New York: Palgrave Macmillan, 2015.

Charon, Rita, and Martha Montello, eds. *Stories Matter: The Role of Narrative in Medical Ethics*. New York: Routledge, 2002.

Charon, Rita, Nellie Hermann, and Michael Devlin. "Close Reading and Creative Writing in Clinical Education: Teaching Attention, Representation, and Affiliation." *Academic Medicine: Journal of the Association of American Medical Colleges* 91, no. 3 (2016): 345–50.

Chen, Pauline. *Final Exam: A Surgeon's Reflections on Mortality*. New York: Vintage, 2008.

Churchill, Larry. "Narrative Awareness in Ethics Consultations: The Ethics Consultant as Story-Maker." *Hastings Center Report* 44, no. 1 (2014): S36–S39.

Chute, Hillary L., and Alison Bechdel. "An Interview with Alison Bechdel." *MFS: Modern Fiction Studies* 52, no. 4 (2006): 1004–13.

Cimino, James J. "Improving the Electronic Health Record—Are Clinicians Getting What They Wanted?" *Journal of the American Medical Association* 309, no. 10 (2013): 991–92.

Cixous, Hélène. "The Laugh of the Medusa." Translated by Keith Cohen. *Signs* 1, no. 2 (1976): 875–93.

Clark, Phillip G. "Emerging Themes in Using Narrative in Geriatric Care: Implications for Patient-Centered Practice and Interprofessional Teamwork." *Journal of Aging Studies* 34 (2015): 177–82.

Clark, Phillip G. "Narrative in Interprofessional Education and Practice: Implications for Professional Identity, Provider-Patient Communication and Teamwork." *Journal of Interprofessional Care* 28, no. 1 (2014): 34–39.

Clifton, Lucille. "the death of fred clifton." 1987. In *The Collected Poems of Lucille Clifton, 1965– 2010.* Rochester, NY: BOA Editions, Ltd., 2012.

Clouser, K. Danner. "Common Morality as an Alternative to Principlism." *Kennedy Institute of Ethics Journal* 5, no. 3 (1995): 219–36.

Clouser, K. Danner. "Veatch, May, and Models: A Critical Review and a New View." In *The Clinical Encounter: The Moral Fabric of the Patient–Physician Relationship*, edited by Earl E. Shelp, 89–104. Dordrecht: D. Reidel Publishing, 1983.

Clouser, K. Danner, and Bernard Gert. "A Critique of Principlism." *Journal of Medicine and Philosophy* 15, no. 2 (1990): 219–36.

Clouser, K. Danner, and Bernard Gert. "Morality vs. Principlism." In *Principles of Health Care Ethics*, edited by Raanan Gillon, 251–66. New York: John Wiley, 1994.

Cole, Thomas R., Thelma Jean Goodrich, and Ellen R. Gritz, eds. *Faculty Health in Academic Medicine: Physicians, Scientists, and the Pressures of Success.* New York: Humana Press, 2009.

Conway, Kathlyn. *Beyond Words: Illness and the Limits of Expression.* Albuquerque: University of New Mexico Press, 2007.

Coulehan, John L., and Marian R. Block. *The Medical Interview: Mastering Skills for Clinical Practice.* 5th ed. Philadelphia: F. A. Davis, 2006.

Couric, Katie. "*Orange is the New Black*'s Laverne Cox." *The Katie Couric Show.* Posted 2014. https://www.youtube.com/watch?v=sMH8FH7O9xA.

Couser, G. Thomas. *Recovering Bodies: Illness, Disability and Life Writing.* Madison: University of Wisconsin Press, 1997.

Cross, F. L., and E. A. Livingstone, eds. *The Oxford Dictionary of the Christian Church.* New York: Oxford University Press, 2005.

Culler, Jonathan. *On Deconstruction: Theory and Criticism after Structuralism.* Ithaca, NY: Cornell University Press, 1982.

Culler, Jonathan. *Structuralist Poetics: Structuralism, Linguistics, and the Study of Literature.* Ithaca, NY: Cornell University Press, 1975.

Czarniawska, Barbara. *Narratives in Social Science Research.* Los Angeles, CA: Sage Publications, 2004.

Damasio, Antonio. *Descartes' Error: Emotion, Reason, and the Human Brain.* New York: Penguin Books, 2005.

DasGupta, Sayantani. "Decentering the Doctor-Protagonist: Personal Illness Narratives in the Narrative Medicine Classroom." In *Keeping Reflection Fresh*, edited by Allan Peterkin and Pamela Brett-MacLean. Kent: Kent State University Press, 2016 (in press).

DasGupta, Sayantani. "Medicalization." In *Keywords for Disability Studies*, edited by Rachel Adams, Benjamin Weiss, and David Serlin, 120–121. New York: New York University Press, 2014.

DasGupta, Sayantani. "Narrative Humility." *Lancet* 371, no. 9617 (2008): 980–1.

DasGupta, Sayantani. "Narrative Humility." *TEDx Sarah Lawrence College.* April 2012. http://tedxtalks.ted.com/video/Narrative-Humility-Sayantani-Da.

DasGupta, Sayantani. "Teaching Medical Listening Through Oral History." *NYU Literature, Arts and Medicine Blog.* January 2009. http://medhum.med.nyu.edu/blog/?p=126.

DasGupta, Sayantani, and Rita Charon. "Personal Illness Narratives: Using Reflective Writing to Increase Empathy." *Academic Medicine* 79, no. 4 (April 2004): 351–56.

Davis, Kate. *Southern Comfort.* Q Ball Productions, 2001. DVD.

Davis, Philip. *Reading and the Reader.* New York: Oxford University Press, 2013.

Dehaene, Stanislas. *Reading in the Brain: The Science and Evolution of a Human Invention.* New York: Viking, 2009.

Delbanco, Tom, Jan Walker, Sigall K. Bell, Jonathan D. Darer, Joann G. Elmore, Nadine Farag, Henry J. Feldman, Roanne Mejilla, Long Ngo, James D. Ralston, Stephen E. Ross, Neha Trivedi, Elisabeth Vodicka, and Suzanne G. Leveille. "Inviting Patients to Read Their Doctors' Notes: A Quasi-experimental Study and a Look Ahead." *Annals of Internal Medicine* 157 (2012): 461–70.

Denzin, Norman K., and Yvonna S. Lincoln. *Handbook of Qualitative Research.* 2nd ed. Thousand Oaks, CA: Sage Publications, 2009.

Derrida, Jacques. *Of Grammatology.* Translated by Gayatri Chakravorty Spivak. Baltimore: Johns Hopkins University Press, 1976.

Descartes, René. *Discourse on Method and Meditations on First Philosophy.* Translated by Donald A. Cress. Indianapolis: Hackett, 1998.

Descartes, René. *The Philosophical Works of Descartes.* Translated by E. S. Haldane and G. R. T. Ross. London: Cambridge University Press, 1931.

Devlin, Michael, Boyd Richards, Hetty Cunningham, Urmi Desai, Owen Lewis, Andrew Mutnick, Mary Ann Nidiry, Prantik Saha, and Rita Charon. "'Where Does the Circle End?': Representation as a Critical Aspect of Reflection in Teaching Social and Behavioral Sciences in Medicine." *Academic Psychiatry* 39, no. 6 (2014): 669–77.

Dewey, John. *Art as Experience.* New York: Perigee Books, 1980.

Diabetes Australia. "A New Language for Diabetes." July 7, 2011. https://static.diabetesaustralia. com.au/s/fileassets/diabetes-australia/9864613f-6bc0-4773-9337-751e953777cd.pdf.

Diabetes UK. "Author Guidelines." *Diabetic Medicine.* http://onlinelibrary.wiley.com/journal/10.1111/%28ISSN%291464-5491/homepage/ForAuthors.html. Accessed May 4, 2016.

Djikic, Maja, Keith Oatley, and Mihnea C. Moldoveanu. "Reading Other Minds." *Scientific Study of Literature* 3, no. 1 (2013): 28–47.

Donald, Anna. "The Words We Live In." In *Narrative Based Medicine,* edited by Trisha Greenhalgh and Brian Hurwitz, 17–26. London: BMJ Books, 1998.

Donzelli, Gianpaolo, Erika Maria Paddeu, Francesca D'Alessandro, and Alessandro Nanni Costa. "The Role of Narrative Medicine in Pregnancy after Liver Transplantation." *Journal of Maternal-Fetal and Neonatal Medicine* 28, no. 2 (2015): 158–61.

Dostoevksy, Fyodor. *Notes from Underground.* Translated and edited by Michael R. Katz. Norton Critical Editions. New York: W. W. Norton, 1989.

Dreifus, Claudia. "Chloe Wofford Talks About Toni Morrison." *New York Times Magazine,* September 11, 1994. http://www.nytimes.com/1994/09/11/magazine/chloe-wofford-talks-about-toni-morrison.html.

DuBose, Edwin R., Ronald P. Hamel, and Laurence J. O'Connell, eds. *A Matter of Principles? Ferment in U.S. Bioethics.* Valley Forge, PA: Trinity Press International, 1994.

Edson, Margaret. *W;t: A Play.* New York: Faber and Faber, 1999.

Eliot, T. S. "Tradition and the Individual Talent." In *The Sacred Wood: Essays on Poetry and Criticism,* 47–59. London: Methuen, 1920.

Empson, William. *Seven Types of Ambiguity.* New York: New Directions, 1947.

Eng, David, Judith Halberstam, and José Esteban Muñoz. "What's Queer About Queer Studies Now?" *Social Text* 23, no. 3–4 (2005): 84–85.

Engel, George. "The Need for a New Medical Model: A Challenge for Biomedicine." *Science* 196 (1977): 129–36.

Euripides. *The Trojan Women.* Translated by Gilbert Murray. London: George Allen, 1905.

Fanon, Franz. *Black Skin, White Masks.* Rev. ed. New York: Grove Press, 2008.

Fantuzzi, Giamila. "The Sound of Health." *Frontiers in Immunology* 5 (July 21, 2014). doi:10.3389/fimmu.2014.00351.

Felski, Rita. *Uses of Literature.* Malden, MA: Wiley-Blackwell, 2008.

Ferguson, Frances. "Now It's Personal: D. A. Miller and Too-Close Reading." *Critical Inquiry* 41, no. 3 (Spring 2015): 521–40.

Ferry, David. *Bewilderment: New Poems and Translations*. Chicago: University of Chicago Press, 2012.

Finkelstein, Peter. "Studies in the Anatomy Laboratory: A Portrait of Individual and Collective Defense." In *Inside Doctoring: Stages and Outcomes in the Professional Development of Physicians*, edited by Robert H. Coombs, D. Scott May, and Gary W. Small, 22–42. New York: Praeger, 1986.

Fish, Stanley. *Is There a Text in This Class? The Authority of Interpretive Communities*. Cambridge, MA: Harvard University Press, 1980.

Flexner, Abraham. *Medical Education in the United States and Canada, Bulletin Number Four*. New York: Carnegie Foundation for the Advancement of Teaching, 1910.

Fludernik, Monica. "Metaphor and Beyond: An Introduction." *Poetics Today: Special Issue on Metaphor* 20, no. 3 (Fall 1999).

Flynn, Elizabeth A., and Patricinio P. Schweickart. *Gender and Reading: Essays on Readers, Texts, and Contexts*. Baltimore: Johns Hopkins University Press, 1986.

Fon, Vincy, and Francesco Parisi. "Reciprocity-Induced Cooperation." *Journal of Institutional and Theoretical Economics* 159, no. 1 (2003): 76–92.

Forster, E. M. *Aspects of the Novel*. San Diego, CA: Harcourt Brace Jovanovich, 1985.

Fortin, Auguste, Francesca C. Dwamena, Richard M. Frankel, and Robert C. Smith. *Smith's Patient Centered Interviewing: An Evidence-Based Approach*. Dubuque, IA: McGraw-Hill Education, 2012.

Foucault, Michel. *The Archaeology of Knowledge*. Translated by Alan Sheridan. New York: Pantheon Books, 1972.

Foucault, Michel. *The Order of Things: An Archaeology of the Human Sciences*. New York: Random House, 1970.

Foucault, Michel. "Of Other Spaces." Translated by Jay Miskowiec. *Diacritics* 16, no. 1 (Spring 1986): 22–27. doi:10.2307/464648. Originally published in *Architecture, Mouvement, Continuité*, no. 5 (October 1984): 46–49.

Frank, Arthur. *The Wounded Storyteller: Body, Illness, Ethics*. Chicago: University of Chicago Press, 1995.

Frank, Arthur W. "Narrative Ethics as Dialogical Story-Telling." *Narrative Ethics: The Role of Stories in Bioethics*, special report, *Hastings Center Report* 44 (2014): S16–S20.

Frank, Arthur W. "Why Study People's Stories? The Dialogical Ethics of Narrative Analysis." *International Journal of Qualitative Methods* 1, no. 1 (2002): 109–17.

Freire, Paulo. *Pedagogy of the Oppressed*. Translated by Myra Ramos. 30th Anniversary ed. New York: Continuum, 2000.

Gadamer, Hans-Georg. *Truth and Method*. Translated by Joel Weinsheimer and Donald G. Marshall. New York: Continuum International, 2004.

Gallagher, Ann. "Slow Ethics: A Sustainable Approach to Ethical Care Practices?" *Clinical Ethics* 8, no. 4 (2013): 98–104.

Gallop, Jane. "The Historicization of Literary Studies and the Fate of Close Reading." *Profession* 2007: 181–86.

Garrison, David, Jeffrey M. Lyness, Julia B. Frank, and Ronald M. Epstein. "Qualitative Analysis of Medical Student Impressions of a Narrative Exercise in the Third-Year Psychiatry Clerkship." *Academic Medicine* 86, no. 1 (2011): 85–89.

Gass, William. *Finding a Form: Essays*. Ithaca, NY: Cornell University Press, 1997.

Gawande, Atul. *Being Mortal*. New York: Henry Holt, 2014.

Geertz, Clifford. "Thick Description: Toward an Interpretive Theory of Culture." In *The Interpretation of Cultures: Selected Essays*, 3–30. New York: Basic Books, 1973.

Geisler, Sheryl L. "The Value of Narrative Ethics to Medicine." *Journal of Physician Assistant Education* 17, no. 2 (2006): 54–57.

Genette, Gérard. *Narrative Discourse: An Essay in Method.* Translated by Jane E. Lewin. Ithaca, NY: Cornell University Press, 1980.

Gerrig, Richard J. *Experiencing Narrative Worlds: On the Psychological Activities of Reading.* New Haven, CT: Yale University Press, 1993.

Gert, Bernard. *Morality: A New Justification of the Moral Rules.* New York: Oxford, 1988.

Gilligan, Carol. *In a Different Voice: Psychological Theory and Women's Development.* Cambridge, MA: Harvard University Press, 1982.

Gold, Hannah. "Narrative Medicine Isn't the Same Old Story." *Truthout*, April 30, 2014. www. truth-out.org/news/item/23398-narrative-medicine-isnt-the-same-old-story.

Goleman, Daniel. *Emotional Intelligence.* New York: Bantam Dell, 1995.

Goodman, Nelson. *Languages of Art: An Approach to a Theory of Symbols.* Indianapolis: Hackett Publishing, 1976.

Goyal, Rishi, and Rita Charon. "In Waves of Time, Space, and Self: The Dwelling-Place of Age in Virginia Woolf's *The Waves.*" In *Storying Later Life: Issues, Investigations, and Interventions in Narrative Gerontology*, edited by Gary Kenyon, Ernst Bohlmeijer, and William L. Randall, 66–83. New York: Oxford University Press, 2011.

Graham, Lori, Courtney West, and David Bauer. "Faculty Development Focused on Team-Based Collaborative Care." *Education in Primary Care* 25, no. 4 (2014): 227–29.

Greenhalgh, Trisha, and Brian Hurwitz, eds. *Narrative Based Medicine: Dialogue and Discourse in Clinical Practice.* London: BMJ Books, 1998.

Greer, Annette G., Maria Clay, Amy Blue, Clyde H. Evans, and David Garr. "The Status of Interprofessional Education and Interprofessional Prevention Education in Academic Health Centers: A National Baseline Study." *Academic Medicine* 89, no. 5 (2014): 799–805.

Gregory, Marshall. *Shaped by Stories: The Ethical Power of Narratives.* Notre Dame, IN: University of Notre Dame Press, 2009.

Grossman, David. "Desire to be Gisella." In *Writing in the Dark: Essays on Literature and Politics*, 29–58. New York: Picador, 2009.

Grossman, David. "Individual Language and Mass Language." In *Writing in the Dark: Essays on Literature and Politics*, 69–86. New York: Picador, 2009.

Grosz, Elizabeth. *Volatile Bodies: Toward a Corporeal Feminism.* Bloomington: Indiana University Press, 1994.

Guillemin, Marilys, and Lynn Gillam. "Emotions, Narratives, and Ethical Mindfulness." *Academic Medicine* 90, no. 6 (2015): 726–31.

Habermas, Jürgen. *Knowledge and Human Interests: A General Perspective.* Translated by Jeremy J. Shapiro. Boston: Beacon Press, 1971.

Haggerty, Kevin D., and Richard V. Ericson. "The Surveillant Assemblage." *British Journal of Sociology* 51, no. 4 (2000): 605–22.

Hale, Dorothy J. "Fiction as Restriction: Self-Binding in New Ethical Theories of the Novel." *Narrative* 15, no. 2 (2007): 187–206.

Hale, G. E., and Rosemary D. Hale. "Reciprocity under the Antitrust Laws: A Comment." *University of Pennsylvania Law Review* 113, no. 1 (1964): 69–76.

Hamkins, SuEllen. *The Art of Narrative Psychiatry: Stories of Strength and Meaning.* New York: Oxford University Press, 2013.

Hankinson, R. James. "Galen's Anatomy of the Soul." *Phronesis* 36, no. 2 (1991): 197–233.

Harkin, Patricia. "The Reception of Reader-Response Theory." *College Composition and Communication* 56, no. 3 (2005): 410–25.

Harries, Karsten. "Metaphor and Transcendence." In *On Metaphor*, edited by Sheldon Sacks, 71–88. Chicago: Chicago University Press, 1979.

Hartman, Geoffrey. *Scars of the Spirit: The Struggle against Inauthenticity.* New York: Palgrave Macmillan, 2002.

Hedgecoe, Adam M. "Critical Bioethics: Beyond the Social Sciences Critique of Applied Ethics." *Bioethics* 18, no. 2 (2004): 120–43.

Hellerstein, David. "'The City of the Hospital': On Teaching Medical Students to Write." *Journal of Medical Humanities* 36, no. 4 (2015): 269–89.

Hemon, Aleksander. "The Aquarium." *New Yorker*, June 13 and 20, 2011: 50–62. Reprinted in Aleksander Hemon, *The Book of My Lives*, 185–212. New York: Farrar, Straus and Giroux, 2013.

Herman, David. *Story Logic: Problems and Possibilities of Narrative.* Lincoln: University of Nebraska Press, 2002.

Herman, David, Manfred Jahn, and Marie-Laure Ryan, eds. *Routledge Encyclopedia of Narrative Theory.* London: Routledge, 2005.

Hermann, Nellie. *The Cure for Grief.* New York: Scribner, 2008.

Ho, Kendall, Sandra Jarvis-Selinger, Francine Borduas, Blye Frank, Pippa Hall, Richard Handfield-Jones, David F. Hardwick, Jocelyn Lockyer, Doug Sinclair, Helen Novak Lauscher, Luke Ferdinands, Anna MacLeod, Marie-Anik Robitaille, and Michel Rouleau. "Making Interprofessional Education Work: The Strategic Roles of the Academy." *Academic Medicine* 83, no. 10 (2008): 934–40.

Hojat, Mohammadreza, Michael J. Vergare, Kaye Maxwell, George Brainard, Steven K. Herrine, Gerald A. Isenberg, Jon Veloski, and Joseph S. Gonnella. "The Devil is in the Third Year: A Longitudinal Study of Erosion of Empathy in Medical School." *Academic Medicine* 84, no. 9 (2009): 1182–91.

Holland, Norman N. *The Dynamics of Literary Response.* New York: Columbia University Press, 1968.

Holland, Norman N. *5 Readers Reading.* New Haven, CT: Yale University Press, 1975.

hooks, bell. *Feminist Theory: From Margin to Center.* London: Pluto Press, 2000.

hooks, bell. *Teaching to Transgress: Education as the Practice of Freedom.* New York: Routledge, 1994.

hooks, bell. *Yearning: Race, Gender, and Cultural Politics.* Boston: South End Press, 1999.

Hunter, Billie. "The Importance of Reciprocity in Relationships between Community-based Midwives and Mothers." *Midwifery* 23 (2006): 308–22.

Hunter, Kathryn Montgomery. *Doctors' Stories: The Narrative Structure of Medical Knowledge.* Princeton, NJ: Princeton University Press, 1991.

Hurwitz, Brian. "Form and Representation in Clinical Case Reports." *Literature and Medicine* 25, no. 2 (Fall 2006): 216–40.

Hurwitz, Brian, Trisha Greenhalgh, and Vieda Skultans. *Narrative Research in Health and Illness.* Malden, MA: Blackwell Publishing, 2004.

Huyler, Frank. "The Woman in the Mirror: Humanities in Medicine." *Academic Medicine* 88, no. 7 (2013): 918–20.

Hwang, David Henry. *M. Butterfly.* New York: New American Library, 1988.

Iaquinta, Salvatore. *The Year They Tried to Kill Me: Surviving a Surgical Internship Even If the Patients Don't.* E-Book, Version 4.1. Self-published, 2012.

Ikoku, Alvan. "Refusal in 'Bartleby, the Scrivener': Narrative Ethics and Conscientious Objection." *American Medical Association Journal of Ethics* 15, no. 3 (2013): 249–56.

Institute of Medicine. *Crossing the Quality Chasm: A New Health System for the 21st Century.* Washington, DC: National Academy Press, 2001.

Interprofessional Education Collaborative Expert Panel. "Core Competencies for Interprofessional Collaborative Practice: Report of an Expert Panel." Washington, DC: Interprofessional Education Collaborative, 2011. https://ipecollaborative.org/uploads/IPEC-Core-Competencies.pdf.

Inwood, Brad, and Lloyd P. Gerson. *The Epicurus Reader.* Indianapolis: Hackett Publishing, 1994.

Irvine, Craig. "The Ethics of Self Care." In *Academic Medicine: In Sickness and in Health*, edited by T. Cole, T. J. Goodrich, and E. Gritz, 127–46. New York: Humana Press, 2009.

Irvine, Craig. "The Other Side of Silence: Levinas, Medicine and Literature." *Literature and Medicine* 24, no. 1 (2005): 8–18.

Iser, Wolfgang. *The Act of Reading: A Theory of Aesthetic Response.* Baltimore: Johns Hopkins University Press, 1978.

Ishiguro, Kazuo. *Never Let Me Go.* New York: Alfred A. Knopf, 2011.

Jackson, Tony E. "Issues and Problems on the Blending of Cognitive Science, Evolutionary Psychology, and Literary Study." *Poetics Today* 23, no. 1 (2002): 161–79.

Jakobson, Roman, and Morris Halle. *Fundamentals of Language.* The Hague: Mouton, 1956.

James, Henry. "The Art of Fiction." In *Partial Portraits,* 375–408. London: MacMillan and Company, 1984.

James, Henry. "The Novels of George Eliot." *Atlantic Monthly* 18 (108) (October 1866): 479–92.

James, Henry. Preface to *The Ambassadors.* In *The Novels and Tales of Henry James: The New York Edition,* vol. 21. New York: Charles Scribner's Sons, 1909.

James, Henry. *Portrait of a Lady.* In *Novels and Tales of Henry James: The New York Edition,* vol. 3. New York: Charles Scribner's Sons, 1909.

James, Henry. *What Maisie Knew.* In *The Novels and Tales of Henry James: The New York Edition,* vol. 11. New York: Charles Scribner's Sons, 1909.

Jameson, Fredric. *The Political Unconscious: Narrative as a Socially Symbolic Act.* Ithaca, NY: Cornell University Press, 1981.

Jaspers, K. *Philosophy and the World: Selected Essays and Lectures.* Translated by E. B. Ashton. Chicago: Hegnery Regnery, 1963.

Johnson, T. R. "Writing as Healing and the Rhetorical Tradition." In *Writing and Healing: Toward an Informed Practice,* edited by Charles Anderson and Marian MacCurdy, 85–114. Urbana, IL: National Council of Teachers of English, 2000.

Jones, Anne Hudson. "Literature and Medicine: Narrative Ethics." *Lancet* 349, no. 9060 (1995): 1243–46.

Jones, Tess, Delese Wear, and Lester J. Friedman. *Health Humanities Reader.* New Brunswick, NJ: Rutgers University Press, 2014.

Jonsen, Albert R. "Casuistry: An Alternative or Complement to Principles?" *Kennedy Institute of Ethics Journal* 5, no. 3 (1995): 237–51.

Jonsen, Albert R., Mark Siegler, and William J. Winslade. *Clinical Ethics: A Practical Approach to Ethical Decisions in Clinical Medicine.* 8th ed. New York: McGraw Hill, 2015.

Jonsen, Albert R., and Stephen Toulmin. *The Abuse of Casuistry: A History of Moral Reasoning.* Berkeley: University of California Press, 1988.

Josiah Macy, Jr. Foundation. *2012 Annual Report: Accelerating Interprofessional Education.* New York: Josiah Macy Jr. Foundation, 2012. www.macyfoundation.org/docs/annual_reports/macy_AnnualReport_2012.pdf.

Jurecic, Ann. *Illness as Narrative.* Pittsburgh, PA: University of Pittsburgh Press, 2012.

Kandel, Eric R. *The Age of Insight: The Quest to Understand the Unconscious in Art, Mind, and Brain.* New York: Random House, 2012.

Kearney, Michael K., Radhule B. Weininger, Mary L. S. Vachon, Richard L. Harrison, Balfour M. Mount. "Self-care of Physicians Caring for Patients at the End of Life." *JAMA* 301, no. 11 (2009): 1155–64.

Keen, Suzanne. *Empathy and the Novel.* New York: Oxford University Press, 2007.

Kenyon, Gary, Brian de Vries, and Phillip Clark, eds. *Narrative Gerontology: Theory, Research, and Practice.* New York: Springer, 2001.

Kenyon, Gary, Ernst Bohlmeijer, William L. Randall. *Storying Later Life: Issues, Investigations, and Interventions in Narrative Gerontology.* New York: Oxford University Press, 2011.

Keohane, Robert O. "Reciprocity in International Relations." *International Organization* 40, no. 1 (Winter 1986): 1–27.

Kermode, Frank. *The Sense of an Ending: Studies in the Theory of Fiction.* London: Oxford University Press, 1966.

Kidd, David Comer, and Emanuele Castano. "Reading Literary Fiction Improves Theory of Mind." *Science* 342, no. 6156 (October 18, 2013): 377–80.

Kinnell, Galway. "Wait." In *Mortal Acts, Mortal Words,* 15. New York: Houghton Mifflin Harcourt, 1980.

Kleinman, Arthur. *The Illness Narratives: Suffering, Healing and the Human Condition.* New York: Basic Books, 1989.

Knight, Isobel. "The Role of Narrative Medicine in the Management of Joint Hypermobility Syndrome/Ehlers-Danlos Syndrome, Hypermobility Type." *American Journal of Medical Genetics, Part C (Seminars in Medical Genetics)* 169, no. 1 (2015): 123–29.

Koski, C. *The Autobiography of Medical Education: Anatomy of a Genre.* Knoxville: University of Tennessee Press, 2002.

Kreiswirth, Martin. "Merely Telling Stories? Narrative and Knowledge in the Human Sciences." *Poetics Today* 21, no. 2 (2000): 293–318.

Kreiswirth, Martin. "Trusting the Tale: The Narrativist Turn in the Human Sciences." *New Literary History* 23 (1992): 629–57.

Kristeva, Julia. *Desire in Language: A Semiotic Approach to Literature and Art.* Translated by Thomas Gora, Alice Jardine, and Leon S. Roudiez. Edited by Leon S. Roudiez. New York: Columbia University Press, 1980.

Kuiken, Don, Leah Phillips, Michelle Gregus, David S. Miall, Mark Verbitsky, and Anna Tonkonogy. "Locating Self-Modifying Feelings Within Literary Reading." *Discourse Processes* 38, no. 2 (2004): 267–86.

Lacan, Jacques. *Écrits: A Selection.* Translated by Alan Sheridan. New York: W. W. Norton, 1977.

Lakoff, George, and Mark Johnson. *Metaphors We Live By.* Chicago: University of Chicago Press, 1980.

Lane, Harlan. "Constructions of Deafness." In *The Disability Studies Reader,* 3rd ed., edited by Lester J. Davis. New York: Routledge, 2010.

Latour, Bruno, and Steve Woolgar. *Laboratory Life: The Construction of Scientific Facts.* 2nd ed. Princeton, NJ: Princeton University Press, 1986.

Laub, Dori. "Bearing Witness, or the Vicissitudes of Listening." In Shoshana Felman and Dori Laub, *Testimony: Crises of Witnessing in Literature, Psychoanalysis, and History,* 57–74. New York: Routledge, 1992.

Launer, John. *Narrative-based Primary Care: A Practical Guide.* Oxon, UK: Radcliffe Medical Press, 2002.

Leder, Drew. *The Absent Body.* Chicago: University of Chicago, 1990.

Leder, Drew. "A Tale of Two Bodies: The Cartesian Corpse and the Lived Body." In *The Body in Medical Thought and Practice,* edited by Drew Leder, 17–35. Boston: Kluwer Academic Publishers, 1992.

Lee, Keekok. *The Philosophical Foundations of Modern Medicine.* New York: Palgrave Macmillan, 2012.

Leeuw, Sarah de, Margot W. Parkes, and Deborah Thien. "Questioning Medicine's Discipline: The Arts of Emotions in Undergraduate Medical Education." *Emotion, Space and Society* 11 (2014). www.elsevier.com/locate/emospa.

Lentricchia, Frank, and Andrew DuBois, eds. *Close Reading: The Reader.* Durham, NC: Duke University Press, 2003.

Levi, Primo. *Survival in Auschwitz.* Translated by Stuart Woolf. New York: Simon and Schuster, 1996.

Levi-Strauss, Claude. *Structural Anthropology, Vol. 2.* Translated by Monique Layton. Chicago: University of Chicago Press, 1976.

Lewis, Bradley. "Narrative Medicine." In *Narrative Psychiatry: How Stories Can Shape Clinical Practice,* 18–31. Baltimore: Johns Hopkins University Press, 2011.

Lewis, Bradley. "Narrative Medicine and Healthcare Reform." *Journal of Medical Humanities* 32, no. 9 (2011): 9–20.

Leys, Ruth. "The Turn to Affect: A Critique." *Critical Inquiry* 37, no. 3 (Spring 2011): 434–72.

Liben, Stephen, Kevin Chin, J. Donald Boudreau, Miriam Boillat, and Yvonne Steinert. "Assessing a Faculty Development Workshop in Narrative Medicine." *Medical Teacher* 34, no. 12 (2012): e813–e819.

Lieberman, Matthew D., Ruth Gaunt, Daniel T. Gilbert, and Yaacov Trope. "Reflexion and Reflection: A Social Cognitive Neuroscience Approach to Attributional Inference." *Advances in Experimental Social Psychology* 34 (2002): 199–249.

Lindemann Nelson, Hilde. *Damaged Identities, Narrative Repair.* Ithaca, NY: Cornell University Press, 2001.

Lipkin, Mack, Samuel Putnam, and Aaron Lazare, eds. *The Medical Interview: Clinical Care, Education, and Research.* New York: Springer-Verlag, 1995.

Loewald, Hans. "On the Therapeutic Action of Psycho-Analysis." *International Journal of Psychoanalysis* 41 (1960): 16–33.

Lorde, Audre. "The Master's Tools Will Never Dismantle the Master's House." In *Sister Outsider: Essays and Speeches,* 110–113. Berkeley, CA: Crossing Press, 1984.

Lövtrup, Michael. "Here, The Patient Is Part of the Team." [in Swedish] *Läkartidningens: Journal of the Swedish Medical Assocation* 111 (2014). http://www.lakartidningen.se/Aktuellt/Nyheter/2014/06/Har-ar-patienten-del-i-teamet/.

Lorde, Audre. "A Burst of Light: Living with Cancer." In *Feminist Theory and the Body,* edited by Janet Price and Margrit Shildrick, 149–52. New York: Routledge, 1999.

Louth, Andrew. *The Origins of the Christian Mystical Tradition: From Plato to Denys.* Oxford: Oxford University Press, 1983.

"Love and Knowledge." *PBS NewsHour with Jim Lehrer.* April 14, 1999. Transcript. http://www.pbs.org/newshour/bb/entertainment-jan-june99-edson_4-14/.

Lubbock, Percy. *The Craft of Fiction.* London: Jonathan Cape, 1921.

Lyotard, Jean-François. *The Postmodern Condition: A Report on Knowledge.* Translated by Geoffrey Bennington and Brian Massumi. Minneapolis: University of Minnesota Press, 1984.

Lukács, Georg. *The Theory of the Novel: A Historico-philosophical Essay on the Forms of Great Epic Literature.* Translated by Anna Bostock. Cambridge, MA: MIT Press, 1971.

MacCormack, Geoffrey. "Reciprocity." *Man,* New Series 11, no. 1 (1976): 89–103.

MacIntyre, Alasdair. *After Virtue: A Study in Moral Theory.* Notre Dame, IN: University of Notre Dame Press, 1981.

MacIntyre, Alasdair. *Against the Self-Images of the Age: Essays on Ideology and Philosophy.* Notre Dame, IN: University of Notre Dame Press, 1978.

Mackenzie, Catriona, and Natalie Stoljar. "Introduction: Autonomy Refigured." In *Relational Autonomy: Feminist Perspectives on Autonomy, Agency, and the Social Self.* New York: Oxford University Press, 2000.

Mahr, Greg. "Narrative Medicine and Decision-Making Capacity." *Journal of Evaluation in Clinical Practice.* 21 (2015): 503–7.

Mailer, Norman. "At the Point of My Pen." In *Why I Write: Thoughts on the Craft of Fiction,* edited by Will Blythe, 3–4. Boston: Back Bay Books, 1999.

Maitland, Sara. "Forceps Delivery." In *Women Fly When Men Aren't Looking,* 165–73. New York: Random House, 1993.

Mann, Karen, Jill Gordon, and Anna MacLeod. "Reflection and Reflective Practice in Health Professions Education: A Systematic Review." *Advances in Health Science Education* 14 (2009): 595–621.

Marck, Patricia. "Therapeutic Reciprocity: A Caring Phenomenon." *Advances in Nursing Science* 13, no. 1 (1990): 49–59.

Marcum, James A. *An Introductory Philosophy of Medicine: Humanizing Modern Medicine.* Philosophy and Medicine series. Dordrecht: Springer, 2008.

Marcus, Eric R. *Psychosis and Near Psychosis: Ego Function, Symbol Structure, and Treatment.* 2nd ed. Madison, CT: International Universities Press, 2003.

Martin, Wallace. *Recent Theories of Narrative.* Ithaca, NY: Cornell University Press, 1986.

Martinez, Cecilia. "Feeding the Soul with Words: Narrative Medicine in Pediatrics Helps Doctors, Patients with Treatment." *Connections: Columbia Women's and Children's Health* (Spring 2015): 12–13.

Marx, Karl. *Grundrisse*. Foundations of the Critique of Political Economy (Rough Draft). London: Penguin Books, 1973.

Mateu-Gelabert, Pedro, M. Bolyard, C. Maslow, M. Sandoval, P. L. Flom, and S. R. Friedman. "For the Common Good: Measuring Residents' Efforts to Protect Their Community from Drug- and Sex-Related Harm." *Journal of Social Aspects of HIV/AIDS* 5, no. 3 (September 2008): 144–57.

Maxwell, William. *So Long, See You Tomorrow*. New York: Vintage/Random House, 1996.

May, Rollo. *The Courage to Create*. New York: W. W. Norton, 1994.

McAdams, Dan P. "The Role of Narrative in Personality Psychology Today." *Narrative Inquiry* 16 (2006): 11–18.

McEwan, Ian. *Saturday*. New York: Anchor, 2006.

McKechnie, Claire Charlotte. "Anxieties of Communication: The Limits of Narrative in the Medical Humanities." *Medical Humanities* 40 (2014): 119–24.

McNaughton, Nancy. "Discourse(s) of Emotion within Medical Education: The Ever-present Absence." *Medical Education* 47, no. 1 (January 2013): 71–79.

Merleau-Ponty, Maurice. *Phenomenology of Perception*. Translated by Donald A. Landes. London: Routledge, 2014.

Metzl, Jonathan M. "Structural Competency." *American Quarterly* 64, no. 2 (2012): 213–18.

Miller, D. A. "Hitchcock's Understyle: A Too-Close View of *Rope*." *Representations* 121, no. 1 (Winter 2013): 1–30.

Miller, Eliza, Dorene Balmer, Nellie Hermann, Gillian Graham, and Rita Charon. "Sounding Narrative Medicine: Studying Students' Professional Development at Columbia University College of Physicians and Surgeons." *Academic Medicine* 89, no. 2 (2014): 335–42.

Miller, Henry. "Reflections on Writing." In *Wisdom of the Heart*. New Directions, 1960.

Miller, J. Hillis. *The Ethics of Reading: Kant, de Man, Eliot, Trollope, James, and Benjamin*. New York: Columbia University Press, 1987.

Miller, J. Hillis. *Literature as Conduct: Speech Acts in Henry James*. New York: Fordham University Press, 2005.

Miller, J. Hillis. *Reading for Our Time: "Adam Bede" and "Middlemarch" Revisited*. Edinburgh: Edinburgh University Press, 2012.

Mishler, Elliot G. *Research Interviewing: Context and Narrative*. Cambridge, MA: Harvard University Press, 1986.

Mitchell, Stephen A. "Attachment Theory and the Psychoanalytic Tradition: Reflections on Human Relationality." *British Journal of Psychotherapy* 15, no. 2 (1998): 177–93.

Mitchell, Stephen A. *Relationality: From Attachment to Intersubjectivity*. Hillsdale, NJ: Analytic Press, 2000.

Mitchell, W. J. T. *On Narrative*. Chicago: University of Chicago Press, 1981.

Mohanty, Chandra Talpade. *Feminism without Borders: Decolonizing Theory, Practicing Solidarity*. Chapel Hill, NC: Duke University Press, 2003.

Molm, Linda D. "The Structure of Reciprocity." *Social Psychology Quarterly* 73, no. 2 (2010): 119–31.

Montello, Martha, ed. *Narrative Ethics: The Role of Stories in Bioethics*. Special report of *Hastings Center Report* 44, no. 1 (2014).

Montgomery, Kathryn. "Literature, Literary Studies, and Medical Ethics: The Interdisciplinary Question." *Hastings Center Report* 31, no. 3 (2001): 36–43.

Montross, Christine. *Body of Work: Meditations on Mortality From the Human Anatomy Lab*. New York: Penguin Books, 2007.

Moody, Michael. "Serial Reciprocity: A Preliminary Statement." *Sociological Theory* 26, no. 2 (2008): 130–51.

Moore, Lorrie. "People Like That Are the Only People Here: Canonical Babbling in Peed Onk." In *Birds of America: Stories*, 212–50. New York: Picador, 1999.

Moran, Judith. "Families, Law, and Literature: The Story of a Course on Storytelling." *University of San Francisco Law Review* 49, no. 1 (2015): 1–56. http://papers.ssrn.com/sol3/papers.cfm?abstract_id=2596782.

Morrison, Toni. *Home*. New York: Vintage Books, 2013.

Munro, Alice. "Floating Bridge." In *Hateship, Friendship, Courtship, Loveship*, 55–85. New York: Alfred A. Knopf, 2001.

Munro, Alice. *Selected Stories*. New York: Vintage Books, 1997.

Murdoch, Iris. *The Black Prince*. New York: Penguin Classics, 2003.

Murdoch, Iris. "The Sublime and Beautiful Revisited." *The Yale Review* 49 (1959): 247–77.

Nancy, Jean-Luc. *The Inoperative Community*. Minneapolis: University of Minnesota Press, 1991.

National Commission for the Protection of Human Subjects of Biomedical and Behavioral Research, Department of Health, Education and Welfare. *The Belmont Report*. DHEW pub. No. (OS) 78-0012. Washington, DC: United States Printing Office, 1978.

National Endowment for the Arts and Santa Fe Institute, eds. "How Creativity Works in the Brain: Insights from a Santa Fe Institute Working Group, co-sponsored by the National Endowment for the Arts." Washington, DC: National Endowment for the Arts. http://arts.gov/publications/how-creativity-works-brain. Accessed May 4, 2016.

Nelson, Hilde Lindemann. "Feminist Bioethics: Where We've Been, Where We're Going." *Metaphilosophy* 31, no. 5 (2000): 492–508.

Nelson, Hilde Lindemann. *Stories and their Limits: Narrative Approaches to Bioethics*. New York: Routledge, 1997.

Newell, Robert. *Interviewing Skills for Nurses and Other Health Care Professionals: A Structured Approach*. New York: Taylor and Francis, 1994.

Newton, Adam Zachary. *Narrative Ethics*. Cambridge, MA: Harvard University Press, 1995.

Ng, Stella I., Elizabeth A. Kinsella, Farah Friesen, and Brian Hodges. "Reclaiming a Theoretical Orientation to Reflection in Medical Education Research: A Critical Narrative Review." *Medical Education* 49 (2015): 461–75.

Nistelrooij, Inge van, Petruschka Schaafsma, and Joan C. Tronto. "Ricoeur and the Ethics of Care." *Medical Health Care and Philosophy* 17 (2014): 485–91.

Noddings, Nel. *Caring: A Feminine Approach to Ethics and Moral Education*. Berkeley: University of California Press, 1984.

North, Joseph. "What's 'New Critical' about 'Close Reading?': I. A. Richards and His New Critical Reception." *New Literary History* 44 (2015): 141–57.

Novak, Joseph D. "A Theory of Education: Meaningful Learning Underlies the Constructive Integration of Thinking, Feeling, and Acting Leading to Empowerment for Commitment and Responsibility." *Meaningful Learning Review* 1, no. 2 (2011): 1–14.

Nowaczyk, Malgorzata J. M. "Narrative Medicine in Clinical Genetics Practice." *American Journal of Medical Genetics Practice Part A*, 158A (2012): 1941–47.

Nowak, Martin A., and Sébastian Roch. "Upstream Reciprocity and the Evolution of Gratitude." *Proceedings: Biological Sciences* 274, no. 1610 (March 7, 2007): 605–9.

Nussbaum, Martha C. *Love's Knowledge: Essays on Philosophy and Literature*. New York: Oxford University Press, 1990.

Nussbaum, Martha. Introduction. In *The Black Prince*, by Iris Murdoch, vii–xxvi. New York: Penguin Classics, 2003.

Oatley, Keith. "Fiction Hones Social Skills." *Scientific American Mind* 22, no. 5 (November/December 2011). http://www.scientificamerican.com/article/in-the-minds-of-others/.

Oatley, Keith. "In the Minds of Others." *Scientific American Mind* 22, no. 5 (November/December 2011): 62–67.

Oatley, Keith. *Such Stuff as Dreams: The Psychology of Fiction*. Oxford, UK: Wiley Blackwell, 2011.

Odegaard, C. E. *Dear Doctor: A Personal Letter to a Physician.* Menlo Park, CA: H. J. Kaiser Family Foundation, 1986.

Ofri, Danielle. "The Passion and the Peril: Storytelling in Medicine." *Academic Medicine* 90, no. 8 (2015): 1005–6.

Ofri, Danielle. *What Doctors Feel: How Emotions Affect the Practice of Medicine.* Boston: Beacon Press, 2013.

Ogden, Charles Kay, and Ivor Armstrong Richards. *The Meaning of Meaning: A Study of the Influence of Language upon Thought and of the Science of Symbolism.* New York: Harcourt, Brace and World, 1923.

Oliver, Kelly. "Witnessing and Testimony." *Parallax* 10, no. 1 (2004): 78–87.

Olson, Bonnie McDougall. "Narrative Medicine: Recovery of Soul through Storytelling of the Chronically Mentally Ill." *National Association of Catholic Chaplains Vision Online* 22, no. 5, September–October 2012. http://www.nacc.org/vision/backissues/.

O'Mahoney, Seamus. "Against Narrative Medicine." *Perspectives in Biology and Medicine* 56, no. 4 (2014): 611–19.

Orr, Gregory. *Poetry as Survival.* Athens: University of Georgia Press, 2002.

O'Toole, John. "The Story of Ethics: Narrative as a Means for Ethical Understanding and Action." *JAMA* 273, no. 17 (1995): 1387–90.

Ozick, Cynthia. "The Moral Necessity of Metaphor: Rooting History in a Figure of Speech." *Harper's*, May, 1986: 62–68.

Palmer, Alan. *Social Minds in the Novel.* Columbus: The Ohio State University Press, 2010.

Parisi, Peter. "Close Reading, Creative Writing, and Cognitive Development." *College English* 41, no. 1 (1979): 57–67.

Paulsen, Jens Erik. "A Narrative Ethics of Care." *Health Care Analysis: Journal of Health Philosophy* 19 (2011): 28–40.

Pauly, Bernadette M., Colleen Varcoe, and Jan Storch. "Framing the Issues: Moral Distress in Health Care." *HEC Forum* 24 (2012): 1–11.

Peabody, Francis W. "The Care of the Patient." *JAMA* 88, no. 12 (1927): 877–82.

Pearson, A. Scott, Michael P. McTigue, and John L. Tarpley. "Narrative Medicine in Surgical Education." *Journal of Surgical Education* 65 (2009): 99–100.

Pellegrino, Edmund D. *The Philosophy of Medicine Reborn: A Pellegrino Reader.* Notre Dame Studies in Medical Ethics. Notre Dame, IN: University of Notre Dame Press, 2008.

Pellegrino, Edmund D. "Toward a Reconstruction of Medical Morality." *American Journal of Bioethics* 6, no. 2 (2006): 65–71.

Pellegrino, Edmund. "Toward a Virtue-Based Normative Ethics for the Health Professions." *Kennedy Institute of Ethics Journal* 5, no. 3 (1995): 253–77.

Pellegrino, Edmund D., and David C. Thomasma. *A Philosophical Basis of Medical Practice: Toward a Philosophy and Ethic of the Healing Professions.* New York: Oxford University Press, 1981.

Percy, Walker. "Metaphor as Mistake." *Sewanee Review* 66, no. 1 (Winter 1958): 79–99.

Peters, Kyle R. "'Diabetic' and 'Noncompliant Diabetic': Terms That Need to Disappear." *Clinical Diabetes* 30, no. 3 (2012): 89–91.

Peters, Michael A., and Tina Besley. "The Narrative Turn and the Poetics of Resistance: Towards a New Language for Critical Education Studies." In *The Last Book of Postmodernism*, 155–71. New York: Peter Lang, 2011.

Phelan, James. "Dual Focalization, Discourse as Story, and Ethics: *Lolita.*" In *Living to Tell About It: A Rhetoric and Ethics of Character Narration*, 98–131. Ithaca, NY: Cornell University Press, 2005.

Phelan, James. *Living to Tell About It: A Rhetoric and Ethics of Character Narration.* Ithaca, NY: Cornell University Press, 2005.

Phelan, James. "Rhetoric, Ethics, and Narrative Communication: Or, from Story and Discourse to Authors, Resources, and Audiences." *Soundings* 94, nos. 1–2 (2011): 55–75.

Plato. *The Collected Dialogues of Plato*. Edited by E. Hamilton and H. Cairns. Princeton, NJ: Princeton University Press, 1989.

Plato. "Phaedo." In *Plato, Complete Works*, edited by John M. Cooper and D. S. Hutchinson, translated by G.M.A. Grubel, 49–100. Cambridge, MA: Hackett, 1997.

Plato. *The Republic*. Translated by Allan Bloom. New York: Basic Books, 1968.

Plato. *Symposium*. Translated by Seth Benardete. Chicago: University of Chicago Press, 2001.

Plato. "Timaeus." In *Plato, Complete Works*, edited by John M. Cooper and D. S. Hutchinson, translated by Donald J. Zeyl, 1224–91. Cambridge, MA: Hackett, 1997.

Poirier, Suzanne. *Doctors in the Making: Memoirs and Medical Education*. Iowa City: University of Iowa Press, 2009.

Poland, Warren S. "The Analyst's Witnessing and Otherness." *Journal of the American Psychoanalytic Association* 48, no. 1 (2000): 17–34.

Portelli, Alessandro. "Research as an Experiment in Equality." In *The Death of Luigi Trastulli and Other Stories: Form and Meaning in Oral History*. Albany: State University of New York Press, 2001.

Poulet, Georges. "Criticism and the Experience of Interiority." In *The Structuralist Controversy: The Languages of Criticism and the Sciences of Man*, edited by Richard A. Macksey and Eugenio Donato, 56–72. Baltimore: Johns Hopkins University Press, 1972.

Powers, Richard. "Richard Powers." *The Believer* February 2007. http://www.believermag. com/issues/200702/?read=interview_powers

Puig, Manuel. *Kiss of the Spider Woman*. Translated by Thomas Colchie. New York: Random House, 1991.

Rabinowitz, Peter J. "The Rhetoric of Reference; Or, Shostakovich's Ghost Quartet." *Narrative* 15, no. 2 (2007): 239–56.

Rankine, Claudia. *Citizen: An American Lyric*. Minneapolis, MN: Graywolf Press, 2014.

Ransom, John Crowe. *The New Criticism*. Norfolk, CT: New Directions, 1941.

Rawlinson, Mary. "The Concept of a Feminist Bioethics." *Journal of Medicine and Philosophy* 26, no. 4 (2001): 405–516.

Reddy, William. *The Navigation of Feeling: Framework for the History of Emotions*. Cambridge, UK: Cambridge University Press, 2001.

Reed, Esther D., Rob Freathy, Susannah Cornwall, and Anna Davis. "Narrative Theology in Religious Education." *British Journal of Religious Education* 35, no. 3 (2013): 297–312.

Reeves, Scott, Merrich Zwarenstein, Joanne Goldman, Hugh Barr, Della Freeth, Marilyn Hammick, and Ivan Koppell. "Interprofessional Education: Effects on Professional Practice and Health Care Outcomes." *Cochrane Database Systematic Reviews* 1 (2008). Article No: CD002212. doi:10.1002/14651858.CD002213.pub2.

Reeves, Scott, Simon Lewin, Sherry Espin, and Merrick Zwarenstein. *Interprofessional Teamwork for Health and Social Care*. Oxford: Blackwell Publishing, 2010.

Reis, Shmuel, Adriaan Visser, and Richard Frankel. "Health Information and Communication Technology in Healthcare Communication: The Good, the Bad, and the Transformative." *Patient Education and Counseling* 93 (2013): 350–62.

Relman, Arnold S. *When More Is Less: The Paradox of American Health Care and How to Resolve It*. New York: W. W. Norton, 1997.

Riach, Kathleen. "Exploring Participant-Centered Reflexivity in the Research Interview." *Sociology* 43, no. 2 (2009): 356–70.

Rian, Johanna, and Rachel Hammer. "The Practical Application of Narrative Medicine at Mayo Clinic: Imagining the Scaffold of a Worthy House." *Culture, Medicine, and Psychiatry* 37 (2013): 670–80.

Richards, Ivor Armstrong. *Principles of Literary Criticism*. New York: Harcourt, Brace and Company, 1928.

Richards, Ivor Armstrong. *Practical Criticism: A Study of Literary Judgment*. New York: Harcourt, Brace and Company, 1929.

Richards, Ivor Armstrong. *Richards on Rhetoric.* Edited by Ann E. Berthoff. New York: Oxford University Press, 1991.

Richardson, Brian. *Unnatural Voices: Extreme Narration in Modern and Contemporary Fiction.* Columbus: The Ohio State University Press, 2010.

Ricoeur, Paul. *Freud and Philosophy: An Essay on Interpretation.* Translated by Denis Savage. New Haven, CT: Yale University Press, 1970.

Ricoeur, Paul. "Life in Quest of Narrative." In *On Paul Ricoeur: Narrative and Interpretation,* edited by David Wood, 20–33. London: Routledge, 1991.

Ricoeur, Paul. *Oneself as Another.* Chicago: University of Chicago Press, 1992.

Ricoeur, Paul. *Time and Narrative.* Translated by Kathleen McLaughlin and David Pellauer (vols. 1 and 2). Translated by Kathleen Blamey and David Pellauer (vol. 3). Chicago: University of Chicago Press, 1984–1988.

Riese, Walther. "Descartes as a Psychotherapist. The Uses of Rational Philosophy in the Treatment of Discomfort and Disease; Its Limitations." *Medical History* 10, no. 3 (1966): 237–44.

Riessman, Catherine Kohler. *Narrative Methods for the Human Sciences.* Los Angeles, CA: Sage Publications, 2008.

Riska, Elianne, Adele E. Clarke, Laura Mamo, Jennifer Ruth Fosket, Jennifer R. Fishman, and Janet K. Shim. *Biomedicalization: Technoscience, Health, and Illness in the U.S.* Chapel Hill, NC: Duke University Press, 2009.

Robinson, Alan. *Narrating the Past: Historiography, Memory and the Contemporary Novel.* London: Palgrave MacMillan, 2011.

Rosenberg, C. E. "The Tyranny of Diagnosis: Specific Entities and Individual Experience." *Milbank Quarterly* 80, no. 2 (2002): 237–60.

Rosenblatt, Louise M. *Literature as Exploration.* 5th ed. New York: Modern Language Association of America, 1995.

Ross, Fiona C. *Bearing Witness: Women and the Truth and Reconciliation Commission in South Africa.* London: Pluto Press, 2003.

Royle, Nicholas. *Veering: A Theory of Literature.* Edinburgh: Edinburgh University Press, 2011.

Rudnytsky, Peter, and Rita Charon, eds. *Psychoanalysis and Narrative Medicine.* Albany: State University of New York Press, 2008.

Russell, Bertrand. "On the Experience of Time." *Monist* 25 (1915): 212–33.

Ryan, Marie-Laure. *Possible Worlds, Artificial Intelligence, and Narrative Theory.* Bloomington: Indiana University Press, 1991.

Said, Edward. "The Music Itself: Glenn Gould's Contrapuntal Vision." In *Music at the Limits,* 3–10. New York: Columbia University Press, 2007.

Said, Edward W. *Orientalism.* New York: Vintage Books, 1979.

Sandhu, Sima, Eleonora Arcidiacono, Eugenio Aguglia, and Stefan Priebe. "Reciprocity in Therapeutic Relationships: A Conceptual Review." *International Journal of Mental Health* (2015). doi:10.1111/inm.12160.

Sands, Stephen, Patricia Stanley, and Rita Charon. "Pediatric Narrative Oncology: Interprofessional Training to Promote Empathy, Build Teams, and Prevent Burnout." *Journal of Supportive Oncology* 6 (2008): 307–12.

Scarry, Elaine. *The Body in Pain.* New York: Oxford University Press, 1985.

Schafer, Roy. *Retelling a Life: Narration and Dialogue in Psychoanalysis.* New York: Basic Books, 1992.

Schalk, Susan. "Coming to Claim Crip: Disidentification With/in Disability Studies." *Disability Studies Quarterly* 33, no. 2 (2013). http://dsq-sds.org/article/view/3705/3240.

Schneider, Pat. *How The Light Gets In: Writing as a Spiritual Practice.* New York: Oxford University Press, 2013.

Scholes, Robert, James Phelan, and Robert Kellogg. *The Nature of Narrative.* 40th ed. New York: Oxford University Press, 2006.

Schön, Donald. *The Reflective Practitioner: How Professionals Think in Action.* New York: Basic Books, 1983.

Schultz, Dawson Stafford, and Lydia Victoria Flasher. "Charles Taylor, Phronesis, and Medicine: Ethics and Interpretation in Illness Narrative." *Journal of Medicine and Philosophy* 36 (2011): 394–409.

Schweizer, Harold. *On Waiting.* London: Routledge, 2008.

Scully, Jackie Leach, Laurel E. Baldwin-Ragavan, and Petya Fitzpatrick, eds. *Feminist Bioethics: At the Center, On the Margins.* Baltimore: Johns Hopkins University Press, 2010.

Sedgwick, Eve Kosofsky. *Touching, Feeling: Affect, Pedagogy, Performativity.* Durham, NC: Duke University Press, 2003.

Sember, Robert, and D. Rhine (writing for Ultra-red). *Ten Preliminary Theses on Militant Sound Investigation.* Artists and Activists Series, no. 5. New York: Printed Matter, 2008.

Shapiro, Johanna. "Movies Help Us Explore Relational Ethics in Health Care," In *The Picture of Health: Medical Ethics and the Movies,* edited by Henri Colt, Silvia Quadrelli, and Lester Friedman, New York: Oxford University Press, 2011: 19–28.

Shapiro, Johanna. "The Feeling Physician: Educating the Emotions in Medical Training." *European Journal for Person Centered Healthcare* 1, no. 2 (2013): 310–16.

Shapiro, Johanna, Deborah Kasman, and Audrey Shafer. "Words and Wards: A Model of Reflective Writing and Its Uses in Medical Education." *Journal of Medical Humanities* 27 (2006): 231–44.

Shem, Samuel. "Fiction as Resistance." *Annals of Internal Medicine* 137, no. 11 (2002): 934–37.

Shem, Samuel, with introduction by John Updike. *The House of God.* New York: Delta Trade Paperbacks, 2003.

Sherwin, Susan. "Whither Bioethics? How Feminism Can Help Reorient Bioethics." *International Journal of Feminist Approaches to Bioethics* 1, no. 1 (2008): 7–27.

Singer, Janet, Stephen Fiascone, Warren J. Huber, Tiffany C. Hunter, and Jeffrey Sperling. "Four Residents' Narratives on Abortion Training." *Obstetrics and Gynecology* 126, no. 1 (2015): 56–60.

Soja, Edward W. *Thirdspace.* Malden, MA: Blackwell, 1996.

Spencer, Danielle. "All Creatures Great and Small." *Lancet* 386 (2015): 22–23.

Spivak, Gayatri Chakravorty. "Can the Subaltern Speak?" In *Marxism and the Interpretation of Culture,* edited by Cary Nelson and Lawrence Grossberg, 271–313. Basingstoke, UK: MacMillan Education, 1988.

Starr, Paul. *The Social Transformation of American Medicine: The Rise of a Sovereign Profession and the Making of a Vast Industry.* New York: Basic Books, 1982.

Stein, Leo. *Appreciation: Painting, Poetry, and Prose.* Lincoln, NE: University of Nebraska Press, 1947.

Steinmetz, Katy. "The Transgender Tipping Point." *Time Magazine,* May 29, 2014.

Stempsey, William E. "Plato and Holistic Medicine." *Medicine, Health Care and Philosophy* 4, no. 2 (2001): 201–9.

Stevens, Wallace. *The Necessary Angel: Essays on Reality and the Imagination.* New York: Random House, 1965.

Stockwell, Peter. *Cognitive Poetics: An Introduction.* London: Routledge, 2002.

Stoller, Paul. *Sensuous Scholarship.* Philadelphia: University of Pennsylvania Press, 1997.

Strand, Mark. "Mark Strand on Edward Hopper." *The New York Review of Books,* June 25, 2015: 40–41.

Street, Richard L., Jr., Howard Gordon, and Paul Haidet. "Physicians' Communication and Perceptions of Patients: Is It How They Look, How They Talk, or Is It Just the Doctor?" *Social Science and Medicine* 65 (2007): 586–98.

Stringfellow, William. *Count It All Joy: Reflections on Faith, Doubt, and Temptation, Seen through the Letter of James.* Eugene, OR: Wipf and Stock Publishers, 1999.

Sue, Derald Wing. *Race Talk: and the Conspiracy of Silence.* Hoboken, NJ: John Wiley and Sons, 2015.

Svenaeus, Fredrik. *The Hermeneutics of Medicine and the Phenomenology of Health: Steps Towards a Philosophy of Medical Practice*. International Library of Ethics, Law, and the New Medicine, vol. 5. Dordrecht: Kluwer Academic Publishers, 2000.

Taylor, Charles. *Sources of the Self: The Making of Modern Identity*. Cambridge, UK: Cambridge University Press, 1989.

Tervalon, Melanie, and Jan Murray-Garcia. "Cultural Humility Versus Cultural Competence: A Critical Distinction in Defining Physician Training Outcomes in Multicultural Education." *Journal of Health Care for the Poor and Underserved* 9 (1998): 117–25.

Thistlewaite, Jill. "Interprofessional Education: A Review of Context, Learning and the Research Agenda." *Medical Education* 46 (2012): 58–70.

Tóibín, Colm. "One Minus One." In *Mothers and Sons: Stories*, 271–88. New York: Scribner, 2007.

Tompkins, Jane, ed. *Reader-Response Criticism: From Formalism to Post-Structuralism.* Baltimore: Johns Hopkins University Press, 1980.

Toombs, S. Kay. "Illness and the Paradigm of Lived Body." *Theoretical Medicine* 9 (1988): 201–26.

Toombs, S. Kay. *The Meaning of Illness: A Phenomenological Account of the Different Perspectives of Physician and Patient*. Dordrecht: Kluwer Academic Publishers, 1993.

Toombs, S. Kay. *Handbook of Phenomenology and Medicine*. Philosophy and Medicine series. Dordrecht: Springer, 2001.

"This is the Voice I Want to Use." In *Transamerica*, directed by Duncan Tucker. 2005. New York: Weinstein Company, 2006. DVD.

Tronto, Joan. *Moral Boundaries: A Political Argumentation for an Ethics of Care.* New York: Routledge, 1993.

Truog, Robert D., Stephen D. Brown, David Browning, Edward M. Hundert, Elizabeth A. Rider, Sigall K. Bell, and Elaine C. Meyer. "Microethics: The Ethics of Everyday Clinical Practice." *Hastings Center Report* 45, no. 1 (2015): 11–17.

Tsevat, Rebecca, Anoushka Sinha, Kevin Gutierrez, and Sayantani DasGupta. "Bringing Home the Health Humanities: Narrative Humility, Structural Competency, and Engaged Pedagogy." *Academic Medicine* 90, no. 11 (2015): 1462–5.

Turner, Mark. "The Cognitive Study of Art, Language, and Literature." *Poetics Today* 23, no. 1 (2002): 9–20.

Vanhoutte, Jacqueline. "Cancer and the Common Woman in Margaret Edson's 'W;t'," *Comparative Drama* (2002): 391–410.

Vannatta, Seth, and Jerry Vannatta. "Functional Realism: A Defense of Narrative Medicine." *Journal of Medicine and Philosophy* 38 (2013): 32–49.

Vico, Giambattista. *The New Science*. 1744. Translated by Thomas G. Bergin and Max H. Fisch, 2nd ed. Ithaca, NY: Cornell University Press, 1968.

Viederman, Milton. "Active Engagement in the Consultation Process." *General Hospital Psychiatry* 24 (2002): 93–100.

Viederman, Milton. "The Induction of Noninterpreted Benevolent Transference as a Vehicle for Change." *American Journal of Psychotherapy* 65, no. 4 (2011): 337–54.

Viederman, Milton. "A Model of Interpretative Supportive Dynamic Psychotherapy." *Psychiatry* 71, no. 4 (2008): 349–58.

Viederman, Milton. "The Therapeutic Consultation: Finding the Patient." *American Journal of Psychotherapy* 60, no. 2 (2006): 153–59.

Vogel, Elizabeth. "What We Talk About When We Talk About Emotion: The Rhetoric of Emotion in Composition." Unpublished dissertation, University of North Carolina at Greensboro, 2008.

Von Tevenar, Gudrun. "Gratitude, Reciprocity, and Need." *American Philosophical Quarterly* 43, no. 2 (2006): 181–88.

Wald, Hedy S., Jeffrey Borkan, Julie Scott Taylor, David Anthony, and Shmuel P. Reis. "Fostering and Evaluating Reflective Capacity in Medical Education: Developing the REFLECT Rubric for Assessing Reflective Writing." *Academic Medicine* 97 (2012): 355.

Wald, Hedy S., Stephen W. Davis, Shmuel Reis, Alicia D. Monroe, and Jeffrey M. Borkan. "Reflecting on Reflections: Enhancements of Medical Education Curriculum with Structured Field Notes and Guided Feedback." *Academic Medicine* 84 (2009): 830–37.

Wallace, David Foster. *Infinite Jest.* New York: Little, Brown and Company, 1996.

Walzer, Richard. *Greek into Arabic: Essays in Islamic Philosophy.* Columbia, SC: University of South Carolina Press, 1962.

Wear, Delese, and Therese Jones. "Bless Me Reader for I Have Sinned: Physicians and Confessional Writing." *Perspectives in Biology and Medicine*, 53, no. 2 (2010): 215–30.

Wear, Delese, Joseph Zarconi, Rebecca Garden, and Therese Jones. "Reflection in/ and Writing: Pedagogy and Practice in Medical Education." *Academic Medicine* 87 (2012): 603–9.

Wearden, Graeme. "178 Oxfam Briefing Paper." *The Guardian*, January 20, 2014.

Weaver, Sallie J., Rebecca Lyons, Deborah DiazGranados, Michael A. Rosen, Eduardo Salas, James Oglesby, Jeffrey S. Augenstein, David J. Birnbach, Donald Robinson, and Heidi B. King. "The Anatomy of Health Care Team Training and the State of Practice: A Critical Review." *Academic Medicine* 85, no. 11 (November 2010): 1746–60.

Weil, Simone. *Waiting for God.* Translated by Emma Crauford with an introduction by Leslie A. Fiedler. New York: Harper and Row, 1973.

Weil, Simone. *Waiting for God.* Translated by Emma Crauford. New York: Perennial Classics, 2001.

Wells, Kathleen. *Narrative Inquiry.* New York: Oxford University Press, 2011.

West, Courtney, Michael Veronin, Karen Landry, Terri Kurz, Bree Watzak, Barbara Quiram, and Lori Graham. "Tools to Investigate How Interprofessional Education Activities Link to Competencies." *Medical Education Online* 20: 28627 (2015). http://dx.doi.org/10.3402/meo.v20.28627.

Westfall, Richard. *The Construction of Modern Science: Mechanisms and Mechanics.* Cambridge, UK: Cambridge University Press, 1977.

White, Hayden. *Metahistory: The Historical Imagination in Nineteenth Century Europe.* Baltimore: Johns Hopkins University Press, 1973.

White, Michael. *Narrative Practice and Exotic Lives: Resurrecting Diversity in Everyday Life.* Adelaide: Dulwich Centre Publication, 2004.

White, Michael. "Working with People Who Are Suffering the Consequences of Multiple Trauma: A Narrative Perspective." *The International Journal of Narrative Therapy and Community Work* 1 (2004): 44–75.

White, Michael, and David Epston. *Narrative Means to Therapeutic Ends.* New York: W. W. Norton, 1990.

Williams, Ian. *The Bad Doctor.* University Park: Pennsylvania State University Press, 2015.

Williams, Raymond. *Marxism and Literature.* Oxford: Oxford University Press, 1977.

Wimsatt, William K., and Monroe C. Beardsley. *The Verbal Icon: Studies in the Meaning of Poetry.* Lexington: University of Kentucky Press, 1954.

Winkel, Abigail Ford, Nellie Hermann, Mark J. Graham, and Rini B. Ratan. "No Time to Think: Making Room for Reflection in Obstetrics and Gynecology Residency." *Journal of Graduate Medical Education* 2 (2010): 610–15.

Winnicott, Donald W. *Playing and Reality.* London: Routledge, 2005.

Winnicott, Donald W. *The Maturational Processes and the Facilitating Environment.* New York: International University Press, 1965.

Woods, Angela. "The Limits of Narrative: Provocations for the Medical Humanities." *Medical Humanities* 37 (2011): 73–78.

Woolf, Virginia. "How Should One Read a Book?" In *The Second Common Reader*, 234–45. New York: Harcourt Brace Jovanovich, 1932.

Woolf, Virginia. "On Rereading Novels." In *The Moment and Other Essays*, 155–66. New York: Harcourt Brace Jovanovich, 1948.

Woolf, Virginia. "Reading." In *The Captain's Deathbed and Other Essays*, 151–79. San Diego, CA: Harcourt Brace Jovanovich, 1950.

World Health Organization. *Learning Together to Work Together for Health*. Geneva: WHO, 1988.

World Health Organization. *Framework for Action on Interprofessional Education and Collaborative Practice*. Geneva: WHO, 2010.

Worsham, Lynn. "Coming to Terms: Theory, Writing, Politics." In *Rhetoric and Composition as Intellectual Work*, edited by Gary A. Olson. Carbondale: Southern Illinois University Press, 2002.

Yancy, George. *Black Bodies, White Gazes*. New York: Rowan and Littlefield, 2008.

Zaner, Richard. *Context of Self: Phenomenological Inquiry*. Series in Continental Thought. Columbus: Ohio University Press, 1981.

Zaner, Richard M. *Conversations on the Edge: Narratives of Ethics and Illness*. Washington, DC: Georgetown University Press, 2004.

Zaner, Richard M. *Ethics and the Clinical Encounter*. Englewood Cliffs, NJ: Prentice Hall, 1988.

Zaner, Richard M. "Examples and Possibles: A Criticism of Husserl's Theory of Free-Phantasy Variation." *Research in Phenomenology* 3, no. 1 (1973): 29–43.

Zaner, Richard M. "Medicine and Dialogue." *Journal of Medicine and Philosophy* 15, no. 3 (1990): 303–25.

Zaner, Richard M. "The Phenomenon of Vulnerability in Clinical Encounters." *Human Studies* 29, no. 3 (2006): 283–94.

Zunshine, Lisa. *Why We Read Fiction: Theory of Mind and the Novel*. Columbus: Ohio State University Press, 2006.

INDEX

Johnson, Mark, 207n49
Johnson, T. R., 222
Jonsen, Albert, 117
Josiah Macy, Jr. Foundation, 299
Joyce, James, 186
Justice, 4, 115, 118, 172

Kant, Immanuel, 159
Kermode, Frank, 185
Kincaid, Jamaica, 238
Kinnell, Galway, 197–199
Kiss of the Spider Woman (Manuel Puig),
    202–204
Kleinman, Arthur, 67, 72, 101
Kristeva, Julia, 161

Lacan, Jacques
    critique of the Enlightenment
        subject by, 29
    and hermeneutics of suspicion, 25
    impact of, 161
Lakoff, George, 207n49
La Mettrie, Julian Offray de, 81
Language
    as bodily expression, 89–92
    in creative writing, 223, 225
    elements of, 168
    in psychoanalysis, 282
Laub, Dori, 305
Law schools, 4
Law studies, 285
Leder, Drew, 72–73, 81
Leeuw, Sarah de, 40
Lentricchia, Frank, 162, 164
Leonardo da Vinci, 81
Leriche, René, 279, 292
Levi, Primo, 304–305
Levinas, Emmanuel, 31, 147
Levi-Strauss, Claude, 161
The Life of the Mind (Hannah Arendt), 287
Liling, Song, 146–147
Lincoln, Yvonna S., 260–261
Linguistics
    and close reading, 158
    cognitive, 89
    influence of, 1, 161
Listening
    attentive, 157, 166–169, 293–294
    in qualitative research, 267
Literary criticism, 157
Literary studies, 121–125
Literary theory, 1
Liver transplants, 295
Loewald, Hans, 282
Lorde, Audre

and dualism, 63–65, 68
    on the master's tools, 143
    and philosophy, 92, 98, 101
Love's Knowledge (Martha Nussbaum), 123
Lubbock, Percy, 185
Lukács, George, 185
Lyotard, Jean-François, 161

M. Butterfly (David Henry Hwang), 146–147
MacCurdy, Marian, 221
MacIntyre, Alisdair, 21, 72, 87, 118
Maitland, Sara, 64, 68
Mar, Raymond, 224
Marcus, R. Eric, 2
Marcus, Sharon, 162
Mariceau, Francois, 64
Marx, Karl, 260, 264, 265
Marxist theories, 161, 162
Master narratives, 98
Materiality, 263
Maxwell, William, 286–287
May, Rollo, 212, 214
McEwan, Ian, 104
McGann, Tara, 2
Meaning-making, 123
The Meaning of Meanings (I. A. Richards &
    C. K. Ogden), 159
Medical education
    attitudes toward emotions in,
        38–42, 54–56
    emotional regulation in, 38–40, 68–69
Medicalization, 140–141
Medical paternalism, 64, 98
Meditations on First Philosophy (René
    Descartes), 104
Mentally ill patients, 68
Meretoja, Hanna, 125
Merleau-Ponty, Maurice, 79, 87–93
Metaphor, 200–205
Metaphors We Live By (George Lakoff & Mark
    Johnson), 207n49
Metonymy, 201
Microethics, 128
Miller, D. A., 163
Miller, Henry, 228
Miller, J. Hillis, 122
Milne, A. A., 27
Mind/body relation. *See* Dualism
Minorities, 68
Mishler, Elliot, 284
Mitchell, Stephen A.
    on affective experience, 37
    and close reading, 175
    and relationality in literature, 15, 16, 19, 34
Modern Language Association, 164
Mohanty, Chandra Talpade, 137, 138, 142–143